This is an admirably concise and clear guide to fundamental concepts in physiology relevant to clinical practice. It covers all the body systems in an accessible style of presentation. Bulleted checklists and boxed information provide an easy overview and summary of the essentials. By concentrating on the core knowledge of physiology, it will serve as a useful revision aid for all doctors striving to achieve postgraduate qualification, and for anyone needing to refresh their knowledge base in the key elements of clinical physiology.

The author's own experience as an examiner at all levels has been distilled here for the benefit of postgraduate trainees and medical and nursing students.

Dr Ashis Banerjee is Consultant in Emergency Medicine and serves as Examiner for those undertaking their MB, BS, MRCS and MFAEM examinations.

Clinical Physiology

An Examination Primer

Ashis Banerjee

Consultant in Emergency Medicine, Lewisham University Hospital

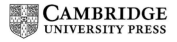

CAMBRIDGE
UNIVERSITY PRESS

CAMBRIDGE UNIVERSITY PRESS
Cambridge, New York, Melbourne, Madrid, Cape Town, Singapore, São Paulo

CAMBRIDGE UNIVERSITY PRESS
The Edinburgh Building, Cambridge CB2 2RU, UK

Published in the United States of America by Cambridge University Press, New York

www.cambridge.org
Information on this title: www.cambridge.org/9780521542265

First published 2005

Printed in the United Kingdom at the University Press, Cambridge

A catalogue record for this publication is available from the British Library

ISBN-13 978-0-521-54226-5 paperback
ISBN-10 0-521-54226-X paperback

Cambridge University Press has no responsibility for the persistence or accuracy of URLs
for external or third-party internet websites referred to in this publication, and does not
guarantee that any content on such websites is, or will remain, accurate or appropriate.

Contents

Preface   page   vii

1   Cell physiology   1
2   Water and electrolyte balance   19
3   Acid–base balance   31
4   Renal physiology   44
5   Temperature regulation   66
6   Cardiovascular system   71
7   Respiratory system   115
8   Blood   140
9   Neurophysiology   177
10 Endocrine physiology   258
11 Gastrointestinal physiology   316

Index   349

Preface

The teaching of physiology at the undergraduate level often fails to provide its students with any enthusiasm or lasting zeal for the subject. This is regrettable because a good knowledge of normal human physiology is critically important in understanding the effects of organ dysfunction secondary to disease. Adequate treatment of the multiple insults to the body in the seriously ill patient requires a good understanding of the underlying pathophysiological mechanisms. Undoubtedly, the gradual demise of academic physiology in the United Kingdom has contributed to the current state of affairs. This book explains the basic concepts of physiology in a succinct and didactic fashion. Its aim is to aid the medical student and the junior doctor in obtaining a good understanding of the homeostatic mechanisms of the human body so that the effects of dysfunction of these mechanisms can be better understood. It is also designed to aid with the basic science component of the various royal college examinations that are required to be passed prior to entering specialist training in the United Kingdom.

Ashis Banerjee

Cell physiology

■ Introduction

The cell is the **structural and functional unit of life**. Bounded by a cell membrane, which maintains the homeostasis of the cell interior, it contains various membrane-bound compartments or **organelles** within, which subserve specialised functions. These membrane-bound organelles are characteristic of all eukaryotic cells, including those in humans.

■ Cell membrane

The **cell membrane** bounds all cells in the human body, forming a dynamic interface between the intracellular and extracellular environments.

It serves, or facilitates, the following **functions**:

- The maintenance of **cell shape and structure**. This is achieved by the presence of anchoring sites for cytoskeletal filaments and extracellular matrix components.
- A **transport** function. This is brought about by selective permeability to ions and macromolecules, allowing the maintenance of cytosolic ionic composition, osmotic pressure and pH (around 7.2–7.4).
- **Intercellular communication**, involving signal transduction, i.e. the detection of chemical signals (messengers) from other cells. These signals mediate nerve transmission, hormone release, muscle contraction and the stimulation of growth. This is the result of the binding of signalling molecules by transmembrane receptors.
- **Intercellular adhesion**. This is brought about by the fusion of the membrane with other cell membranes via specialised junctions.
- Directed **cell movement**.

Structure of cell membranes

The thickness of cell membranes ranges from 6–10 nm, typically being about 7.5 nm.

● One nanometre is equal to 10^{-9} metre.

Cell membranes are composed primarily of lipids and proteins. Lipids are the major components of membranes, including glycerophospholipids (phosphoglycerides), sphingolipids (sphingomyelin) and cholesterol. Cephalin (phosphatidylethanolamine) and lecithin (phosphatidylcholine) are the most common glycerophospholipids in membranes. Membrane lipids form **self-sealing bilayers**. They are amphipathic molecules, with hydrophobic and hydrophilic moieties. The hydrophobic groups, the long fatty acyl side chains, form the core, with the polar hydrophilic groups lining both surfaces.

Carbohydrates comprise 5%–10% of cell membranes. They consist of glycolipids and glycoproteins and form the **glycocalyx** coat on the surface of the plasma membrane. This layer is responsible for the immunological characteristics of the cell and carries surface receptors that are involved in molecular recognition.

According to the **fluid mosaic model** of Singer and Nicolson cell membranes possess fluid structures, being considered as two-dimensional solutions of oriented globular proteins and lipids. They take the form of a continuous fluid but stable lipid bilayer, studded with an array of membrane-associated or membrane-spanning proteins. The fluidity of the membrane is determined by the degree of unsaturation of the constituent fatty acids. The lipids and proteins can undergo rotational and lateral movement.Membranes are **structurally and functionally asymmetrical**. This is due to asymmetrical orientation of integral and peripheral membrane proteins, laterally and transversely. Membranes are also **electrically polarised**, with the inside being negative with respect to the exterior.

On electron microscopy, a **trilaminar structure** is evident. This consists of two dark outer bands, representing the polar heads of the membrane phospholipids and protein molecules on the inner and outer surfaces of the membrane, and an inner lighter band due to the nonpolar tails of the lipid molecules.

Membrane proteins

Classification of membrane proteins

Membrane proteins can be classified according to their structural relationship to the lipid bilayer into:

Integral proteins, which penetrate the lipid bilayer;

Peripheral or extrinsic proteins, which are located outside the lipid bilayer;

Membrane protein functions

Transport carriers in facilitated diffusion processes;

Ion channels;

Pumps involved in active transport;

Receptors for hormones and neurotransmitters, e.g. G-proteins, which act as molecular switches: signal transduction;

Cell to cell recognition and interaction;

Junctional proteins in intercellular junctions: cell adhesion molecules;

Second messenger enzymes.

Lipid-anchored proteins, which lie outside the lipid bilayer but are covalently linked to lipid molecules within the bilayer.

Properties of integral membrane proteins

Integral membrane proteins demonstrate asymmetrical orientation in the membrane. They are amphipathic, with both hydrophobic and hydrophilic regions. If they span the membrane, they are known as transmembrane proteins. Removal from the membrane can be achieved by denaturation of the membrane, using either a detergent, e.g. ionic detergent sodium tetradecyl sulphonate, or the non-ionic detergent Triton X-100, or an organic solvent. Examples of integral membrane proteins include hormone receptors, ion channels, gap junction proteins, Na^+/K^+-ATPase and histocompatibility antigens.

Classification of cell membrane receptors

Cell membrane receptors are classified according to the signal transduction mechanism involved into:

● Ion channel-linked (ionotropic) receptors, which are coupled directly to ligand-gated ion channels. Examples include nicotinic acetylcholine receptors, ionotropic glutamate receptors, and gamma-aminobutyric acid (GABA) A receptors.

● Catalytic receptors, which possess a cytoplasmic catalytic region that usually behaves as a tyrosine kinase.

● G-protein-linked receptors, which are further discussed in the chapter on endocrine physiology (see p. 258).

Cell membrane receptors structurally comprise the following groups, depending on the number of times they span the membrane:

● **Single trans-luminal domain receptors**, which are directly or indirectly coupled to intracellular kinase enzymes.

> **Tyrosine kinase receptors** consist of a tyrosine kinase domain, a hormone-binding domain, and a carboxy-terminal segment with multiple tyrosines for auto-phosphorylation.
> The activation of signalling by tyrosine kinase receptors involves:
>   Ligand-induced oligomerisation of the receptor;
>   Trans-phosphorylation of the activation loop;
>   Phosphorylation of additional sites and recruitment of proteins to the receptor complex;
>   Phosphorylation of substrates.

Tyrosine kinase receptor family, which includes epithelial growth factors, fibroblast growth factors and insulin-like growth factors;

Cytokine receptor superfamily;

Serine-threonine kinase receptor family;

Guanyl cyclase receptor family;

Phosphotyrosine phosphatase family.

- **Seven transmembrane domain receptors**, associated with GTP-activated protein (G-protein)-coupled receptors.
- **Four transmembrane domain receptors**, that form ligand- or transmitter-gated ion channels.

■ Intercellular junctions

Types of intercellular junctions

- **Adherent junctions**, which hold epithelial cells, as well as cardiac muscle cells, together. This is achieved by connecting cytoskeletal elements of the cells.
- **Tight (occluding) junctions**, which segregate the apical and basolateral domains of the cell membrane by sealing the lateral intercellular junctions. They prevent pericellular diffusion of water and ions, thereby performing a barrier function.
- **Gap (communicating) junctions**, which allow intercellular diffusion of ions and signalling molecules. These are composed of hexagonal arrays of identical and tightly packed connexins or gap junction channel proteins, each of which shows a central pore of an approximate diameter of 1.5 nm. They form a connexon. Gap junctions permit electrical coupling between cells.

Types of adherent junctions

Actin filament (microfilament) attachments
Cell-to-cell: adherens junctions: cadherins
Cell-to-extracellular matrix: focal adhesions: integrins

Intermediate filament attachment sites
Cell-to-cell: desmosomes (spot and belt): cadherins
Cell-to-extracellular matrix: hemi-desmosomes: integrins

Cell–cell signalling mechanisms may be:

Endocrine: inter-glandular or inter-structure, i.e. hormones produced by an endocrine gland act on target cells at a distant body site.

Paracrine: local intercellular, i.e. act on neighbouring target cells.

Autocrine: intracellular, i.e. act on the cell responsible for production.

Cell adhesion molecules

Surface molecules involved in cell–cell interactions (**cell adhesion molecules**) are integral membrane proteins with extracellular, transmembrane and cytoplasmic domains. They mediate cell adhesion by forming non-covalent bonds with corresponding surface molecules of neighbouring cells.

Adhesion molecules can be classified as being involved in:

• **Cell body to cell body adhesion**:

Calcium-dependent adhesion molecules: **cadherins** (classic cadherins; desmosomal cadherins). Cadherins are involved in homophilic cell-to-cell adhesion in the presence of calcium ions. They are cell surface adhesion molecules that interact with the intracellular actin cytoskeleton via plakoglobulin and catenin molecules. Neural (N)-cadherins, placental (P)-cadherins, and epithelial (E)-cadherins are recognised.

Calcium-independent adhesion molecules, which belong to the immunoglobulin superfamily including intercellular adhesion molecules (ICAMs) and neural cell adhesion molecules(N-CAMs).

Cell to cell surface carbohydrate ligand-binding proteins: selectins, which are divalent cation-dependent glycoproteins.

• **Cell to extracellular matrix adhesion**: the **integrins**. Integrins are a family of transmembrane proteins that act as receptors for extracellular matrix molecules, integrating the matrix and the cytoskeleton functionally and structurally. They are non-covalently attached heterodimeric glycoproteins, composed of alpha and beta subunits.

The role of cell adhesion molecules

Cell–cell recognition
Cell signalling
Cell growth
Cell migration
Embryogenesis
Information transfer from the extracellular matrix to the cell
Establishment of the blood–brain barrier
Cancer metastasis

■ Cell membrane transport

Classification of transport mechanisms

Membrane transport mechanisms can be **classified** as:

- **Passive diffusion**: along an electrochemical gradient. Diffusion refers to the random movement of particles in solution from an area of higher concentration to one of lower. This may involve either dissolution and diffusion in membrane lipid, or passage through ion channels. **Ion channels** may be permanently open (non-gated, passive, or leakage) or be gated, i.e. can be opened or closed: e.g., voltage-gated; extracellular or intracellular ligand-gated; mechanically gated (mechanical deformation); ion-gated; or gap junction activation. Voltage-gated channels are found in neurons and muscle cells. Mechanical gating is exemplified by the mechanical deformation of cilia of the hair cells of the inner ear brought about by sound waves.

- **Facilitated transport**: aided by membrane **transporters (carrier proteins)** in the direction of the electrochemical gradient. The process is more rapid than simple diffusion. Carriers must be able to recognise the substance transported, to permit translocation, followed by release of the substance with recovery of the carrier.

- **Active transport**: an energy requiring process operating against an electrochemical gradient. The process can be mediated by:

  Primary ATPases: Na^+/K^+-ATPase; H^+-ATPase; K^+/H^+-ATPase; Ca^{2+}-ATPase: these transporters are known as pumps.

  Adenosine 5′-triphosphate (ATP)-binding cassette proteins, which bind ATP and use the free energy from ATP hydrolysis to selectively transport materials, e.g. the cystic fibrosis transmembrane conductance regulator. These

Steps in receptor-mediated endocytosis

Specific binding of ligand to high-affinity receptor, which is clustered in pits coated with clathrin.

Internalisation of the receptor in its coated pit, forming a coated vesicle.

Coated vesicles lose their clathrin coats after endocytosis, and fuse with other vesicles to form early endosomes.

The receptors are recycled to the surface in vesicles that fuse with the cell membrane.

The process is used in cellular uptake of cholesterol (via the low density lipoprotein (LDL) receptor) and of iron, among other substances.

proteins comprise a ligand-binding domain at one surface and an ATP-binding domain at the other.

Secondary mechanisms, being coupled to Na^+ or H^+ transport. The mechanism can be either a **co-transport (symport)** or a **counter-transport (antiport system)**: K^+/H^+-ATPase or proton pump.

● **Osmosis**: the passage of water from a region where its concentration is high, through a semi-permeable membrane, into a region where its concentration is lower.

● **Vesicular transport**, which can be classified as:

Endocytosis:

Pinocytosis: the plasma membrane forms vesicles that trap extracellular fluid;

Phagocytosis;

Receptor-mediated endocytosis.

Exocytosis: fusion of membrane-bound vesicles with the plasma membrane, allowing their contents to be released into the extracellular space.

Diffusion across a membrane

This depends on:

The concentration gradient of the solute across the membrane;

The permeability of the membrane to the solute;

The transmembrane voltage gradient;

The molecular weight of the solute;

The membrane surface area;

The distance over which diffusion occurs.

The rate of diffusion is proportional to the cross-sectional area and to the change in concentration per unit distance, i.e. the concentration gradient across the membrane (**Fick's law**). Fick's law may be stated as:

$Q = - \times AD \, (dc/dx)$

Where Q = the rate of flow of solute at right angles to the interface between two
solutions (mg/s)

dc/dx = the concentration gradient (mg/ml) across the interface

A = the area of the interface (cm)

D = the diffusion coefficient (sq cm/s)

The permeability constant $P = D/d$, where D is the diffusion coefficient and d
is the width of the membrane

Facilitated transport

Facilitated transport demonstrates the following characteristics:

Specificity for the transported solute;

Movement along an electrochemical gradient;

Saturation kinetics: saturation at high substrate concentrations owing to the
limited number of binding sites on the carrier;

Inhibition by structurally similar substrates;

No energy expenditure.

Active transport

Active transport demonstrates the following characteristics:

Specificity for the transported solute.

Movement against an electrochemical gradient.

Saturation kinetics: saturation at high substrate concentrations.

Metabolic energy requirement. Energy dependence leads to active transport
being substrate and oxygen dependent. Inhibition by metabolic poisons
such as cyanide and dinitrophenol may occur. Profound inhibition may
result from lowering of ambient temperature.

Competition for uptake by similar substrates.

Kinetic characteristics shared by facilitated diffusion and active transport processes

These include:

- **Stereochemical specificity**. Thus amino acid transport systems of cell membranes are much more active with L-amino acids than the D isomers.
- **Saturation**, i.e. the transport system can become saturated with the substance being transported. Plots of the rate of transport against substrate concentration usually show a hyperbolic curve approaching a maximum at which the rate is zero order with respect to substrate concentration.

- **Competitive inhibition** by other transported species (structurally related compounds).
- **Non-competitive inhibition by carrier poisons**, which can block or alter specific functional groups of proteins.

Ion channels

Ion channels are integral membrane proteins that form aqueous (water-filled) macromolecular membrane-spanning pores in the plasma membrane. They are involved in the generation and propagation of nerve impulses, synaptic transmission, muscle contraction, salt balance and hormone release.

The advantages of ion channel transport

- High selectivity for specific ion species (**substrate specificity**).
- The **ability to be gated**. The gating mechanism is a regulatory system controlling the opening and closing of gates in ion channels. Gating is a process of transition through open (conducting), closed and inactive states accompanied by conformational changes in the ion channels. Forward and backward rate constants for the transitions determine the likelihood of the various channel states.
- The ability to allow very large ion fluxes in short time periods, i.e. a **very high catalytic power** to substantially increase the flow rate of ions over the free diffusion rate in water.

Ion channel flow rates

The **rate of ion flow** through an open ion channel depends on:

The concentration gradient across the plasma membrane.

The voltage gradient across the plasma membrane.

The conductance of the ion channels, which is expressed in units of charge/ second per volt. A high conductance channel allows more ionic flow for a given driving voltage than a low conductance channel.

Opening may lead to either inward current generation, leading to depolarisation; outward current generation, leading to hyperpolarisation; or increased conductance, leading to stabilisation of membrane potential.

Closure may lead to either switching off of the inward current, leading to hyperpolarisation; switching off of the outward current, leading to depolarisation; or reduced conductance, leading to increased sensitivity of the cell to other components.

Classification of ion channels

Ion channels are classified according to their electrophysiological properties, drug sensitivity, and by molecular cloning.

- **Ligand (agonist)-gated ion channels** (direct-coupled; G-protein-coupled; second messenger-coupled), which include acetylcholine receptors (muscle (nicotinic); neural), glycine receptors, GABA A receptors and glutamate receptors.

- **Calcium channels** are present in cell membranes in smooth muscle, cardiac muscle and other tissues, and in cellular organelle membranes such as the sarcoplasmic reticulum and mitochondria. Calcium functions as a primary generator of the cardiac action potential and as an intracellular second messenger. Calcium channels are further subdivided into three subgroups based on their threshold for activation and on the spread of inactivation:

   L-type (long-lasting): slowly inactivating; high threshold calcium conductance; sensitive to dihydropyridines; involved in excitation–contraction coupling in smooth and cardiac muscle (where they carry current in the plateau phase of the action potential), and in excitation-secretion coupling in endocrine cells and in some neurons.

   T-type (transient): low voltage activated, rapidly inactivated.

   N-type (neuronal): transient, high threshold calcium conductance; blocked by omega-conotoxin

   The T and L channels are located in smooth and cardiac muscle tissue, whereas the N channels are located only in neuronal tissue.

   Calcium channel blockers interact with the L-type calcium channel and consist of four classes of drugs: the 1,4-dihydropyridine derivatives (nifedipine, nimodipine, amlodipine), the phenylalkyl-amines (verapamil), the benzothiazepines (diltiazem), and a diarylaminopropylamine ether (bepridil).

- **Potassium channels** are tetrameric and composed of four identical peptide subunits (alpha subunits) that are symmetrically arranged to form a conical pore that spans the cell membrane. Many potassium channels also contain auxiliary proteins, beta subunits, that may alter electrophysiological or biophysical properties, expression levels or expression patterns. They are divided into:

   Six transmembrane-helix voltage-gated channels, which are activated by membrane depolarisation.

   Two transmembrane-span G-protein-coupled inward rectifying channels, which favour the influx rather than efflux of potassium ions.

   Calcium-activated channels, which are sensitive to intracellular calcium concentrations:

   Large conductance: blocked by charybdotoxin and iberiotoxin;

   Small conductance: blocked by apamin.

Leak channels, with an apparent lack of gating control.

- **Sodium channels** are discrete, four domain, transmembrane glycoprotein complexes. Each complex consists of four alpha subunits around the central channel and a beta 1 and beta 2 subunit peripherally.

DNA cloning has identified three types in central neurons (I, II and III), m1 in skeletal muscle, and h and I in cardiac muscle.

Sodium channels are blocked by tetrodotoxin (produced by puffer fish), geographotoxin and by lipid-soluble amines used as local anaesthetic agents. They are activated by ciguatoxins, pyrethrin and low molecular weight polypeptide toxins from scorpions and sea anemones.

- **Chloride channels** play an important role in stabilisation of the membrane potential, regulation of cell volume, transepithelial transport and secretion of fluid from secretory glands.

Activation of chloride channels can be achieved by:

Extracellular ligands

Intracellular calcium

Cyclic AMP

G-proteins

Mechanical stretch

Cell swelling

Transmembrane voltage

Methods for the study of ion channel structure

Physical conformation
   High resolution electron microscopy;
   Electron diffraction;

Molecular structure
   Isolation of channel proteins by biochemical methods;
   Molecular cloning to determine amino acid sequences of proteins;
   Site-directed mutagenesis to alter sequences at selected sites;
   Expression of channel proteins in host cells, e.g. Xenopus oocytes.

Ion channel disorders

   Calcium channels: malignant hyperthermia
   Chloride channel: cystic fibrosis
   Sodium channels: Liddle's syndrome (aldosterone-activated sodium channels in the collecting ducts)
   Mutant sodium channels: long QT syndrome; Brugada syndrome
   Potassium channels: isolated deafness syndrome

■ Subcellular organelles

Nucleus

The nucleus is the most prominent cellular organelle, and contains the cell's database or genome, which is encoded in DNA. It comprises the following components:

Nuclear envelope.

Outer membrane, which is continuous with the endoplasmic reticulum membrane.

Inner membrane.

Pore complex: nuclear pores connect the inner and outer membranes. This is a gated channel through which ribonucleoproteins are transported to the cytoplasm.

Nucleolus: which is associated with ribonucleic acid (RNA) processing and ribosome synthesis. It is not bounded by a membrane.

Fibrous matrix: the structural skeleton of the nucleus.

Deoxyribonucleic acid (DNA)-protein complex: The nucleus contains all chromosomal DNA, the genetic material of the cell.

Functions of the nucleus

The **functions of the nucleus** include:

Synthesis of new DNA, involving DNA replication during mitosis.

Synthesis of ribosomal RNA, messenger RNA, and transfer RNA. The nucleolus is the site of messenger RNA transcription and processing, and of ribosome assembly.

A key role in cell division.

Endoplasmic reticulum

The endoplasmic reticulum comprises two morphologically distinct systems that are interconnected to form a single membrane system. The functions of the system broadly consist of synthesis, storage, transport and detoxification. The endoplasmic reticulum consists of membrane-enclosed branching tubules and flattened sacs (cisternae) and vesicles, which intercommunicate throughout the cytosol forming an intracellular transport network. The cisternal space is enclosed within. The endoplasmic reticulum is the largest subcellular organelle.

The **rough endoplasmic reticulum** contains ribosomes and is the site of protein synthesis, being involved in translation of messenger RNA into protein.

Functions of smooth endoplasmic reticulum

Site of mixed function oxidase systems in the liver, which detoxify various organic compounds.

The site of glucose release from glucose-6-phosphate in the liver via glucose 6-phosphatase.

In muscle it forms the T-system of sarcoplasmic reticulum, which is involved in calcium sequestration.

The **smooth endoplasmic reticulum** does not contain ribosomes and is the site of lipid (fatty acids and phospholipids) and steroid synthesis. This includes the synthesis of steroid hormones in the adrenal cortex and the gonads.

Golgi apparatus

The Golgi apparatus is an organelle involved in the modification of complex molecules. There are three levels of organisation:

Cisternae: flattened sac-like membranes

Dictyosomes: stacks of cisternae

Golgi complex: an association of dictyosomes

A Golgi apparatus usually contains a stack of four to six cisternae with an entry (cis) and an exit (trans) surface. The Golgi apparatus distributes newly synthesised proteins and lipids from the endoplasmic reticulum to the plasma membrane, lysosomes and secretory vesicles for export. It is concerned with post-translational modification of proteins, including:

O-glycosylation to form glycoproteins;

Proteoglycan formation;

Sulphation of sugars and tyrosine residues.

The effects of Golgi apparatus function involve the sorting of molecules for transport out of the cell by exocytosis, incorporation in the cell membrane as integral membrane proteins, or intracellular transport to lysosomes for digestion.

Mitochondria

These are the respiratory organelles of the cell. Mitochondria are about 2 μm long and 0.5–1 μm in diameter. A mitochondrion comprises:

- A smooth **outer membrane**, which recognises and translocates mitochondrial proteins.
- A highly folded **inner membrane** with invaginations, called **cristae**, projecting into the inner matrix. The spaces between the cristae are narrow. The inner

membrane contains five complexes of integral membrane proteins: nicotin-amide adenine dinucleotide (NAD)H dehydrogenase, succinate dehydrogen-ase, cytochrome c reductase, cytochrome c oxidase and ATP synthase. These are involved in oxidative phosphorylation.

- An internal gel-like **matrix space**, which contains:
  Enzymes of the tricarboxylic acid cycle;
  Enzymes involved in beta oxidation of fatty acids;
  Enzymes involved in urea formation;
  Gluconeogenesis enzymes;
  Ribosomes.
- An **inter-membrane space**.

The mitochondria synthesise ATP by the process of oxidative phosphorylation. Mitochondrial content is highest in cells with a high energy expenditure.

The **mitochondrial genome** consists of 5–10 identical circular double-stranded DNA molecules, which encode for two ribosomal RNA molecules; 22 transfer RNA molecules; and 13 polypeptides of complexes I, III, IV and V of the respiratory chain. Mitochondria replicate, transcribe and translate their DNA independently of nuclear DNA. Mitochondrial DNA is inherited maternally and does not recom-bine. Each mitochondrion acts as an individual unit, because there is no evidence of transfer of mitochondrial proteins or DNA between mitochondria. Thus a mixture of normal and mutant mitochondrial DNA can coexist within the same cell.

Mitochondrial diseases are disorders of energy metabolism, including defects of pyruvate metabolism, the Krebs cycle, respiratory chain, oxidative phospho-rylation and fatty acid oxidation. Over 90% of mitochondrial disorders are caused by mutations in nuclear genes. Mitochondrial DNA, however, mutates more than ten times as frequently as nuclear DNA. As mitochondrial DNA does not possess any introns, a random mutation affects a coding DNA sequence. Furthermore, mitochondrial DNA lacks protective histones or other effective repair systems.

Lysosomes

Lysosomes are vesicular structures limited by a single smooth membrane, com-prising the intracellular digestive system. Their **functions** include:

  Intracellular digestion of proteins, carbohydrates, lipids and nucleic acids.
  Autophagy: the destruction of unwanted subcellular organelles.
  Autolysis: the digestion of cells after death.
  The handling of the products of receptor-mediated endocytosis.
  The release of enzymes by exocytosis in the extracellular environment to
    digest external material.

Lysosomes contain hydrolytic enzymes, the **lysosomal acid hydrolases**, which require an acidic pH (around 4.8–5.0) to function. They include:

Proteases

Lipases

Phospholipases

Nucleases

Phosphatases

Polysaccharidases

Oligosaccharidases

Glucosaminoglycan (GAG)-hydrolysing enzymes

Lysosomal storage diseases are caused by defects of lysosomal enzymes resulting in intracellular accumulation of non-degraded substances.

Lysosomal storage diseases

Mucopolysaccharidoses: I to VII

Glycoproteinoses

Sphingolipidoses: Gaucher's disease, metachromatic leukodystrophy

Gangliosidoses

Neutral sphingolipidoses: Fabry disease, Niemann-Pick disease

Neutral lipid-storage diseases: Wolman disease, cholesterol ester storage disease

Peroxisomes (microbodies)

Peroxisomes are round or oval membrane-bound organelles, with an average diameter of 0.5 μm. They contain high concentrations of oxidative enzymes, i.e. catalase, D-amino oxidase and urate oxidase. Peroxisomes are abundant in the liver and kidneys.

Their **functions** include:

Synthesis of plasmalogens, important in cell membranes and myelin;

Cholesterol synthesis;

Bile acid synthesis;

Beta oxidation of fatty acids: the peroxisomal oxidation of ultra long-chain fatty acids is defective in X-linked adrenoleukodystrophy;

Conversion of amino acids into glucose;

The reduction of hydrogen peroxide, preventing tissue damage;

The prevention of excess synthesis of oxalate.

Cytoskeleton

The cytoskeleton is responsible for:

- Maintaining cell shape by mechanically strengthening it;

Classification of peroxisomal disorders

Peroxisomal structural defects, with generalised peroxisomal disorders
Zellweger syndrome (cerebro-hepato-renal syndrome)
Infantile Refsum disease

Single enzyme deficiencies with an intact peroxisomal structure
X-linked adrenoleukodystrophy
Hyperoxaluria type 1

- Cell polarity;
- Directional cell motility;
- Intracellular movements, including organelle, protein and vesicle transport;
- Providing the structural backbone of cilia and flagella, which produce beating movements on cell surfaces;
- The structure of the axoneme in the flagellum of spermatozoa;
- Spindle assembly and chromosome movement during mitosis;
- Phagocytosis;
- Cell–cell and cell–extracellular matrix adherence.

Components of the cytoskeleton

The cytoskeleton comprises:

Microfilaments (8 nanometre diameter) containing polarised alpha-helical double-stranded polymers of actin. The two ends of the polymer are not equivalent.

Intermediate filaments (10 nanometre diameter), which are tissue-specific.

Microtubules (25 nanometre diameter) containing tubulin monomers.

The power for motility is provided by **molecular motor proteins**, the myosins (which move along actin microfilaments) and the dyneins and kinesins (which move along actin microfilaments and along microtubules). They are homologous proteins, containing core structures of the P-loop NTPase superfamily which undergo change in conformation in response to nucleoside triphosphate binding and hydrolysis.

Functions of microfilaments

Specific functions mediated by actin microfilaments include:

Phagocytosis;

Linkage of transmembrane proteins to cytoplasmic proteins;

Amoeboid motility of macrophages and neutrophils;

The **intermediate filament proteins** include:
Cytokeratin – epithelial cells
Glial fibrillary acidic protein – glial cells
Desmin – muscle cells
Vimentin – mesenchymal cells
Peripherin
Alpha-internexin
Neurofilament proteins: NF-L, NF-M, NF-H – nerve cells
Lamin

Interaction with myosin (thick) filaments in skeletal muscle fibres to allow skeletal muscle contraction;
Anchoring of centrosomes at opposite poles of the cell during mitosis;
Contraction of intestinal microvilli;
Change in shape of activated platelets;
Outgrowth of dendrites and axons in developing neuroblasts.
The **functions of the intermediate filaments** include:
Anchoring of thick and thin filaments in skeletal muscle cells;
Mechanical strengthening of axons;
Anchoring the nucleus in the cells, which is achieved by keratins.

Microtubule structure

Thirteen lobular tubulin subunits form the walls of a hollow cylindrical or tubular structure. The tubular structure is stabilised by microtubule-associated proteins, including capping proteins.

There are two families of microtubule motor proteins, dyneins and kinesins. They translocate along the microtubules in opposite directions. Microtubule-based structures include cilia, axons and mitotic spindles.

Structure of cilia

The **core** or **axoneme** of each cilium comprises two single central and nine peripheral pairs (doublets) of microtubules, composed of tubulins. This is referred to as a $9 + 2$ array. Each **peripheral microtubule pair** possesses an inner and an outer cross-arm composed of dyneins. Each pair is connected by a series of radial spokes with the central pair, preventing buckling when the cilium bends. The dynein arms possess ATPase activity and an affinity for tubulin. The peripheral microtubule pairs are connected by **interdoublet links**.

Ciliary disorders

Primary: primary ciliary dyskinesia is associated with abnormal ciliary activity, defective or absent muco-ciliary transport and abnormal ciliary ultrastructure. Kartagener's syndrome is associated with the triad of sinusitis, bronchiectasis and situs inversus.

Secondary(acquired):

Drugs

Toxins

Environmental factors

Microbial pathogens

The immotile cilia syndrome is associated with lack of dynein cross-arms or radial spokes.

■ Cell polarity

Epithelial cells demonstrate structural and functional polarity, with:

An **apical domain**, which may bear cilia, microvilli, or stereocilia. This domain is the interface with the external environment.

A **basolateral domain**, which contains junctional complexes and cell adhesion molecules. This domain is the interface with the internal environment.

BIBLIOGRAPHY

Danielli, J. F. & Davson, H. A contribution to the theory of permeability of thin films. *J. Cell. Comp. Physiol.*, **5** (1935), 495–508.

Singer, S. J. & Nicolson, G. The fluid mosaic model of the structure of cell membranes *Science*, **175** (1972), 720–31.

RECOMMENDED FURTHER READING

Alberts, B., Johnson, A., Lewis, J., Raff, M., Roberts, K. & Walter, P. *Molecular Biology of The Cell*, 4th ed. New York: Garland Science (Taylor Francis Group). 2003.

Bolsover, S., Hyams, J., Shephard, E., White, H. & Wiedemann, C. *Cell Biology. A Short Course*. Hoboken, NJ: John Wiley & Sons, Inc. 2004.

Hille, B. *Ion Channels of Excitable Membranes*. Sunderland, MA: Sinauer Associates, Inc. 2001.

Pollard, T. D. & Earnshaw, W. C. *Cell Biology*. Philadelphia: W. B. Saunders, 2002.

Water and electrolyte balance

■ Water balance

In most steady state situations, water intake matches water losses through all sources. Water balance involves adjusting the effects of intake, which is determined by thirst; renal dilution or concentration of urine; and losses, via the skin, kidney, gastrointestinal tract, respiratory tract.

The usual **sources of water intake** are ingested liquids, foods (fruits and vegetables) and endogenous metabolic water production.

The **sources of water output** comprise:

Sensible losses: urine, stools and sweat. The ability to dilute and to concentrate urine allows for a wide flexibility in urine flow.

Insensible losses: skin loss (insensible perspiration); exhaled air from the respiratory tract.

Mechanisms of water homeostasis

The **mechanisms contributing to water balance** can be outlined as:

Afferent mechanisms, involving hypothalamic osmoreceptors; non-osmotic arginine vasopressin sensors, activated by pain, stress, vomiting and extracellular fluid changes; and thirst sensors.

Efferent mechanisms, including arginine vasopressin release, and increased thirst.

Osmolality and tonicity

The total solute concentration (**tonicity**) of body fluids is maintained virtually constant. Body fluid **osmolality** is defined by the ratio of total body solute to total body water. It is regulated at 280–95 mOsm/l. Osmolality is a colligative property, depending on the number of dissolved solute particles, and not on size or structure of the particles. The maintenance of osmolality is achieved primarily through the regulation of water balance.

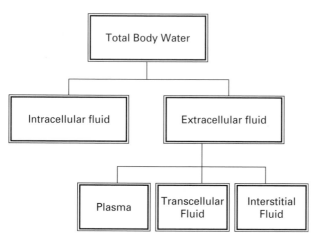

Figure 2.1 Body fluid compartments.

Body fluid compartments

In a 75 kg man
    Total body water = 55%–65% body weight = 45 litres
    Extracellular fluid = 15 litres; intravascular fluid = 5 litres
    Interstitial fluid = 10 litres
    Intracellular fluid = 30 litres
    Transcellular compartment = 1 litre

Osmolality (in mOsm/l) = n x molar concentration (mmol/l of water)

Plasma osmolality (in mOsm/kg) = $2(Na^+) + 2(K^+) + (glucose) + urea$ (all in mmol/l)

Osmolar gap = measured plasma osmolality – calculated plasma osmolality

The osmolar gap is a measure of unmeasured osmotically active molecules, such as mannitol and alcohols.

Components of extracellular fluid

Extracellular fluid comprises:
    Blood plasma.
    Lymph.
    Transcellular fluids: intra-ocular, pericardial, peritoneal, pleural and synovial fluids. These are separated from plasma by an additional epithelial layer.
    Cerebrospinal fluid.
    Glandular secretions.

Normal blood volume

Preterm: 90–105 ml/kg
Term infant: 85 ml/kg
>1 month age: 75 ml/kg
>1 year age: 67–75 ml/kg
Adult: 55–75 ml/kg

Measurement of body fluid compartments

The volume of body fluid compartments is measured by the dilution of indicators, which must fulfil the following requirements:

All the indicator administered remains in the volume to be measured;

Uniform distribution of the indicator follows an adequate time for mixing;

The indicator does not alter the volume of the compartment;

The indicator does not enter the system by another route.

The volume of the compartment = (The amount of the indicator administered – the amount of indicator excreted)/Concentration of indicator in the volume being measured.

Indicators for measurement of body compartments

Plasma volume

Uses a substance that binds to plasma albumin:

Evans Blue (T-1124)

Indocyanin green

Radiolabelled albumin(^{131}I)

Radiolabelled erythrocytes

Total body water:

Uses a substance that diffuses freely into all fluid compartments:

Radioactive water

Deuterium oxide

Tritiated water

Extracellular fluid volume

Non-metabolised substances

Mannitol

Inulin

Sucrose

Raffinose

Daily fluid requirements

Premature infant (<2 kg birth weight)	150 ml/kg
Neonates and infants (2–10 kg)	100 ml/kg for the first 10 kg
Infants and children (10–20 kg)	1000 ml/kg + 50 ml/kg for every kg 10–20 kg
Children (>20 kg)	1500 ml/kg + 20 ml/kg for every kg > 20 kg

Normal water losses

Urine 1.0–1.5 l/24 h

Stool 0.2–0.4 l/24 h

Insensible loss 0.6–0.8 l/24 h

Diffusible ions

Sulphate

Thiocyanate

Thiosulphate

Chloride

Bromide

Sodium

Extracellular fluid volume assessment and replacement

Extracellular fluid volume status can be assessed by:

Level of consciousness;

The presence of thirst;

Moistness of mucosal surfaces;

Skin turgor;

Heart rate;

Supine and standing blood pressure;

Urine output.

Options for extracellular fluid volume replacement

Colloids

Smaller infusion volume required, with more rapid resuscitation;

Prolonged plasma volume expansion;

Better oxygen delivery;

Minimal peripheral oedema;

Lower intracranial pressure;

Reduced risk of thromboembolism;

Higher cost;

Risk of coagulopathy;

Production of osmotic diuresis;

Pulmonary oedema in capillary leak states, owing to increased total lung water.

Crystalloids

Require a larger volume to reach similar end-points;

Short-lived plasma volume expansion;

Risk of peripheral oedema and pulmonary oedema;

Lower cost;

Raised glomerular filtration rate;

Replaces interstitial fluid.

In general, water will equilibrate across the intravascular, intracellular and interstitial spaces, while sodium equilibrates across the intravascular and interstitial spaces. Large molecules tend to be retained, for the major part, in the intravascular space.

■ Water reabsorption

Water reabsorption of 65% to 75% takes place in the proximal convoluted tubule, accompanying sodium and other solutes. Further reabsorption occurs in the descending limb of the loop of Henle and, finally, in the collecting ducts, via water channels or pores.

Properties of arginine vasopressin (antidiuretic hormone; ADH)

Arginine vasopressin is a nine amino acid peptide, comprising a six-membered disulphide ring and a tail of three amino acid residues on which the C-terminal carboxy group is amidated. It is synthesised in magnocellular neural cells in the supraoptic and paraventricular nuclei of the hypothalamus, in proximity to the osmoreceptors. The **osmotic threshold for thirst** is at 290–5 mOsm/kg H_2O, and is above the threshold for vasopressin release, which is 280–90 mOsm/kg.

The synthesised peptide is enzymatically cleaved from the prohormone and transported to the posterior pituitary, where it is stored in neurosecretory granules. Release into the bloodstream is triggered by specific stimuli, i.e. osmoreceptor stimulation by thirst, and by hypovolaemia. It has a short half-life of 15–20 minutes and is rapidly metabolised in the liver and kidneys.

Arginine vasopressin acts via V1 receptors in vascular tissue, which are responsible for vasopressor effects, and V2 receptors in the kidneys, which are

Renal aquaporins (water channel proteins)

Aquaporin	Renal localisation
AQP1	Proximal tubule, thin descending limb
AQP2	Collecting duct apical membrane and subapical vesicles. Regulated by vasopressin
AQP3	Collecting duct basolateral membrane
AQP4	Inner medullary collecting duct basolateral membrane

Factors that control arginine vasopressin release:

Stimulation

Increased extracellular fluid (plasma) tonicity (osmolarity): hypothalamic osmoreceptors

Reduced extracellular fluid volume

Plasma volume contraction: cardiovascular volume receptors

Fall in arterial blood pressure: cardiovascular baroreceptors

Hormonal: beta-adrenergic stimulation

    angiotensin II

    hypothyroidism

    hypoadrenalism

Drugs: nicotine

    barbiturates

    vincristine

Miscellaneous: nausea and vomiting

    hypoglycaemia

    stress

    heat

Inhibition

Decreased tonicity of the extracellular fluid

Extracellular fluid volume: volume expansion

    rise in blood pressure

Hormonal: alpha-adrenergic stimulation

Drugs: ethanol

Miscellaneous: cold

responsible for antidiuretic effects. The **V1 receptor** is a 394 amino acid protein with 7 transmembrane domains. The **V2 receptor** is a 370 amino acid protein, coupled to adenyl cyclase by a Gs protein.

Antidiuretic effects of arginine vasopressin

Arginine vasopressin increases water reabsorption in the collecting ducts of the kidney. This is achieved by binding to the G-protein-coupled V2 receptor in the basolateral membrane of the collecting duct cells. This stimulates adenyl cyclase and increases intracellular adenosine-3′-5′- monophosphate (cyclic AMP) levels.

Cyclic AMP activates one or more cyclic AMP-dependent protein kinases, including protein kinase A, which phosphorylates proteins, alters the cytoskeleton and allows subapical vesicles containing **aquaporins** to fuse with the apical plasma membrane, increasing water permeability. The aquaporins are a family of water channel proteins, which are membrane bound and comprise approximately 260 amino acids.

■ Sodium

Sodium is the principal extracellular cation. The total body sodium is around 5000–6000 mmol in a 70 kg adult. Only 2/3 of the total body sodium is exchangeable, the remainder being bound in bone. Regulation of sodium content is achieved through a balance between intake, absorption and excretion (in the urine, sweat and faeces).

Physiological role of sodium

Osmotic skeleton of extracellular fluid. Maintains plasma and extracellular fluid osmolality by virtue of being the principal osmotically active solute. Maintains intravascular and extracellular (interstitial) fluid volumes. Increases or decreases in total body sodium tend to increase or decrease the extracellular fluid and plasma volume.

Causes **transmembrane potential differences** that are responsible for excitability in nerve, muscle and other cells.

Permits movement of water and thereby influences cell volume.

Ensures potassium supply to intracellular fluid.

Permits dilution of urine.

Facilitates defence against hyperkalaemia.

By co-transport, facilitates both enteric uptake of solutes such as glucose and amino acids, along with their renal reabsorption.

By counter-transport, influences concentration of other cations, e.g. Ca^{2+}, in intracellular fluid and may therefore influence, e.g., response of arterioles to vasoconstrictor tone.

Rates of sodium transport potentially affect a variety of metabolic pathways because Na^+K^+-ATPase is a major consumer of ATP.

Sodium homeostasis

Sodium balance is maintained by a variety of mechanisms, outlined below:

- **Afferent mechanisms**

  Arterial baroreceptors in the carotid sinus;

  Renal baroreceptors in the juxtaglomerular apparatus;

  Cardiac sensors in the atria and ventricles;

  Hepatic vascular sensors;

  Hypothalamic sensors.

- **Efferent mechanisms**

  Renal: glomerular filtration rate; physical forces in the proximal tubule; distal nephron.

  Neurohumoral: sympathetic nervous system activity; renin–angiotensin–aldosterone system; prostaglandins E2 and I2, nitric oxide, atrial natriuretic peptide, arginine vasopressin.

Abnormalities in sodium metabolism

The serum sodium level is normally maintained between 135 and 145 mmol/l. The level normally reflects total body water content. Abnormalities in serum sodium levels need to be interpreted in relation to the extracellular fluid volume status.

   Hyponatraemia refers to a serum sodium level under 130 mmol/l. The pathophysiological mechanisms responsible for a low level can be enumerated as follows:

- **Pseudo-hyponatraemia**, accompanied by normal osmolality and tonicity of the extracellular fluid: severe hyperproteinaemia; hypertriglyceridaemia.

- **True hyponatraemia**

  Hypovolaemic hyponatraemia, which is due to a disproportionately greater reduction in total body sodium than in total body water, and is accompanied by features of extracellular fluid depletion. This can be due to renal losses (e.g. from diuretics), gastrointestinal losses, skin losses, and intraperitoneal losses.

  Euvolaemic hyponatraemia, which is associated with increased total body water and normal total body sodium (dilutional hyponatraemia). This can be due to arginine vasopressin excess or a reset osmostat.

  Hypervolaemic hyponatraemia, which is associated with a disproportionately greater reduction in total body water than in total body sodium, and is accompanied by features of expanded extracellular fluid volume. Oedematous states responsible may be due to congestive heart failure, cirrhosis of the liver, nephrotic syndrome or renal failure.

Redistributional hyponatraemia, which is secondary to water shifts from the intracellular to the extracellular compartment, and associated with normal total body water and total body sodium. The extracellular fluid osmolality and tonicity are high. This can be associated with severe hyperglycaemia.

Sodium deficit can be calculated by the formula: (Desired Na^+ minus actual Na^+) $\times$ body weight (kg) $\times$ total body water (l/kg)

Hypernatraemia refers to a serum sodium level greater than 150 mmol/l, and is always indicative of an absolute or relative water deficit. It is associated with the following pathophysiological mechanisms:

Hypovolaemic hypernatraemia, which is due to a total body water deficit that is disproportionately greater than total body sodium deficit. This is associated with renal losses (e.g., osmotic diuresis), skin losses, or gastrointestinal losses (e.g. secretory diarrhoea). Renal water loss can be evaluated by measuring urine osmolality.

Hypervolaemic hypernatraemia, which is due to an increase in total body sodium that is disproportionately greater than the increase in total body water. This is either iatrogenic and caused by hypertonic saline or sodium bicarbonate, or associated with primary hyperaldosteronism.

Euvolaemic hypernatraemia. This is caused by either renal water losses (diabetes insipidus) or increased insensible water losses, and is associated with a normal total body sodium content.

■ Potassium

Potassium is the major cation in the intracellular fluid. Daily dietary intake ranges from 40–120 mmol. The serum level ranges between 3.5 and 5 mmol/l. The total body potassium is around 3500 mmol in a 70 kg adult, representing around 50 mmol/kg.

Ninety-eight percent of the total body potassium is intracellular. Cellular uptake is achieved by stimulation of the cell membrane Na^+/K^+-ATPase. Ninety per cent of the daily load is excreted by the kidneys; the remainder by the gastrointestinal tract. Renal excretion depends on renal blood flow, sodium delivery to the distal tubule, urine output, aldosterone, antidiuretic hormone, and acid–base balance.

Functions of potassium

Generation of transmembrane potentials, thereby affecting the electrical excitability of tissues. It is responsible for the resting membrane potential, which is set by the equilibrium potential for potassium. It also prolongs the plateau of the action potential, initiates repolarisation and is responsible for diastolic depolarisation in cardiac pacemaker cells.

A cofactor in enzymatic reactions.

Responsible for normal cell volume by virtue of being the predominant intra-cellular solute

Maintenance of cell polarity.

Receptor-mediated endocytosis.

RNA synthesis and processing.

Protein synthesis.

Hormone secretion.

Vascular reactivity.

Maintenance of acid–base balance.

Apoptosis.

Potassium balance

Potassium homeostasis is maintained by a balance between intake, excretion, and cellular uptake and efflux. Ninety per cent of the total body potassium is available for exchange, allowing for major **translocations** or shifts between body compartments.

Factors stimulating K$^+$ entry into cells

Alkalosis, mainly metabolic;

Hormonal: insulin, beta-adrenergic agonists (catecholamines);

High extracellular potassium concentration;

Hyperosmolarity of the extracellular fluid.

Factors stimulating exit from cells

Acidosis, mainly respiratory;

Low osmolarity of the extracellular fluid;

Hormonal: glucagon, beta-adrenergic blockade; alpha-adrenergic agonists (catecholamines);

Cell injury.

Renal excretion of potassium

This depends on the net effect following:

Reabsorption in the proximal convoluted tubule and in the ascending limb of the loop of Henle.

Secretion, which depends on the basolateral Na^+K^+ -ATPase, and the luminal voltage-gated potassium channels.

Abnormalities in potassium homeostasis

Serum potassium is normally maintained between 3.5 and 5.0 mmol/l. A reduction of 1 mmol/l reflects a deficit of 150–400 mmol in total body potassium.

Hypokalaemia can be related to the following pathophysiological mechanisms:

- **Redistribution** due to transcellular shifts: alkalosis, beta 2-adrenergic stimulation, insulin, rapid cell growth in acute anabolic states.
- **True hypokalaemia**:

  Renal losses, associated with urine potassium greater than 20 mmol in 24 hours. This can be produced by diuretics, mineralocorticoids, high dose glucocorticoids, or in states of osmotic diuresis.

  Gastrointestinal losses: malabsorption; secretory diarrhoea; laxative abuse; cation-binding resins; villous adenoma.

Hyperkalaemia can be related to:

- **Pseudohyperkalaemia**: improper blood collection with haemolysis; marked leukocytosis; marked thrombocytosis.
- **True hyperkalaemia:**

  Reduced excretion: acute renal failure; potassium-sparing diuretics.

  Increased intake or release: potassium supplements; rhabdomyolysis; haemolytic states.

  Transcellular shifts of potassium: acidosis; beta blockers; cell destruction (tumour lysis).

■ Magnesium

Magnesium is the second most abundant intracellular cation. The total body content in an adult is around 2000 mmol (24 g). Sixty per cent is contained in bone, and 20% in muscle. The normal calcium: magnesium ratio in bone is 50:1, the ratio being higher in trabecular than in cortical bone. Only 1% is contained in the extracellular fluid.

Daily intake is around 10–12 mmol. Requirements are increased in childhood, pregnancy, critical illness and in magnesium-losing states (renal, gastrointestinal or cutaneous). The serum concentration ranges from 0.8–1.2 mmol/l. 25%–30% is protein bound, 10%–15% is complexed and 50%–60% (the physiologically active fraction) is ionised. The intracellular concentration is around 40 mmol/l.

Functions of magnesium

Regulator or cofactor for a number of enzymes, including phosphatases and phosphokinases involved in energy storage and utilisation:

Na^+K^+ -ATPase: the sodium pump

Ca^{2+}-ATPase

Proton pumps

Protein synthesis

Adenyl cyclase: involved in cyclic AMP production

Glycolytic enzymes

Regulator of slow calcium channels.

Mediates hypocalcaemia-induced parathyroid hormone (PTH) release and is involved in maintenance of end-organ sensitivity to PTH and vitamin D.

Acts as an endogenous calcium antagonist, competing with calcium for intra-cellular entry via cytoplasmic channels and by activating cell membrane pumps that actively pump out calcium.

Neuromuscular transmission.

Muscle contraction.

Membrane stabilisation: regulator of membrane excitability.

Structural component of cell membranes and the cytoskeleton.

Cell division.

Hypomagnesaemia

This is associated with

Reduced intake.

Renal losses: acute tubular necrosis; post-obstructive diuresis; diuretics; renal tubular acidosis.

Gastrointestinal losses: malabsorption; secretory diarrhoea.

Redistribution into cells.

BIBLIOGRAPHY

King, L. S., Agre, P. Pathophysiology of the aquaporin water channels. *Annu. Rev. Physiol.*, **58** (1996), 619–48.

Acid–base balance 3

■ Introduction

Acid–base homeostasis is essential to allow normal tissue and organ system function. Specifically, intracellular enzyme systems require an appropriate pH for maintenance of activity. Extracellular fluid pH is normally maintained around a level of 7.35–7.45. This is achieved through reversible chemical buffer systems and through homeostatic responses mediated by the lungs and the kidneys.

■ The pH scale

This scale for measurement was introduced by Sorenson in 1909 to facilitate dealing with hydrogen ion concentrations. This avoids the need to deal with negative indices and to accommodate the very wide range of H^+ and OH^- solutions that are encountered in acid–base reactions, when measured in nanomoles per litre.

The pH is the negative logarithm to base 10 of H ion activity. Acidic solutions always have a pH less than 7.0. The pH scale is an exponential scale, where a 0.3 unit fall in pH reflects a doubling of hydrogen ion concentration.

■ Bronsted–Lowry definitions

An **acid** is a proton donor to a base.

A **base** is a proton acceptor from an acid.

Acid–base reactions are **proton transfer reactions**.

An acid losing a proton to a base forms a base itself.

A base accepting a proton forms an acid.

Every acid has its conjugate base, and every base its conjugate acid.

An acid–base reaction is a dynamic equilibrium between two conjugate acid–base pairs.

Table 3.1. Relation of pH to hydrogen ion activity

pH	H ion activity(nmol/l)
6.90	126
7.0	100
7.10	79
7.20	63
7.30	50
7.40	40
7.50	32
7.60	25
7.70	20
7.80	16

A substance that can act as both an acid and as a base is called an **amphoteric** substance. Water has amphoteric properties.

The **strength of an acid** is specified by its **dissociation constant**.

A strong acid has a dissociation constant greater than that of H_3O^+ and is almost completely ionised in aqueous solutions. A weak acid has a dissociation constant less than that of H_3O^+ (1 in aqueous solutions) and is only partially ionised in aqueous solutions.

■ Factors affecting body acid–base balance

- Body acid production creates a **hydrogen ion load**, mainly from oxidation of proteins, carbohydrates and other organic molecules. This amounts to 50–100 mmol of hydrogen ions per day in the adult, and includes volatile acids (such as carbonic acid) and fixed acids (such as phosphoric and sulphuric acids). The body is a net producer of acid. Acids produced by the body consist of carbonic acid (respiratory acid), and various metabolic acids, including sulphuric acid, phosphoric acid, lactic acid, citric acid, ammonium ions and ketone bodies (acetoacetic acid and beta-hydroxybutyric acid).
- **Buffering of the hydrogen ion load** by extracellular and intracellular buffer systems.
- **Excretion of the hydrogen ion load** due to loss of bicarbonate.

Respiratory regulation of volatile acid excretion by variations in alveolar ventilation affecting the excretion of carbon dioxide. Respiratory compensation is achieved by control of alveolar ventilation through the intervention of:

Peripheral chemoreceptors in the carotid and aortic bodies;

Central chemoreceptors in the ventro-lateral medulla.

Acid production by the body

Volatile: carbonic acid: 15–20 moles per day
Non-volatile or fixed: 80 moles per day
Phosphoric acid: oxidation of phosphoproteins, phospholipids,
phosphoglycerides and nucleic acids
Sulphuric acid: oxidation of methionine and cysteine

Buffers

A **buffer** is a **conjugate acid–base pair**. It is represented by a mixture of substances in aqueous solution, usually a weak acid and its corresponding sodium salt (a conjugate base), which acts as a proton acceptor for the corresponding weak acid. A buffer system can resist changes in H ion concentration when small amounts of strong (completely ionised) acids or bases are added. It can thus be considered as a pair of substances that can donate or accept (reversibly bind) H ions in order to minimise changes in H ion concentration. The body's buffer systems are primarily involved with the neutralisation of acids.

Activity of the buffer system depends on a simple equilibrium constant determined by the unique **dissociation constant** (pK) of the buffer. The system is most effective at a concentration identical to that of the concentration of its conjugate base or acid.

In a mixture of buffer pairs, each buffer pair is in equilibrium with all others at a given pH. By controlling one buffer pair, all pairs in equilibrium with this pair can be controlled, minimising changes in pH. The larger the concentration of acid and conjugate base (or base and conjugate acid) the greater the buffering capacity of the system.

Henderson–Hasselbach equation

The pK of an acid is numerically equal to the pH of the solution when the molar concentrations of the acid and its conjugate base are equal.

$$CO_2 + H_2O = H_2CO_3 = H^+ + HCO_3^-$$
$$(H_2CO_3) = K(H^+)(HCO_3^-)$$
$$I/H^+ = K^+(HCO_3^-)(H_2CO_3)$$

Taking logarithms on both sides,

$$pH = pK + log10(HCO_3^-)(H_2CO_3)$$

By the equation, pH remains constant provided the ratio of HCO_3^-/CO_2 remains constant. The equation can be used to calculate the pH of a buffer solution, the amount of acid or salt required to make a buffer solution of desired pH, or the effect on the pH of a buffer solution when a small amount of acid or base is added.

Physiological buffer systems

Buffer systems comprise the first line of the body's response to changes in pH. They include:

Blood

$NaHCO_3/H_2CO_3$

Haemoglobin and its potassium salt

Plasma proteins: plasma protein and sodium proteinate

Phosphate($H_2PO_4^-$/HPO_4^{2-})

Extracellular fluid and cerebrospinal fluid

HCO_3^-/CO_2

Proteins

Phosphate($H_2PO_4^-$/HPO_4^{2-})

Intracellular fluid

Proteins

Phosphate

Organic phosphates

HCO_3^-/CO_2

Buffering capacity

The **buffering capacity** of a buffer pair depends on their total concentration rather than on their ratio. The pH of a solution containing a buffer pair depends wholly on their ratio, and concentrating or diluting the system does not alter the pH.

Intracellular proteins account for 75% of the body's buffering capacity. The protein and phosphate systems buffer changes in carbon dioxide. The bicarbonate system can only buffer metabolic acids.

Bicarbonate and non-bicarbonate buffer systems are in equilibrium with each other.

The total buffering capacity of blood at a pH of 7.4 and constant $paCO_2$ is about 75 mmol/l. The total **buffer base** is the sum of the concentrations of all buffer anions that can take up H^+ ions, and is about 45 mmol/l.

A scheme for the assessment and management of acid–base abnormalities

- Look at the paO_2.

  Correct rapidly if abnormal, with supplemental oxygen and ventilatory support where appropriate. The paO_2 needs to be interpreted in relation to the inspired oxygen concentration, and calculation of the alveolar–arterial gradient may be necessary to unmask hypoxia under these circumstances.

- Look at the pH: is it life threatening?

  Acidosis: H^+ greater than 44 nmol/l or pH less than 7.35

  Alkalosis: H^+ less than 35 nmol/l or pH greater than 7.45

- Is acidosis respiratory or metabolic?

  Respiratory: $paCO_2$ greater than 45 mm Hg (6 kPa) –the $paCO_2$ reflects alveolar ventilation

  Metabolic: HCO_3 less than 22 mm Hg (2.9 kPa)

- Is alkalosis respiratory or metabolic?

  Respiratory: $paCO_2$ less than 35 mm Hg (4.7 kPa)

  Metabolic: HCO_3 greater than 26 mm Hg (3.5 kPa)

- Is there any compensation?

- Consider the anion gap (indicates presence of non-volatile acids): this is the difference between measured cations and measured anions.

- Check the electrolyte values.

The **alveolar–arterial oxygen gradient** is normally 10 mm Hg (1.33 kPa), with a range from 0.5 to 3 kPa. The alveolar gas equation allows calculation of the alveolar pO_2 from the formula

$PAO_2 = FiO_2 \times 95 - PACO_2 \times 1.25$. The gradient is equal to $PAO_2^- paO_2$. There is no gradient between $PACO_2$ and $paCO_2$. There is a reciprocal relationship between PAO_2 and $PACO_2$. The expected PAO_2 in kPa is approximately equal to the FiO_2 (%) minus 10.

The **base excess** or **base deficit** (negative base excess) is the amount of strong acid or base, respectively, required to restore a litre of whole blood to normal composition with a pH of 7.4 and $paCO_2$ of 5.3 kPa (40 mm Hg) at 37 °C. This reflects the change in buffer base concentration of blood in the presence of excess acid or base, ranging from -2 to $+2$ mmol/l. A normal range of values denotes normal metabolic acid–base status. A base deficit indicates metabolic acidosis, and a base excess metabolic alkalosis. The base deficit x body weight (in kilograms), divided by 4, yields the deficient number of millimoles of HCO_3.

The **standard bicarbonate** is the plasma bicarbonate concentration in fully oxygenated whole blood at 37 °C at a $paCO_2$ of 5.3 kPa (40 mm Hg).

Acid–base disorders

There are four **primary acid–base disorders**, with four secondary compensatory mechanisms

Primary disorder	Compensation
Metabolic acidosis	respiratory alkalosis
Metabolic alkalosis	respiratory acidosis
Respiratory acidosis	metabolic alkalosis

Table 3.2. Primary acid–base disorders

	Plasma pH	pCO_2	HCO_3
Respiratory Acidosis	reduced	increased	increased
Metabolic Acidosis	reduced	normal	reduced
Respiratory Alkalosis	increased	reduced	reduced
Metabolic Alkalosis	increased	normal	increased

Respiratory alkalosis   metabolic acidosis

The four components in the pathophysiology of acid–base disorders can be categorised as:

Generation

Buffering

Compensation

Correction

Compensatory mechanisms always cease before normality is reached. Overcompensation does not occur. In general, increases in HCO_3^- follow increases in pCO_2 and reductions in HCO_3^- follow decreases in pCO_2.

Renal compensation mechanisms

- **Excretion of free acid and base**. This includes Na^+-H^+ exchange across the apical membrane of proximal tubular cells, and direct H^+ ion secretion via the H^+-ATPase of the intercalated cells of the distal tubule and collecting ducts.
- **Excretion of buffered acid and base**
- **Reabsorption and excretion of the filtered HCO_3^- load**. Eighty per cent to 90% of the filtered load is reabsorbed in the proximal tubule. This involves the secretion of hydrogen ions by the proximal tubular cells, which combine with bicarbonate to form carbonic acid. The carbonic acid forms carbon dioxide and water in the tubular lumen. Carbon dioxide diffuses into the proximal tubular cell and re-forms carbonic acid. Hydrogen ions are removed to be secreted into the lumen, facilitating further reabsorption of bicarbonate.
- **Ammonia production** from glutamine and ammonium ion (NH_4^+) secretion into the distal tubule.
- **Excretion of hydrogen ions as titratable acid** in the distal tubule, fixed to phosphate, creatinine and urate.

Urine acidification involves:

Formation of hydrogen ions for exchange of HCO_3 in proximal and distal tubules;

Buffering of certain salts, including Na_2HPO_4, hydroxybutyrate and creatinine;

Ammonium ion formation.

The pH of urine cannot be lowered below 4.4 normally.

Components of an arterial blood gas analyser

Oxygen analysis is achieved by either spectrophotometric or polarographic methods. The Clark or polarographic electrode uses a platinum cathode, a silver/silver chloride anode and a solution of potassium chloride. A small polarising potential is maintained between the cathode and anode. Current flow through the system depends on oxygen tension at the cathode, where oxygen is reduced.

Carbon dioxide analysis is achieved by the use of a Severinghaus carbon dioxide electrode. Carbon dioxide diffusion through a Teflon membrane alters the pH of a test solution.

Measurement of pH is by a pH electrode, which relies on the electrical potential generated by the movement of hydrogen ions between a sample and a reference buffer at known H^+ ion concentration, these being separated by hydrogen-ion sensitive glass. The reference and reading electrodes are both silver/silver chloride electrodes.

A co-oximeter measures the proportions of oxyhaemoglobin, reduced haemoglobin, carboxyhaemoglobin and methaemoglobin.

Derived measurements include:

Serum bicarbonate.

Standard bicarbonate: the serum bicarbonate of a sample in equilibrium with a gas mixture containing PCO_2 at 5.3 kPa and PO_2 at 13.3 kPa at 37° C.

Active acid extruders in the kidney

Transporters
Primary active
Vacuolar H^+-ATPase proximal tubule(PT), collecting duct(CD)
K^+/H^+-ATPase CD
Secondary active
Na-H antiporter   PT, thick ascending limb of loop of Henle (TAL), distal convoluted tubule (DCT)
Base extruders in the kidney
Transporters
$Cl - HCO_3$ exchanger   CD
$Na^+HCO_3^-/CO_2$ co-transporter   PT, TAL

Base excess, which is negative in acidosis and positive in alkalosis. It is a measure of the severity of the abnormality in acid–base balance.

Siggaard–Andersen curve nomogram

The nomogram is useful in determining the presence and nature of acid–base disorder. The PCO_2 is plotted on a logarithmic scale on the vertical axis, whilst pH is plotted on the horizontal axis. Any point to the left of a vertical line through pH 7.40 indicates acidosis. Any point to the right of a vertical line through pH 7.40 indicates alkalosis.

Acidosis

Effects of acid load

The **response to an acid load** consists of:

Extracellular buffering

HCO_3

Intracellular and bone buffering

Proteins

Phosphates

Bone carbonate

Respiratory compensation

Stimulation of central and peripheral chemoreceptors, resulting in an increase in alveolar ventilation (begins within 1–2 hours, reaching its maximum level at 12–24 hours). There is mainly an increase in tidal volume rather than in respiratory rate.

Renal excretion of the H^+ load.

Filtered HCO_3 is reabsorbed

Ninety per cent in the proximal tubule (primarily by Na^+/H^+ exchange).

H^+ secretion via the Na^+/H^+ antiporter leads to carbonic acid formation with the HCO_3^-;

The carbonic acid formed is dehydrated by carbonic anhydrase to form CO_2 and H_2O;

CO_2 diffuses into the cell and combines with OH^- to form HCO_3^-;

HCO_3^- is transported through the basolateral membrane via a Na^+/HCO_3^- co-transporter.

Ten per cent in the distal nephron (by an active H^+-ATPase pump).

The dietary acid load is excreted by the secretion of H^+ ions from the distal tubular cell into the lumen. This is mediated by K^+/H^+-ATPase and H^+-ATPase. The H^+ ions then combine either with the urinary buffers (especially HPO_4^{2-} in a

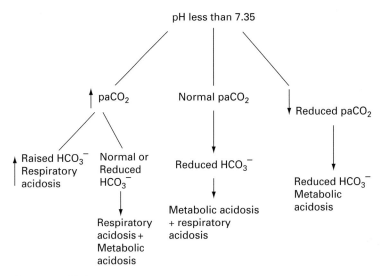

Figure 3.1 Acidosis.

process called titratable acidity) or with NH_3. The ammonium ion is excreted in the urine.

Pathophysiology of metabolic acidosis

Increased hydrogen ion, reduced base, or rapid dilution of base secondary to normal saline infusion;

Hydrogen ions buffered by HCO_3^-;

Reduced HCO_3^- and increased H_2CO_3;

Increased CO_2 and reduced pH stimulate ventilation, reducing plasma CO_2.

The causes of metabolic acidosis can be listed as:

Increased endogenous production or exogenous administration of acid: increased anion gap;

Reduced renal excretion of acid, which fails to match endogenous acid production: normal anion gap;

Metabolic alkali losses: normal anion gap.

Anion gap

The normal range is 8–16 mmol/l. It is equal to $(Na^+ + K^+) + (Cl^- + HCO_3)$, i.e. the difference between measured cations and measured anions. The gap thus represents unmeasured anions, including plasma proteins, phosphates and sulphates. It contributes to the recognition of the cause of the metabolic acidosis.

The causes of an elevated anion gap can be broadly categorised as:

Renal failure.

Ketoacidosis.

Lactic acidosis.

Drugs and toxins: salicylates; ethanol; methanol; ethylene glycol.

Inborn errors of metabolism.

Alkalosis

Respiratory alkalosis is the result of increased alveolar ventilation and is due to:

Increased CNS ventilatory drive;

Increased chemoreceptor stimulation;

Increased mechanical ventilation.

The renal compensatory response involves reduced hydrogen ion secretion into the tubular lumen, reduced reabsorption of bicarbonate and reduction in urine ammonium and titratable acid excretion. The net effect is the production of alkaline urine.

Pathophysiology of metabolic alkalosis

Hydrogen ion loss, as with gastrointestinal (vomiting; nasogastric suction; villous adenoma) or renal losses.

Bicarbonate retention with increased tubular reabsorption; gain of OH^- and HCO_3 ions.

Potassium leaves intracellular stores.

Hydrogen ions enter cells to maintain cationic equilibrium.

Reduced intracellular pH and raised extracellular pH.

Metabolic alkalosis can be caused by:

Alkali gain, e.g. from exogenous administration.

Extracellular fluid compartment contraction, with the loss of HCO_3 poor and Cl^- rich extracellular fluid: this is **volume-responsive alkalosis**, with a urine chloride less than 10 mmol/l.

Mineralocorticoid excess, e.g. with hyperaldosteronism, Cushing's syndrome, Bartter's syndrome: this is not volume-responsive and is associated with a urine chloride greater than 20 mmol/l.

Metabolic alkalosis is maintained by the continued stimulation of HCO_3 from the distal tubule, caused by:

Mechanisms of ketoacidosis

Increase in free fatty acid delivery to the liver due to enhanced lipolysis.

Resetting of hepatocyte function such that the free fatty acids are converted preferentially into ketoacids and not triglycerides.

Factors responsible for the association of hypokalaemia and metabolic alkalosis

Common causes of metabolic alkalosis (vomiting, diuretics, mineralocorticoid excess) directly induce both H and K^+ loss.

Hypokalaemia causes a transcellular shift in which K^+ leaves and H enters the cells, thereby raising the extracellular pH.

Hypokalaemia increases net acid secretion and HCO_3 reabsorption, probably due in part to the associated intracellular acidosis.

Saline replacement can lower the plasma HCO_3 concentration in saline-responsive metabolic alkalosis in three different ways:

By expansion of the extracellular fluid volume;

By removing the stimulus to renal Na retention, thereby permitting $NaHCO_3$ excretion in the urine;

By increasing distal Cl^- delivery, which will promote HCO_3 secretion in the cortical collecting tubule.

Reduced renal perfusion, leading to stimulation of the renin–angiotensin–aldosterone mechanism;

Chloride depletion;

Hypokalaemia.

Relationships of HCO_3 ion with Cl^- ion and of H with body cations (Na and K^+)

Exchange across cell membrane

HCO_3 has a reciprocal relationship with Cl^-;

H and K^+ have a reciprocal relationship in the intracellular fluid.

Mechanisms of exchange in renal tubules

Secretion of H is achieved in exchange for Na or K^+ ions;

Reabsorption of Na in distal tubules takes place in exchange for K^+ and H secretion;

H and K^+ compete for the same carrier mechanisms in the distal tubules.

Evaluation of compensatory mechanisms in metabolic acid–base disorders

Metabolic acidosis

Expected $paCO_2$ in normally compensated metabolic acidosis

$paCO2$ in mm Hg $= 1.5 \times (HCO_3) + 8(+/-2)$
Or
$paCO_2$ in mm Hg is approximately $=$ last two digits of pH
If $paCO_2$ is lower than expected: respiratory alkalosis + metabolic acidosis
If $PaCO_2$ is higher than expected: respiratory acidosis + metabolic acidosis

Metabolic alkalosis

Expected $paCO_2$ in mm Hg in normally compensated metabolic alkalosis
$PaCO_2$ should rise by 6 mm Hg (0.8 kPa) for every 10 mmol/l rise in HCO_3
If $paCO_2$ is lower than calculated: respiratory alkalosis + metabolic alkalosis
If $paCO_2$ is higher than calculated: respiratory acidosis + metabolic alkalosis

Clinical effects of acidosis

CNS: reduced cerebral blood flow; depressed level of consciousness; coma.

Cardiovascular system: impaired myocardial contractility (negative inotropy); reduced cardiac output; arteriolar dilatation and venoconstriction, with centralisation of the blood volume; reduced systemic arterial blood pressure; increased pulmonary vascular resistance; reduced responsiveness to catecholamines; reduction in ventricular fibrillation threshold.

Respiratory system: hyperventilation; fatigue of muscles of breathing; dyspnoea.

Metabolic: hypokalaemia; insulin resistance (e.g., diabetic ketoacidosis); inhibition of anaerobic glycolysis; reduced ATP synthesis; increased protein degradation; increased metabolic demands.

Right shift of the oxyhaemoglobin dissociation curve.

Problems associated with the use of sodium bicarbonate to correct metabolic acidosis

Increased osmolality from the large sodium load, leading to volume expansion;
Increased $paCO_2$ causing respiratory acidosis;
Late metabolic alkalosis;
Paradoxical intracellular acidosis;
Hypokalaemia;
Reduced ionised calcium, leading to neuronal irritability and tetany;
Impaired arterial oxygenation and reduced myocardial oxygen
Consumption, secondary to increased affinity of oxygen for haemoglobin;
Reduced cerebral blood flow.

Clinical effects of alkalosis

CNS: reduced cerebral blood flow; seizures; tetany; lethargy; delirium.

Cardiovascular system: arteriolar constriction; reduced coronary blood flow; reduced angina threshold; predisposition to refractory supraventricular and ventricular arrhythmias.

Respiratory system: compensatory hypoventilation; increased bronchial tone; hypoxia; hypercapnia.

Metabolic: hypokalaemia; hypophosphataemia; hypomagnesaemia; reduced serum ionised calcium; increased anaerobic glycolysis and production of organic acids.

Left shift of oxyhaemoglobin dissociation curve, with reduced oxygen availability to the tissues.

BIBLIOGRAPHY

Astrup, P., Engel, K. & Jorgensen, K. Definitions and terminology in blood acid–base chemistry, *Ann. New York Acad. Sci.*, **133** (1966), 59.

Davenport, H. W. *The ABC of Acid-base Chemistry*, 6th edn. Chicago: University of Chicago Press, 1974

Siggaard-Andersen, O. An acid–base chart for arterial blood with normal and pathophysiological reference areas. *Scand. J. Clin. Lab. Invest.*, **27**: (1971), 239–45.

Renal physiology

■ Introduction to renal structure

The kidneys are primarily responsible for the maintenance of the internal environment of the human body. They share the following **structural features**:

- They are paired retroperitoneal organs.
- They weigh 110–170g each in the adult male, are 10–12 cm long, 5–7.5 cm wide and 2.5–3 cm thick.
- They receive 20%–25% of the cardiac output, which corresponds to 1000–1200 ml/minute, but only account for about 10% of the oxygen consumption of the body.
- The kidneys thereby receive the highest blood flow per gram of organ weight in the human body, while accounting for only 0.4% of the body weight. The entire plasma volume is cycled through the glomerular system 20 times per hour.
- Their internal structure consists of an outer cortex and an inner medulla. The medulla consists of ten pyramids, with their bases near the cortex and apices (papillae) which project into the calyceal sinuses. The pyramids are separated by columnar extensions of the cortex. Ninety per cent of the renal blood supply goes to the cortex.
- The cortex comprises glomeruli and proximal convoluted tubules, while the medulla comprises the loops of Henle, the distal convoluted tubules and the collecting ducts.

Functional components of the kidneys

The functional components of the kidney are the nephrons (each kidney contains one million nephrons), collecting ducts and the microvasculature.

A **nephron**, the structural and functional unit of the kidneys, demonstrates functional segmentation and consists of:

Renal corpuscle, which comprises Bowman's capsule and the glomerular capillary tuft. The glomerular tuft has three cell types: mesangial cells, capillary endothelial cells and podocytes (visceral epithelium of Bowman's capsule).

Renal tubule, which comprises:

Proximal convoluted tubule;

Proximal straight tubule (pars recta);

Descending thin limb of loop of Henle (in long-loop nephrons only);

Medullary thick ascending limb of loop of Henle;

Cortical thick ascending limb of loop of Henle;

Distal convoluted tubule.

The **collecting duct system** comprises the connecting tubule, cortical collecting duct, outer and inner medullary collecting ducts.

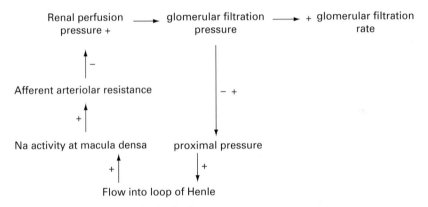

Figure 4.1 Pathway for glomerular feedback.

Types of nephrons

Superficial and mid-cortical nephrons, which comprise 85% of the total. They possess short loops of Henle and their peritubular capillaries carry nutrients to the tubules. Juxtamedullary, which possess long loops of Henle specialised for the concentration of urine. These loops extend into the medulla. The efferent glomerular capillaries form vasa recta, which function as counter-current exchangers.

■ Functions of the kidney

Excretory and regulatory

Removal of water-soluble nitrogenous waste products of metabolism (urea, creatinine, urate) and catabolic turnover of cells, and the elimination of drugs and toxins;

Maintenance of water, electrolyte (ion concentrations) and acid–base balance (pH of body fluids);

Regulation of extracellular fluid volume;

Maintenance of body fluid composition;

Maintenance of blood pressure.

Metabolic

Gluconeogenesis

Endocrine

Renin production;

Erythropoietin production: control of erythropoiesis;

Synthesis of 1,25-dihydroxycholecalciferol;

Catabolism of polypeptide hormones (e.g., parathyroid hormone, insulin);

Prostaglandin synthesis.

Characteristics of erythropoietin

This glycoprotein hormone of molecular weight 34 000 daltons is synthesised by renal cortical interstitial cells, which account for about 80% of the body's production. Production is stimulated by tissue hypoxia.

It is a major regulator of red blood cell production, binding to specific cell surface receptors and promoting erythroid differentiation.

■ The renal circulation

This consists of, in sequence, several orders of branches of the renal artery, including:

Interlobar arteries

Arcuate arteries

Cortical radial (interlobular) arteries

Afferent arterioles

Glomerular capillary tufts

Efferent arterioles

Descending vasa recta

Capillary plexus at medullary level

Ascending vasa recta

Arcuate veins

Interlobular veins

Arcuate veins

Interlobar veins

The kidney is unique in possessing two capillary networks in series, each with a preceding arteriole. These are the glomerular bed and the peritubular capillary bed. The glomerular capillary pressure is much higher than that of any other capillary bed in the body, this being a reflection of its interposition between two arteriolar systems.

Effects of renal circulation on urine production

The renal circulation affects urine formation in the following ways:

The glomerular filtration rate is an important determinant of solute and water excretion.

The peritubular capillaries in the cortex return reabsorbed solutes and water to the systemic circulation and can modulate the degree of proximal tubular reabsorption and secretion.

The vasa recta capillaries return reabsorbed salt and water to the systemic circulation and participate in the counter-current mechanism.

Abnormalities of renal haemodynamics may be involved in the genesis of acute renal failure, associated with a reduction in total renal blood flow and with the redistribution of intrarenal blood flow away from cortical to juxta-medullary nephrons in order to protect the medulla.

Autoregulation

The renal circulation is subject to **autoregulation** by the following mechanisms:

A myogenic response, with arteriolar smooth muscle contraction in response to increased vessel wall tension;

The intranephron tubuloglomerular feedback system, which describes the coupling of distal nephron flow with single nephron glomerular filtration rate.

Humoral influences on the renal vasculature

These are mediated by the following substances:

Vasoconstrictors:

Angiotensin II

Noradrenaline

Thromboxane A2, B2

Leukotrienes D4, C4

Platelet-activating factor

Endothelin-1

Vasopressin

Vasodilators:

Prostaglandins E1, E2, I2

Acetylcholine

Bradykinin

Nitric oxide

Atrial natriuretic peptide (ANP)

■ Processes involved in urine production

- **Glomerular filtration**, which involves the passive formation of an ultrafiltrate (water and crystalloids) of the plasma, which is essentially blood cell and protein macromolecule free, at the glomerulus. Around 180 litres of glomerular filtrate is formed daily, of which 99% is reabsorbed by the tubules. The glomerulus functions as a size-selective, shape-selective and electrical charge-selective barrier for macromolecules. It is normally impermeable to molecules of the size of albumin (69 000 daltons) and larger. Cations are more readily filtered than anions for the same molecular radius.

- **Tubular secretion**, from the peritubular capillary blood to the tubular lumen, which may be active or passive.

- **Tubular reabsorption** from the tubular lumen to the blood, which is either active or passive. About two thirds of the glomerular filtrate is reabsorbed in the proximal tubule. The trans-tubular reabsorption or secretion of ions is facilitated by protein carriers or ion-specific channels.

- Tubular metabolism

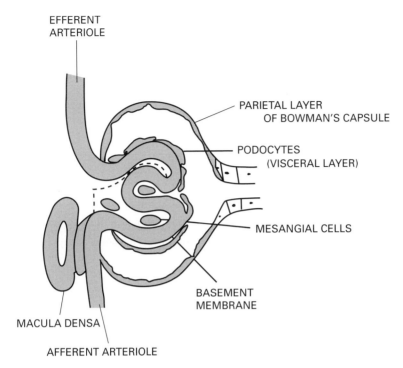

Figure 4.2 Glomerulus and glomerular capillary.

Glomerular filtration

The process of **glomerular filtration** is determined by:

- A balance of Starling forces, i.e. the hydrostatic and colloid osmotic forces acting across the glomerular capillary membrane. Glomerular capillary hydrostatic pressure, which is the main driving force, depends on the systemic arterial blood pressure, afferent arteriolar resistance and efferent arteriolar resistance.
- The capillary filtration coefficient.

Ultrafiltration from the glomerular capillaries into Bowman's membrane occurs through three **filtration barriers**:

Fenestrated **endothelium of the glomerular capillaries**. These are polygonal squamous epithelial cells with large open pores.

Basement membrane of Bowman's capsule. This comprises a lamina densa between two less dense cement layers.

Podocytes, or specialised epithelial cells of Bowman's capsule with numerous foot processes or pedicels that cover the basement membrane. The foot processes are separated by filtration slit diaphragms that contain pores.

Glomerular filtration rate

The **glomerular filtration rate** is determined by the number of functioning glomeruli, which is proportional to kidney size and relates to the glomerular capillary surface area, and by the filtration rate at each single glomerulus.

The determinants for the **single nephron glomerular filtration rate** are:

Mean trans-capillary hydrostatic pressure difference (glomerular capillary hydrostatic pressure minus the pressure in Bowman's space);

Systemic plasma colloid osmotic pressure;

Glomerular plasma flow rate;

Glomerular capillary ultrafiltration coefficient.

The glomerular filtration rate can be represented as the filtration coefficient x the filtration pressure. The **filtration coefficient** is a function of the total capillary surface area and of the permeability per unit of surface area.

The range for the glomerular filtration rate is

60–80 ml/min per m^2 or

100–140 ml/min per 1.73 m^2

The rate falls with increasing age by about 1 ml/min per year beyond the age of 40 years.

The glomerular filtration rate can be measured by **clearance techniques**. The clearance of a marker substance that is not metabolised by the kidneys is a hypothetical measure of the volume of arterial plasma completely cleared of the marker in unit time, usually in one minute. It is a virtual and not a real volume of plasma.

$$\text{Clearance} = \frac{(\text{Urine concentration} \times \text{urine volume per minute})}{\text{Plasma concentration}}$$

A **marker for measurement of glomerular filtration rate** should have the following properties:

Metabolically inert;

Free filtration at the glomerulus, with molecular weight compatible with unimpeded glomerular filtration;

No effect on the glomerular filtration rate;

Not reabsorbed, secreted or metabolised by the renal tubule;

No protein binding;

No extra-renal clearance;

Steady state level in plasma;

Easily measured in serum and urine;

Non-toxic.

Glomerular filtration rate in ml/min can be represented by the formula *UV/P* where

The **Cockcroft–Gault formula** allows calculation of creatinine clearance from plasma creatinine.

$$\text{Creatinine clearance} = \frac{(140 - \text{age in years}) \times \text{lean body weight in kilograms}}{\text{plasmacreatinine} \times 72}$$

In women, the result thus obtained is multiplied by 0.85.

The **filtration fraction** is the ratio of the glomerular filtration rate to the renal plasma flow, and represents the proportion of the renal arterial plasma flow removed by glomerular filtration. The normal value is around 0.2.

$U=$ concentration of marker in urine (mg/ml)

$V=$ flow rate of urine (ml/min)

$P=$ plasma concentration of marker (mg/ml)

The clearance of either inulin or of endogenous creatinine is independent of the plasma concentration and of the rate of urine flow. Glomerular filtration rate can also be measured using chelating agents, such as ^{51}Cr-ethylene diamine tetra-acetic acid (EDTA) and ^{99}Tcm-diethylene triamine penta-acetate (DTPA).

Endogenous creatinine clearance can be measured following collection of a timed overnight urine collection and an early morning blood sample. A 24 hour clearance measurement eliminates errors due to period variable bladder emptying and wash-out effects. One to two per cent of the total muscle creatine pool is converted daily to creatinine. Creatinine clearance is increased in renal failure, leading to an overestimation of glomerular filtration rate.

The measurement of **inulin clearance** is achieved by administration of a bolus dose followed by a constant infusion, until the plasma concentration is almost steady, typically after 90–120 minutes. Moderate diuresis is induced by the regular administration of fluid before and during the test. Timed urine specimens are collected, with blood samples being taken at the mid-points of the collection periods for assay. The glomerular filtration rate is taken as the mean for each period.

Tubular function

The proximal convoluted tubules are lined with cuboidal cells, which possess an inner brush border with microvilli, and possess a high mitochondrial content. The distal convoluted tubules are lined with cuboidal cells, which possess many mitochondria but no microvilli. The tubular cells demonstrate polarity, whereby the apical or luminal membrane and the basolateral or peritubular membrane are structurally and functionally different. The luminal and basolateral aspects of the tubular cell membrane are separated by the tight junction, which is composed primarily of the zona occludens.

The plasma ultrafiltrate is modified in the tubules by the following processes:

Active transport:

Primary active transport: directly coupled to ATP hydrolysis;

Secondary active transport (co-transport): sodium with glucose, amino acids or carboxylic acids.

Simple diffusion using transcellular (through the basolateral or luminal membrane) or paracellular (across tight junctions and lateral intercellular spaces) routes.

Movement via **ion channels**.

Co-transport (symport): carrier-mediated transport.

Counter-transport (antiport): carrier-mediated transport.

Endocytosis.

The transport maximum describes the maximum rate at which a system is able to transport a solute.

The active transport of sodium across the tubular epithelial cells is achieved by the influence of the Na^+/K^+-ATPase, located in the basolateral membrane. This transport is coupled with specific membrane carrier proteins in order to enable the influx (symport) or efflux (antiport) of other molecules. The latter are examples of secondary active transport. Amino acids, glucose, phosphate and chloride can all be co-transported (symport) with sodium entry. Hydrogen and calcium ions can be counter-transported (antiport) against sodium entry.

Mechanisms for reabsorption of sodium

Sodium is the major osmotically active ion in the body and has a major influence on water balance. More than 99% of the filtered sodium load is reabsorbed. There are multiple luminal systems that draw sodium from tubular lumen into tubular cell, acting in conjunction with basolateral systems that convey sodium from the tubular cell into the interstitium and thereby into blood vessels. The basolateral sodium pump produces a favourable electrochemical gradient that facilitates luminal entry of sodium via a variety of mechanisms.

Proximal convoluted tubule (65%–75%)

Luminal systems that draw sodium from the tubular lumen into the cell:

Sodium symport solute co-transport system

Sodium glucose co-transport system

Sodium amino acid co-transport system

Sodium-phosphate co-transport system

Na^+/H^+ exchange system (counter-transporter)

Cl driven sodium reabsorption

A basolateral system that actively pumps sodium from the cell into the interstitium:

Na^+/K^+-ATPase (sodium pump)

Thick ascending limb of the loop of Henle (20%)

Luminal system:

$Na^+/K^+/2Cl^-$ co-transport system: frusemide-sensitive carrier. This is the site of action of loop diuretics. Chloride ion leaves the cell via the basolateral Cl channel or KCl co-transporter.

Basolateral system that actively pumps sodium into the interstitium: Na^+/K^+-ATPase.

Distal convoluted tubule and cortical collecting duct (10%)

Luminal systems:

Na^+/Cl^- co-transport system: thiazide-sensitive carrier

Selective sodium conductive channels, regulated by aldosterone: amiloride-sensitive channel

Basolateral system:

Na^+K^+-ATPase

Renal sodium excretion

This is regulated by:

Glomerular filtration rate

Peritubular and luminal factors

Peritubular capillary Starling forces

Luminal composition

Medullary interstitial composition

Trans-tubular ion gradients

Humoral effector mechanisms

Renin–angiotensin–aldosterone system

Local prostaglandins

Kallikrein–kinin systems

Atrial natriuretic peptide

Other natriuretic hormone(s)

Table 4.1. Renal epithelial co-transporters and antiporters

Co-transporters	Transport substrate	Location	Stoichiometry
	Na^+/glucose	BBM-PCT	1:1
		BBM-PST	1:2
	Na^+/phosphate	BBM-PCT	2:1
	Na^+/Cl^-	apical	
		membrane DCT	1:1
	Na^+/K^+/Cl^-	apical	
		membrane TAL	1:1:2
	Na^+/HCO_3^-	BLM-PCT	1:3
Antiporters			
	Na^+/H^-	BBM-PCT	
		apical membrane TAL	1:1
	Na^+/$Ca2^+$	BLM-PCT	3:2

BBM brush border (apical) membrane
BLM basolateral membrane
DCT distal convoluted tubule
PCT proximal convoluted tubule
PST proximal straight tubule
TAL thick ascending limb

Renal sympathetic nerves, which directly stimulate sodium reabsorption in the proximal tubule and the thick ascending limb of the loop of Henle.

Other proximal tubular reabsorption functions

These relate to:

Water: by osmosis, down the osmotic gradient created by solute reabsorption.

Glucose: carrier-mediated co-transport with sodium across the apical membrane, involving the glucose transporters Na^+-dependent glucose transporter (SLGT)-1 and SLGT-2. Thereafter, facilitated diffusion across the basolateral membrane is mediated by the high affinity GLUT-2 transporter.

Amino acids: seven specific transport systems, including those for neutral, dibasic, dicarboxylic, immunoglycine and beta amino acids.

Proteins: alpha 1-microglobulin; beta 2-microglobulin; retinal-binding protein.

Natriuretic peptides

These are a cardiovascular peptide family, consisting of:

atrial natriuretic peptide (ANP) and brain type natriuretic peptide (BNP, initially isolated from porcine brain): of cardiac myocyte origin

Effects of natriuretic peptides

Kidney: diuresis; natriuresis; inhibition of renin secretion
Adrenal glands: inhibition of aldosterone production
Heart: reduced cardiac output; negative inotropic activity
Vasculature: vasodilatation; increased permeability; antimitogenic effect on vascular smooth muscle cells; release of paracrine vasoactive/antimitogenic agents – nitric oxide; inhibition of release of paracrine mitogenic factors: endothelin.

C-type natriuretic peptide (CNP): of endothelial cell origin

They share a common structure, consisting of a 17 amino acid central disulphide ring, with variable length N-terminal and C-terminal segments. They are synthesised as high molecular weight precursors. Their effects are mediated by cell surface receptors with a guanyl cyclase catalytic domain, with cyclic guanosine monophosphate (GMP) being generated as a second messenger.

The effects of natriuretic peptides

These allow protection against salt and water retention, inhibition of the production of and action of vasoconstrictor peptides, promotion of vascular relaxation and inhibition of sympathetic outflow.

These actions lead to a reduction in arterial blood pressure, most apparent in states of extracellular fluid volume excess. The effects oppose the activity of the renin–angiotensin system.

Atrial natriuretic peptide

It is a 28 amino acid peptide. Secretion by myoendocrine cells in the atrial muscle as a 151 amino acid pre-pro-ANP precursor leads to processing to a 126 amino acid pro-ANP, which is stored in secretory granules. It is primarily released from atria in response to volume expansion, which is sensed as an increase in atrial stretch. The right atrium may be quantitatively more important. Other causes for the stimulation of secretion include angiotensin II, endothelin and beta-adrenergic stimulation.

The end-organ vasoactive, natriuretic and diuretic effects are mediated through binding with guanyl cyclase receptors. Atrial natriuretic peptide promotes natriuresis by causing increased glomerular filtration rate, with simultaneous fall in arterial blood pressure. This is achieved by dilatation of the afferent arteriole and constriction of the efferent arteriole of the glomerulus. Thereby the filtered sodium load is increased. Other actions include:

Inhibition of renin secretion, aldosterone production and vasopressin secretion;
Inhibition of vasopressin-induced water reabsorption in the collecting ducts;

Inhibition of angiotensin-II and aldosterone-induced sodium reabsorption in the distal tubule;

Promotion of arterial vasodilatation;

Increased capillary permeability.

Atrial natriuretic peptide release is increased in any hypervolaemic state, e.g. heart failure, renal failure. Atrial natriuretic peptide resistance does not interfere with the response to chronic volume expansion as induced by oral salt loading or by mineralocorticoid escape.

Measurement of plasma natriuretic peptides is being used clinically for the early diagnosis of heart failure and for the diagnosis of left ventricular dysfunction.

Glomerular balance

Physiological changes in the glomerular filtration rate are offset by parallel changes in proximal tubular function. These are brought about by an increase in the filtered load presented to the proximal tubule and by physical forces

Tubulo-glomerular feedback

This refers to the alterations in glomerular filtration rate that can be induced by changes in tubular flow rate. The ascending limb of the loop of Henle forms an intranephronal anatomical negative feedback loop with the afferent arteriole of the glomerulus at the juxtaglomerular apparatus. This phenomenon is mediated by the effect of the sodium concentration of the tubular fluid perfusing the macula densa cells at the end of the cortical thick ascending limb of the loop of Henle. It plays an important role in autoregulation of renal blood flow, and the stabilisation of single nephron glomerular filtration rate and of tubular flow rate. Eventually, it functions as a regulatory system for extracellular fluid volume.

PATHWAY FOR GLOMERULAR FEEDBACK

Renal perfusion pressure   +   glomerular filtration pressure   + GFR

−

Afferent arteriolar resistance

− +

+

Na activity at macula densa   proximal pressure

+   +

Flow into loop of Henle

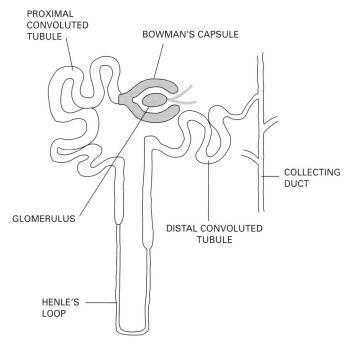

Figure 4.3 The nephron (filtering unit of the kidney).

Juxtaglomerular apparatus

The **juxtaglomerular apparatus** comprises:

The **macula densa cells** which are specialised cells of the end portion of the thick ascending limb of the loop of Henle, located between the afferent and efferent arterioles and the glomerulus. They are polygonal in shape, and are characterised by large nuclei, a luminal membrane with microvilli, an abundance of free ribosomes and lateral intercellular spaces.

The **mesangial cells**, which possess contractile properties and can alter the capillary surface area available for filtration.

The **granular renin-secreting cells** of the terminal afferent arteriole. These are modified smooth muscle cells.

Loop of Henle

The **loop of Henle** comprises:

A **descending thin limb**, which is highly permeable to water and urea, causing it to be in osmotic equilibrium with the interstitial fluid. It is impermeable to sodium.

An **ascending thin limb**, which is permeable to sodium but not to water.

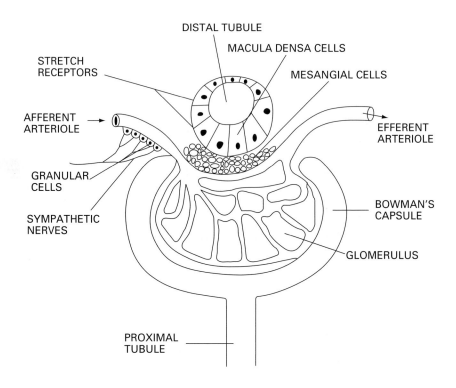

Figure 4.4 Juxtaglomerular apparatus

An **ascending thick limb**, which is involved in the active transport of sodium out of the tubule into the interstitial fluid, mediated by the Na^+K^+-ATPase. It is permeable to sodium, this being mediated by the apical $Na^+/K^+/2Cl^-$ apical carrier. Active sodium and chloride transport generates an osmotic difference between the tubular fluid and the surrounding local interstitium.

Maximum operation of the loop of Henle requires:

Ability of the ascending limb to secrete solute into the interstitium via a sodium pump mechanism

Impermeability of the ascending limb to water

Permeability of the descending limb to water and solute

Overall, 25% of sodium and 15% of water is absorbed in the loop of Henle.

Counter-current multiplier

The process by which the loop of Henle in juxtamedullary nephrons, especially the thick ascending limb, generates a longitudinal hyperosmotic medullary

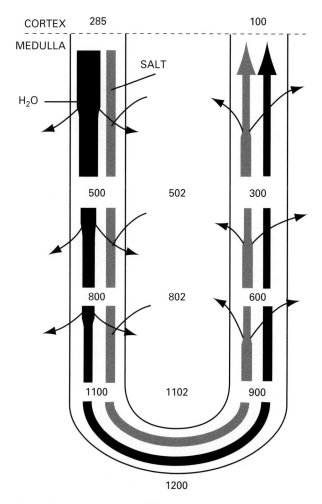

CORTEX 285   100

MEDULLA

SALT

H_2O

500   502   300

800   802   600

1100   1102   900

1200

Figure 4.5 Counter-current multiplier.

interstitial fluid solute concentration gradient. The osmolality of interstitial fluid in medulla progressively increases from the corticomedullary junction (isosmotic) to the tips of the renal papillae. An osmotic gradient exists between the tubular fluid and the interstitial fluid along the entire medullary collecting duct. Osmotic equilibration of the tubular fluid with the hypertonic medullary interstitium forms hypotonic urine.

If two adjacent currents flow in opposite directions in a hairpin loop, then any exchange of material in a transverse direction is multiplied longitudinally as one progresses towards the apex of the loop. The flow (current) in the ascending limb is in the opposite direction (counter) to flow in the descending limb. (U-shaped

Osmolality in the lumen is less than in the interstitium (ascending flows-away from the papillary tip) in:
  Thin ascending limb
  Ascending vasa recta
Osmolality in the lumen is greater than in the interstitium (descending flows-away from the papillary tip) in:
  Thin descending limb
  Inner medullary collecting duct
  Descending vasa recta

counterflow arrangement.) A small transverse osmotic pressure gradient between the ascending and descending limbs of the loop of Henle is thus multiplied into a larger longitudinal gradient.

The ascending limb is water impermeable and actively transports solute (Cl ions actively, followed by Na ions passively) from tubular fluid into the interstitial fluid.

The descending limb is highly permeable to water and solutes and the increased osmolality of medullary interstitium causes water absorption and tubular fluid concentration. The maximal concentration that the urine can attain is equal to that of the medullary interstitium and papilla.

Isosmotic fluid enters the thin descending limbs and is concentrated as it flows down to the bend of the loop of Henle. As it flows up the ascending limbs it is diluted so that the fluid that emerges is hypotonic to plasma.

Elements of urine concentration

The production of a concentrated urine requires:

Hypertonic medullary interstitium (high salt and urea concentration), which is generated and maintained by the counter-current multiplier system in the loop of Henle. The renal medulla is very hypertonic (1200 mOsm/l) compared with the cortex (300 mOsm/l).

Passive reabsorption of water, not solutes, in distal tubule and collecting duct. Removal of water from the papillary and deep medullary interstitium by loops of **vasa recta** (capillary loops descending from the cortex into the medulla), which act as passive counter-current exchangers. Solute entry and water loss in the descending vasa recta is offset by solute loss and water entry in the ascending vasa recta.

■ Renal function tests

These can be categorised as:

Tests of glomerular filtration

- **Blood urea**: this is a poor measure of glomerular filtration rate. Urea is the end product of protein metabolism. It has a molecular weight of 60 daltons, is synthesised primarily by the liver, freely filtered at the glomerulus and undergoes variable tubular reabsorption. The plasma level is affected by dietary protein intake, intravascular volume depletion, gastrointestinal bleeding, liver function and by drug interference with the analytical procedure.
- **Serum creatinine**: creatinine is a metabolic product of both creatine and phosphocreatine. It has a molecular weight of 113 daltons, is freely filtered at the glomerulus and undergoes variable tubular reabsorption. The plasma creatinine level is related to muscle mass and body weight, being derived primarily from synthesis in skeletal muscle. 98% of the total creatine pool is in muscle, with about 1.6%–1.7% being converted to creatinine daily. Glomerular filtration rate in ml/min per 1.73 m^2 body surface area is equal to 40 multiplied by height (cm)/plasma creatinine (μmol/l).
- Endogenous **creatinine clearance** (110–150 ml/min).
- Isotopic methods to measure clearance of chelating agents: ^{51}Cr-EDTA, ^{99}Tcm-DTPA.
- **Proteinuria**: normal excretion should be less than 150 mg/24 h.

Tests of renal tubular function

- **Urine concentrating ability**, as measured by **specific gravity**, which can range from 1.003–1.030. Specific gravity can be determined by a refractometer, a hygrometer or by urine reagent strips (dipsticks). It is a measure of the weight of the solution compared with that of distilled water, and is determined by the number, relative size and density of solute particles in the urine. It can be affected by the state of hydration. A low fixed urine specific gravity is a feature of chronic renal failure.
- Concentrating ability can be further assessed by **water deprivation** or by the administration of vasopressin or the synthetic vasopressin analogue, DDAVP (1-desamino-8-D-arginine vasopressin).
- **Diluting ability** can be assessed in response to a water load.
- **Urine osmolality** depends on the number of particles in solution only and is not affected by size, charge or density of the particles. Osmolality is measured by freezing point depression of urine below that of distilled water. An osmolality of 600 mOsm/l or more on the first urine sample voided in the early morning after fluid restriction to bedtime indicates an adequate urine concentrating ability.

Excessive concentration of relatively insoluble urine constituents;
Physiological changes in urine: volume, pH;
Nucleus or nidus forming material;
Congenital or acquired deformities of the urinary tract, especially causing stasis;
Iatrogenic.

- **Urine sodium**: normally less than 40 mmol/l.
- **Glycosuria**: glucose is not normally detected in the urine by glucose oxidase reagent strips until the plasma glucose exceeds 10 mmol/l, the renal threshold for glucose. Glycosuria at lower thresholds is indicative of a tubular transport defect.
- **Markers of tubular damage**: the detection of low molecular weight proteins (<20 000 daltons), such as β2-microglobulin or α1-microglobulin, indicates failure of proximal tubular reabsorption. The presence of N-acetyl-β-glucosaminidase indicates release secondary to proximal tubular cell injury.

Renal blood flow measurement

- **Clearance techniques**: organic anions (para-aminohippurate or PAH; ortho-aminohippurate or Hippuran). Substances completely cleared by the kidney in a single pass have a clearance that is equal to the renal plasma flow. Indicators should be freely filtered at the glomerulus and secreted by the tubules, but not reabsorbed, metabolised or synthesised by the kidneys. The excretion ratio of PAH is high provided the plasma concentration is kept low. By the application of the Fick principle, flow = removal rate/arteriovenous difference.
- **Isotope washout techniques**: xenon, krypton

■ Diuretics

Mechanisms of diuretic action can be categorised primarily by site of action:
Loop of Henle (thick ascending limb)
    Inhibition of $Na^+/K^+/2Cl^-$ carrier
Distal tubule and connecting segment
    Inhibition of Na^+/Cl^- carrier
Cortical collecting tubule
    Inhibition of Na channel

Classes of diuretics

Proximal tubule

Carbonic anhydrase inhibitors: block reabsorption of Na and HCO_3 from proximal tubule.

Osmotic diuretics: block water reabsorption in proximal tubule and descending loop of Henle.

Loop of Henle

Loop diuretics: block Na and Cl reabsorption in thick ascending loop of Henle by inhibition of the $Na^+/K^+/2Cl^-$ apical carrier.

Distal nephron

Thiazide diuretics: block Na and Cl reabsorption in the early distal tubule. Potassium-sparing diuretics: block Na reabsorption in the late distal tubule and in the collecting duct. Spironolactone is a competitive antagonist of aldosterone, blocking Na reabsorption and K^+ and H excretion in the late distal tubule and collecting duct. Amiloride and triamterene inhibit the Na channel in the apical membrane in the late distal tubule and collecting duct.

■ Micturition

Micturition is a local spinal reflex, influenced by descending pathways from the brain. Stretch receptors in the bladder wall initiate the process. The reflex is a positive feedback reflex, with bladder emptying being completed once the reflex has become established. Central control resides in the nucleus coeruleus in the rostral pons.

Micturition requires:

- **Parasympathetic innervation of the detrusor muscle** (a meshwork of interlacing smooth muscle bundles forming three layers and behaving as a functional syncytium) from the intermediolateral grey column at S2–S4, via the preganglionic nervi erigentes.
- **Sympathetic innervation of the bladder neck** and proximal urethra from the intermediolateral column at T10–L2.
- **Somatic innervation** of the bladder, pelvic floor and urethra via the pudendal nerve (S2–S4).
- **Conscious initiation** at a socially acceptable time.

Micturition cycle

Sympathetic activation facilitates storage and parasympathetic activation facilitates voiding.

Filling and storage phase

- The urinary bladder fills with urine by a series of peristaltic contractions at a rate of 0.5–5 ml/min. This is accomplished without a significant increase in intra-vesical pressure and without any involuntary bladder contractions. In other words, the normal bladder is highly compliant over the usual volume range. Compliance is a function of the components of the bladder wall, including elastic tissue and smooth muscle. Intra-vesical pressure depends on the hydrostatic pressure at the bladder neck, bladder wall tension and on the transmission of intra-abdominal pressure.
- The urethra remains closed during the filling and storage phases, and the intra-urethral pressure always exceeds the intra-vesical pressure. Closure is maintained by a number of factors, including:

  Passive and active effects of striated and smooth muscle components.

  Elasticity of the urethra.

  Transmission of intra-abdominal pressure to the proximal urethra by a flutter-valve effect.

  Surface tension of the urethra.

  Submucosal vascularity of the urethra.
- The normal bladder stores 350–500 ml.

Initiation phase

Voiding can be initiated regardless of the actual volume of urine contained in the bladder.

Voiding phase

This entails pelvic floor relaxation, descent of the bladder base, and reduction in intra-urethral pressure, followed by bladder contraction. Relaxation of the bladder neck and urethral smooth muscle is probably mediated by nitric oxide. The functional competence of the bladder neck smooth muscle is also essential to prevent the retrograde emission of semen.

Urodynamic assessment of micturition

Residual volume in bladder: repeated volumes of 100 ml are abnormal. Measurement can be achieved by either ultrasound or by urethral catheterisation.

Urethral pressure profile: 2 ml/min infusion of saline through a side-hole channel of a catheter that is slowly withdrawn, at a rate of 2 mm/s.

Flow rate: the volume of urine voided per unit time.

Cystometry: a pressure-volume study of the bladder.

Pelvic floor or external urethral sphincter electromyography.

Micturating video-cystourethrography.

Antegrade perfusion test of Whitaker to assess the upper urinary tract: continuous saline infusion into the renal pelvis, with simultaneous pressure recording.

Normal bladder function on cystometry

This demonstrates the following features:

Residual urine is less than 50 ml;

The desire to void starts at a capacity of 150–200 ml;

A strong desire to void is associated with a capacity of around 400 ml or over;

The detrusor pressure does not rise on filling;

There are no systolic detrusor contractions;

There is no leakage of urine on coughing;

The rise in detrusor pressure on voiding is less than 50 cm H_2O;

The peak flow rate is greater than 15 ml/s for voided volumes greater than 150 ml;

BIBLIOGRAPHY

Brenner, B. M. *Rector's The Kidney*, 7th edn., vols. 1 and 2. Philadelphia: W.B. Saunders, 2004.

Johnson, R. J. & Feehally, J. (eds.) *Comprehensive Clinical Nephrology*, 2nd edn. St Louis: 2003.

Lote, C. *Principles of Renal Physiology*, 4th edn. Mosby, Dordrecht: Kluwer Academic Publishers, 2000.

Wirz, H., Hargitay, B. & Kuhn, W. (1951). Lokalisation des konzentrierungs-prozesses in der Niene durch direkte kryoskope. *Helv. Physiol. Pharmacol. Acta*, **9**, (1951) 196–207.

5 Temperature regulation

■ Introduction

Humans are homeotherms, with circadian rhythms, wherein the body temperature is lowest in the mornings and highest in the evenings. The normal diurnal temperature variation is 0.5–1 °C and the body core temperature is maintained around 36.2–38.2 °C (96.5–101.8 °F). Temperature is highest during the awake state, at ovulation and during the first trimester of pregnancy.

Body temperature represents a balance between metabolic heat production and heat losses to the environment. This is achieved by the adjustment of central thermogenesis, and by the maintenance of the differential temperature gradient between the body core and periphery. Fever represents a regulated rise to a new set point of body temperature, mediated by pyrogenic cytokines such as interleukin-1, tumour necrosis factor, interferon-gamma and interleukin-6.

Methods for the measurement of core temperature

Tympanic membrane
Rectal
Oesophageal
Sublingual
Bladder
Axillary

The normal rectal or vaginal temperature is 0.5°C higher than the oral temperature. The normal axillary temperature is 0.5°C lower than the oral temperature.

■ Thermoregulatory mechanism

This comprises the system whereby body core temperature is regulated when it rises above or falls below thermoregulatory set points:

An afferent input: thermally sensitive cells, with impulses carried in Aδ (cold) and C (warm) fibres.

Central control: the heat-loss and heat-gain centres in the preoptic area of the anterior hypothalamus, which act as temperature sensors.

Efferent responses: cutaneous vasoconstriction or vasodilatation allowing shunting of blood to the core or the periphery; opening or closure of thermoregulatory arterio-venous shunts; non-shivering thermogenesis; shivering; sweating. Behavioural responses include heat avoidance and external cooling.

Mechanisms of heat loss to the environment

Radiation: transfer of heat between two objects by electromagnetic waves (infrared rays).

Conduction: heat exchange between two surfaces in direct contact with each other along a temperature gradient.

Convection: heat exchange between an exposed body surface and a medium, brought about by the cooling effect of air currents.

Evaporation of sweat: heat loss that accompanies the vaporisation of sweat from a body surface.

Urination and defaecation.

Heat response

The **body response to heat stress** includes:

Thermoregulatory mechanisms;

An acute phase response with cytokine release;

The production of heat-shock or stress proteins.

Mechanisms to reduce body heat

Cutaneous vasodilatation;

Sweating;

Hyperventilation due to respiratory centre stimulation;

Decreased activity to reduce metabolic heat production.

Acclimatisation to heat

This involves:

Altered cardiovascular performance;

Activation of the renin–angiotensin–aldosterone axis;

Salt conservation by the sweat glands and kidneys;

Increased capacity to secrete sweat;

Plasma volume expansion;

Increased glomerular filtration rate.

Cold response

Thermoregulatory responses to the cold

Reduce heat loss

Cutaneous vasoconstriction, with reduced dermal blood flow;

Curling up;

Horripilation.

Increase heat production

Shivering.

Non-shivering thermogenesis: the exothermic hydrolysis of triglycerides in brown fat to free fatty acids and glycerol, occurring in the first few weeks of life. Brown fat is heavily vascularised and rich in mitochondria.

Hunger.

Increased voluntary activity.

Increased catecholamine secretion.

■ Heat production

Sources of body heat production

Basic metabolic processes (metabolic heat production);

Metabolically active tissues: liver, kidneys, brain, heart;

Food intake (specific dynamic action);

Muscular activity.

Measurement of body heat production

Direct calorimetry

Indirect calorimetry

Metabolic rate

This depends on:

Sex
Age
Muscular exertion during or just before measurement
Recent food ingestion
High/low environmental temperature
Height, weight and surface area
Growth
Reproduction
Lactation
Emotional state
Body temperature
Circulating levels of thyroid hormones
Circulating catecholamine levels

Closed-circuit spirometry
Open-circuit spirometry

■ Hypothermia

Effects of hypothermia

CNS: coma.

Metabolic and endocrine: increased metabolic rate with shivering; hyperglycaemia.

Cardiovascular: cardiac dysrhythmias; peripheral vasoconstriction.

Respiratory: reduced minute ventilation.

Blood: granulocytopenia; platelet dysfunction.

Gastrointestinal: ileus; pancreatitis.

Hypothermia can accompany surgery, owing to the following factors:

Low ambient temperature in the operating theatre;

Anaesthetic agents interfere with hypothalamic thermostats;

Heat loss accompanying humidification of inspired gases;

Administration of cool intravenous fluids;

Drug induced vasodilatation;

Exposure of body cavities to low ambient temperatures.

Causes of fever

Infections: bacterial, viral, fungal, parasitic, rickettsial
Tissue necrosis
Specific inflammations
Immune reactions
Malignant neoplasms
Drugs
Foreign proteins
Acute metabolic failure
Endocrine disease: thyrotoxicosis, phaeochromocytoma
Factitious fever

■ Fever

Pathogenesis of fever

Exogenous pyrogens: bacteria (endotoxin); viruses; protozoa; fungi; drugs; hormones; synthetic polynucleotides.

Endogenous pyrogens produced by cells stimulated by exogenous pyrogens: interleukin-1, interleukin-6 and tumour necrosis factor alpha.

Hyperthermia is caused by situations wherein body metabolic heat production or environmental heat load is greater than the normal heat loss capacity. Body temperatures greater than 41°C can cause irreversible brain damage.

Cardiovascular system

6

■ Introduction

The cardiovascular system comprises:

- A **pump**: the heart, which comprises two atria (reservoirs for blood and booster pumps to augment ventricular filling) and two ventricles (pumps). It consists of two pumps in parallel, with synchronised actions.
- A high pressure **distribution circuit**: the elastic arteries, i.e.the aorta and its major branches, serve a transport function. The muscular arteries serve a distributive function.
- **Exchange vessels**: the capillaries, which are 8–10 μ in diameter. Capillaries can possess either continuous endothelium (muscle, heart, liver), fenestrated endothelium (gastrointestinal tract, renal glomeruli), or discontinuous endothelium (liver, spleen).
- A low pressure **collection and return** circuit.

The system allows rapid transport of oxygen, nutrients, hormones and waste products throughout the body. The structure of the components is related to function across the vascular tree.

■ The fetal circulation

This has the following characteristics:

- The right and left ventricles function in parallel;
- The placenta provides for gas and metabolite exchange;
- The parallel circulation is maintained by shunts at the ductus venosus, foramen ovale and the ductus arteriosus.
- Oxygenated blood flows from the placenta via the ductus venosus and inferior vena cava into the right atrium, where it is deflected by the crista dividens and the eustachian valve across the foramen ovale into the left atrium and thence into the left ventricle. It is then ejected into the ascending aorta.

Distribution of blood volume

Systemic circuit 80%
Arteries 10%
Capillaries 5%
Veins and venules 65%
Pulmonary circuit 12%
Heart 8%

- Deoxygenated blood from the superior vena cava flows into the right atrium, being primarily directed into the right ventricle and ejected into the pulmonary artery.
- Mixing of the venous returns occurs.
- The pulmonary circulation is a high-impedance and low-flow system.
- The placental circulation is a low-impedance and high-flow system

At birth, a **transitional circulation** ensues, with the following changes:

A reduction in pulmonary vascular resistance secondary to expansion of the lungs and an increase in arterial pO_2.

An increase in systemic vascular resistance caused by removal of the low resistance placental circulation.

The systemic vascular resistance exceeds the pulmonary vascular resistance.

A left-to-right shunt through the ductus arteriosus, with progressive closure.

Functional closure of the foramen ovale as a result of raised left atrial pressure and volume.

Closure of the ductus venosus as a result of removal of the placenta from the circulation.

The adult circulation consists of two chambers, the right and left ventricles, in series, with two interposed vascular beds (systemic and pulmonary).

■ Control of blood volume

Blood volume control mechanism

Afferent limb
- **Volume sensors**

Low-pressure baroreceptors (venous side stretch receptors)

Cardiac atria
Roots of great veins
Cardiopulmonary receptors

Left ventricle

Pulmonary vascular bed

High-pressure baroreceptors (arterial side stretch receptors)

Carotid sinus (glossopharyngeal nerve)

Aortic arch (vagus nerve)

- Intrarenal baroreceptor system: juxtaglomerular apparatus
- Hepatic and central nervous system(CNS) sensors

Central control system

- Cardiovascular centre

Pressor system: lateral pathway of descending reticular system

Depressor system: medial pathway of descending reticular system

- Nucleus of the tractus solitarius
- Hypothalamus

Efferent mechanisms

Those regulating renal sodium excretion and controlling extracellular fluid volume

- Glomerular filtration rate
- Physical factors

At proximal tubule level

Beyond proximal tubule level

- Humoral effector mechanisms

Renin–angiotensin–aldosterone system

Vasopressin

Catecholamines

Prostaglandins: PGE2, PGI2, thromboxane

Kinin–kallikrein system

Atrial natriuretic peptide (ANP)

Endothelium-derived factors

- Renal sympathetic nerves

Effects of blood loss

The effects of the rapid loss of one litre of blood (20% total blood volume) in an adult can be listed in sequence as consisting of:

- **Blood loss** leading to reduced venous return, reduced right atrial pressure and reduced cardiac output.
- **Immediate baroreceptor reflex activation**. A reduced discharge rate of baroreceptors in carotid sinus and aortic arch leads to reduced afferent input to

the medullary cardiovascular centre causing a reduction in parasympathetic, and increase in sympathetic, activity. This is manifested by tachycardia, increased myocardial contractility and arteriolar constriction.

- **A slower hypothalamic–pituitary–adrenal response**. Reduced renal blood flow stimulates intrarenal baroreceptors with renin release from the juxtaglomerular apparatus. Angiotensin II which results causes arteriolar constriction and stimulates aldosterone and arginine vasopressin (antidiuretic hormone; ADH) release. Arginine vasopressin release is also stimulated by reduced extracellular fluid volume acting via atrial stretch receptors.
- **Redistribution of cardiac output** from skin, muscle, viscera to heart and brain.
- **Starling forces**, which are responsible for tissue fluid reabsorption into the plasma compartment.

  Movement out of capillary:

      Capillary hydrostatic pressure

      Interstitial fluid colloid osmotic pressure

  Fluid retention within the capillary:

      Plasma colloid osmotic pressure

      Interstitial space hydrostatic pressure
- **Carotid chemoreceptor response**: reduced blood flow to the aortic and carotid bodies, with reduced oxygen in the peripheral chemoreceptor tissues, leading to hyperventilation.

■ Blood pressure

Systemic arterial blood pressure is related to cardiac output and to total peripheral resistance (in turn related to the number and calibre of small arteries and arterioles, and to blood viscosity). Arterial hypertension represents a disproportion between these two components.

Blood pressure comprises:

A steady component, **the mean arterial pressure**, which is related to small arterial and arteriolar resistance. This in turn depends on a combination of neural mechanisms (sympathetic and parasympathetic), hormonal mechanisms (renin–angiotensin–aldosterone mechanism) and local transmitters (nitric oxide), all of which affect arteriolar calibre.

A pulsatile component, the **pulse pressure**, which depends on arterial stiffness and the timing of reflected waves. It represents the oscillation around mean pressure, extending from systolic to diastolic pressures.

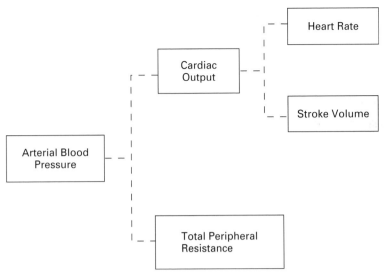

Figure 6.1 Determinants of arterial blood pressure.

Determinants of arterial blood pressure
Physical
Blood volume in arterial system
Elastic characteristics (compliance)
Physiological
Cardiac output
Peripheral resistance

Mean arterial pressure is equal to cardiac output multiplied by total peripheral resistance. Pulse pressure is equal to systolic minus diastolic pressure. It is directly proportional to stroke volume and inversely proportional to compliance. Pulse pressure increases with age due to reduced compliance.

Systolic blood pressure depends on myocardial contractility, the compliance of the great vessels and on diastolic blood pressure. Diastolic blood pressure depends on systemic vascular resistance, peripheral run-off and on heart rate.

Factors regulating blood pressure

Short-term regulation

Baroreceptors comprise a negative feedback system incorporating stretch receptors sensitive to both mean pressure and rate of change of pressure (elevations in blood pressure increase the rate of firing). Under physiological conditions, baroreceptor firing exerts a tonic inhibitory influence on the sympathetic outflow from the medulla oblongata. High-pressure baroreceptors are found in the carotid sinus, at the bifurcation of the common carotid artery and in the aortic sinus in the arch of the aorta.

Hypothalamus.

Arterial chemoreceptors.

Vomiting centre.

Pulmonary stretch receptors.

Ventricular mechanoreceptors.

Atrial stretch receptors.

Longer-term regulation

Alterations in blood volume and osmolality.

Hormonal regulation of blood pressure

This is achieved by a balance of vasopressor and vasodepressor hormones, which include the following:

Vasopressor hormones:

Renin–angiotensin–aldosterone system

Arginine vasopressin

Catecholamines

Endothelins (ETs)

Vasodepressor hormones:

Natriuretic peptides: ANP, brain type natriuretic peptide (BNP)

Kinin–kallikrein system

Prostaglandins (PGI2, prostacyclin)

Medullipine system

Adrenomedullin

Nitric oxide

Endothelins

A family of peptides acting locally as autacoid or paracrine hormones. Three isoforms of the 21 amino acid peptide have been identified: ET-1, ET-2 and ET-3. They are produced by a variety of cells, including endothelial and epithelial cells, macrophages and fibroblasts. Endothelins are characterised by two intra-chain disulphide rings, leading to a hairpin loop configuration, along with six conserved amino acid residues at the C terminus.

Endothelins are synthesised by the proteolysis of large pre-proendothelins, which are cleaved to big endothelins, and then processed to the mature peptide by endothelin-converting enzyme.

Endothelins induce dose-dependent contraction in vascular smooth muscle, ET-1 being the most potent known endogenous vasoconstrictor. Two high affinity endothelin receptors have been recognised, ETA and ETB. They have been characterised as seven transmembrane domain G-protein receptors coupled to phospholipase C. The ETA receptor is the predominant type of receptor.

Valsalva manoeuvre

The **Valsalva manoeuvre** is a global test of cardiovascular responses. It involves forced expiration against a closed glottis
  Effects of the resulting positive intrathoracic pressure include:
  Compression of the lungs
  Blood forced through the pulmonary veins to the left atrium and ventricle
  Increased left ventricular stroke volume
  Transient rise in systemic blood pressure
  Reduced venous return to the heart
  Reduced cardiac output
  Reduced blood pressure

Measurement of arterial blood pressure

Indirect methods
  Sphygmomanometer, using palpation and auscultation, the latter making use of the characteristic sequence of Korotkow sounds.
  Oscillotonometry, which uses a double cuff system, the proximal cuff occluding the arterial pulsations and the distal cuff sensing pulsations. The pulsations are amplified by a pressure-sensitive aneroid chamber.

Direct methods
  Intra-arterial cannula connected to a calibrated pressure transducer.

■ Renin–angiotensin mechanism

This integrated hormonal cascade system regulates arterial blood pressure, intra-vascular volume and electrolyte balance. More broadly, it is a complex autocrine system involved in diverse processes of cellular biology and pathophysiology.

Reduced arterial blood pressure

↓

Renin, a proteolytic enzyme that is synthesised and stored as a precursor in granular juxtaglomerular cells in afferent arteriolar wall of glomerulus (specialised myoepithelial cells in the media). The cells respond to changes in transmural pressure gradient between afferent arteriole and interstitium. They are innervated directly by the sympathetic postganglionic unmyelinated fibres. Renin is a carboxyl-peptidase enzyme acting on plasma alpha-2-globulin

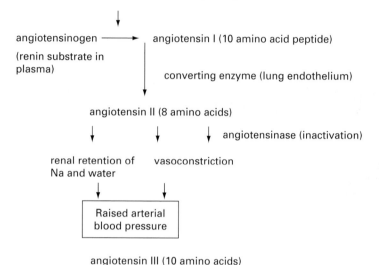

Figure 6.2 Pathway for renin–angiotensin mechanism.

Pathway for renin–angiotensin mechanism

Angiotensin II can also be produced by non-angiotensin-converting enzyme (ACE) pathways, e.g. the chymase pathway.

Angiotensin-converting enzyme is a membrane-bound zinc metallopeptidase localised on the luminal surface of endothelial cells. Plasma levels of ACE are genetically determined. The ACE gene may manifest insertion (I) or deletion (D) polymorphism, with three possible genotypes (DD, DI, II).

Stimulation of the renin–angiotensin–aldosterone mechanism

This is achieved by:

- Increased renal sympathetic nerve activity (beta 1-adrenoreceptor stimulation).
- Fall in afferent arteriolar perfusion pressure (juxtaglomerular cells) (intrarenal baroreceptors).

Renin

This has a circulatory half-life of 40–120 minutes

Release is inhibited by:
Angiotensin II
Angiotensin III
Arginine vasopressin (ADH)
Hypernatraemia
Hyperkalaemia
Atrial natriuretic factor

Causes of increased renin secretion:
Sodium depletion
Diuretics
Hypotension
Haemorrhage
Upright posture
Dehydration
Constriction of renal artery or aorta
Cardiac failure
Cirrhosis

- Reduced sodium load delivered to distal renal tubule (macula densa cells: specialised renal tubular epithelial cells located at the transition between the thick segment of the ascending limb of the loop of Henle and the distal convoluted tubule. They function as chemoreceptors and are stimulated by a decreased Na^+ load).
- Reduction in right atrial pressure.

Effects of angiotensin II

Vasoconstriction: systemic (preferentially coronary and cerebral) and intra-renal vascular smooth muscle constriction;

Increased proximal tubular reabsorption of sodium;

Stimulation of aldosterone release: increased distal tubular reabsorption of sodium;

Arginine vasopressin (ADH) release: water retention;

Stimulation of thirst;

Stimulation of sympathetic nervous system activity;

Augmentation of adrenal medullary catecholamines;

Direct inhibition of renin release in the kidney;

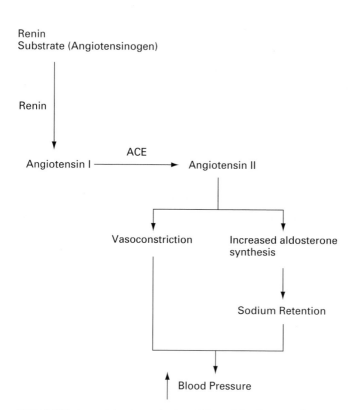

Figure 6.3 Renin–angiotensin mechanism. ACE, angiotensin-converting enzyme.

Positive inotropic action on myocardium;

Increased endothelin secretion;

Stimulation of plasminogen activator inhibitor-1.

Mechanisms for the actions of angiotensin II

Neural mechanisms

Increased central sympathetic outflow;

Presynaptic augmentation of neuronal noradrenaline release;

Augmentation of adrenal adrenaline;

Postsynaptic augmentation of other pressors;

Baroreflex blunting.

Vascular mechanisms

Direct vasoconstriction;

Cellular hypertrophy and hyperplasia (chronic).

Other volume-related mechanisms

Aldosterone release modulation;

Arginine vasopressin (ADH) release modulation;

Increased thirst;

Increased dietary salt intake.

Pharmacological manipulation of the renin–angiotensin mechanism

This can be achieved by the use of angiotensin-converting enzyme inhibitors and angiotensin II-receptor antagonists. Angiotensin-converting enzyme inhibitors have disadvantages relating to the facts that:

Angiotensin-converting enzyme is not a specific enzyme and is involved in the breakdown of other substances, e.g. bradykinin, which results in cough and angio-oedema. Secondary increase in angiotensin I levels due to loss of negative feedback can overcome the ACE blockade, leading to a return of angiotensin II levels to normal with chronic ACE inhibitor use.

Angiotensin II-receptor blockers

Angiotensin II acts on AT1 and AT2 receptors. Angiotensin I receptor stimulation causes vasoconstriction and synthesis and release of aldosterone. Non-peptide angiotensin II antagonists generally act as specific competitive antagonists at the AT1 receptor. They have no intrinsic agonist activity and do not influence pathways outside the renin–angiotensin system such as bradykinin metabolism. The role of the AT2 receptor is yet to be fully elucidated, but it may be involved in the control of growth and differentiation during embryogenic development.

AT2-receptor blockers

Biphenyl tetrazoles
Losartan
Candesartan
Irbesartan
Tasosartan

Non-biphenyl tetrazoles
Eprosartan
Telmisartan

Non-heterocyclic
Valsartan

Classification of antihypertensive agents

Diuretics:
  Thiazides
  Loop diuretics
Beta-adrenergic blockers
  Non-selective: nadolol, propranolol, timolol
Selective: atenolol, metoprolol
Partial agonist: acebutolol, oxprenolol
Alpha blockade + non-selective: labetalol
Non-selective + partial agonist: pindolol
    Angiotensin-converting enzyme inhibitors: captopril, enalapril, lisinopril, ramipril
    Calcium channel blockers: amlodipine, diltiazem, nifedipine, verapamil
Angiotensin II antagonists: losartan, valsartan
Alpha 1-adrenergic blockers: doxazosin, prazosin, terazosin
Central and peripheral sympatholytics: clonidine, methyldopa, reserpine
Direct vasodilators: hydralazine, minoxidil
Adrenergic neuron blockers: guanethidine

Antihypertensive effects of beta blockers

These are achieved by:
  Blockade of beta receptors on the renal juxtaglomerular cells, leading to renin blockade and decreased angiotensin II concentrations.
  Blockade of myocardial beta receptors, leading to reduced cardiac contractility and heart rate.
  Blockade of central nervous system (CNS) beta receptors, leading to reduced sympathetic output from the CNS, and blockade of peripheral beta receptors, reducing noradrenaline concentrations.

Angiotensin II antagonists lower blood pressure by reducing systemic possible vascular resistance, while maintaining cardiac output.

■ Cardiac output

Determinants of cardiac output

The cardiac output is the amount of blood pumped to the peripheral circulation per minute. It depends upon:

Heart rate, which is primarily determined by the rate of spontaneous phase 4 depolarisation of the sino-atrial node pacemaker cells.

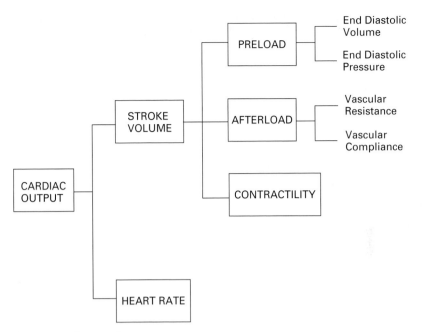

Figure 6.4 Cardiac output.

Stroke volume (end-diastolic volume–end-systolic volume), the amount of blood ejected by the ventricle with each contraction, in turn dependent upon:

- **Preload** (filling pressure) (diastolic myocardial tension or left ventricular (LV) end-diastolic volume) (diastolic stretch), which depends on the initial amount of stretch placed upon LV fibres. End-diastolic volume depends on filling volume, and on factors that impede cavity dilatation (myocardial elasticity and viscoelasticity, wall thickness, and intramyocardial blood volume). Preload is increased by volume loading when LV function is normal, and decreased by diuresis and venodilatation.

- **Afterload** (resistance imposed by the systemic circulation) (systolic myocardial wall tension). Afterload is increased with high intraventricular pressures, increased aortic impedance/systemic vascular resistance, increased ventricular radius and negative intrathoracic pressure, and increased blood viscosity. It is decreased with reduced aortic impedance/systemic vascular resistance, reduced intraventricular pressure, positive intrathoracic pressure and increased ventricular wall thickness.

- **Myocardial contractility** (force of LV contraction independent of preload and afterload) (increased contractility shifts Frank–Starling curve to left). Contractility is increased by inotropic drugs and by the relief of ischaemia and hypoxia. It is decreased by ischaemia, hypoxia and negatively inotropic drugs.

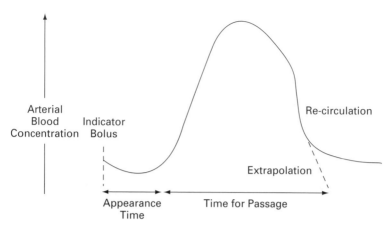

Figure 6.5 Indicator-dilution curve.

Cardiac reserve

Cardiac reserve mechanisms that increase cardiac output in the face of increased demand primarily involve an increase in the heart rate and/or an increase in stroke volume. Other mechanisms that may operate include:

Redistribution of the cardiac output, with differential perfusion of organs;
Cardiac dilatation and hypertrophy, within limits.

Increases in heart rate produce the following effects:

Shortening of systole;
Shortening of diastole, with reduced coronary perfusion time, reduction in ventricular filling and a rate-dependent alteration in stroke volume;
A rate-dependent positive inotropic effect.

Measurement of cardiac output

● **Thermodilution:** The measuring system comprises a disposable insulated syringe, cooling coils and injectate temperature probes with the microprocessor incorporated into a modular physiological monitor. A multilumen balloon catheter with a thermistor near the distal end is inserted via a peripheral vein. The tip is floated into a branch of the pulmonary artery. Ten millilitres crystalloid (ice-cold saline), drawn from a reservoir kept cool by ice, is injected through a proximal opening within the right ventricle. The saline mixes with the blood in the right ventricle. The temperature change is measured by the distal thermistor, which is downstream in the pulmonary artery. The fall in temperature is plotted against time (temperature-dilution curve). The area under the curve correlates with cardiac output.

- **Indicator dye dilution**: Evans blue, indocyanine green

  A dose of indicator dye injected into the superior vena cava or the right atrium will flow as a bolus in the pulmonary circulation and through the left heart and then into the arterial system before it recirculates and completely mixes with the blood.

  If an amount A of suitable indicator is injected into an unknown volume of distribution (V), the V can be estimated from the resultant indicator concentration (C) with the equation: $V = A/C$.

  The flow of a fluid (Q) can be measured if the mean concentration of the indicator is determined for the time (t) required for that indicator to pass a given site. This is measured with the equation: $Q = A / Ct$.

  The dye concentration in arterial blood is plotted on a logarithmic scale against time during the first circulation of the dye bolus on a linear scale.

  The log-linear plot makes the descending limb of the curve a straight line – i.e. the indicator concentration follows an exponential time course, which can be extrapolated to zero concentration. The point of intersection gives the theoretical time taken by the dye bolus to circulate through the lungs and to leave the heart (the duration of indicator passage).

  The average concentration of the dye in the blood is calculated by integration of the area under the curve. Dividing the amount of dye (Q) by the average arterial concentration (C) gives the volume of blood (V) required to carry the dye, i.e. $Q / C = V$

  This volume is the cardiac output during the time given by the curve for one circulation of the dye.

- **Direct Fick principle**: The amount of substance taken up by an organ in a given time is equal to the difference in concentration of that substance between arterial and venous blood, multiplied by the volume of blood flowing through the organ during the same period of time.

$$\text{Cardiac output} = \frac{\text{oxygen consumption (ml/min)}}{\text{arterial oxygen content} - \text{mixed venous oxygen content (ml/100 ml)}} \times 100$$

  The technique for cardiac output measurement requires sampling of systemic arterial blood and of mixed venous blood from a pulmonary artery catheter.

- **Duplex ultrasound**, using an oesophageal Doppler monitor

  Doppler cardiac output (ml/min) = mean aortic blood flow velocity (cm/s) $\times$ aortic cross-sectional area (cm^2) $\times$ 60

- **Thoracic bioimpedance**: this measures stroke volume on a beat-by-beat basis.

Table 6.1. Pressures in the central circulation

Pressures	mm Hg
Central venous pressure	0–5
Right atrium (mean)	0–5
Right ventricle systolic	20–30
diastolic	0–5
Pulmonary artery systolic	20–30
diastolic	8–12
Left atrium (mean)	8–12
Left ventricle systolic	100–150
diastolic	8–12
Aortic systolic	100–150
diastolic	70–90

Derived variables

Cardiac output = stroke volume × heart rate
Cardiac index = cardiac output/body surface area in m^2
$$= 3.0\text{–}4.5\,l/(min/m^2)$$
Left ventricular stroke work = the integral of the LV pressure as a function of volume over the cardiac cycle
Systemic vascular resistance = mean arterial pressure/cardiac output
Left ventricular ejection fraction = stroke volume/end diastolic volume × 100%
$= 55\%\text{–}70\%$
Right ventricular end-diastolic volume = 70–100 ml
Left ventricular end-diastolic volume = 70–100 ml

Starling's law of the heart (length–tension relationship)

'The energy of contraction, however measured, is a function of the initial length of the muscle fibre.' Ventricular performance is a function of the end-diastolic volume (the preload). The concept was introduced into popular practice by Sarnoff and Berglund with the family of **ventricular function curves**. These plots separate the homeometric (at the same sarcomere length) from the heterometric factors (Starling's mechanism) influencing ventricular performance. They represent plots of ventricular mechanical performance against preload.

The curves plot tension (measured by either stroke volume, stroke work or cardiac output) on the ordinate and end-diastolic ventricular fibre length (measured by either LV end-diastolic volume, LV end-diastolic pressure, left atrial pressure, pulmonary artery occlusion pressure) on the abscissa. Left ventricular end-diastolic volume is approximated by LV end-diastolic pressure with normal

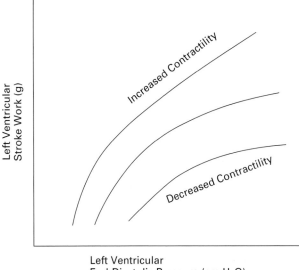

Figure 6.6 Starling curves.

ventricular compliance. Each function curve has an ascending limb, a peak and a descending limb. Volume loading and repeated measurements of cardiac output and arterial blood pressure allow the plotting of stroke work against end-diastolic pressure. A shift of the curve upwards and to the left indicates improved contractility, and downwards and to the right indicates myocardial depression. Similar displacements may be caused by changes in vascular resistance. Alterations in ventricular compliance lead to a situation wherein ventricular end-diastolic pressure may not relate directly to fibre length and ventricular volume.

The **Frank–Starling mechanism** matches cardiac output to venous return (an increase in diastolic filling increases cardiac output) and maintains a precise balance between right ventricular and left ventricular output. Increased venous return increases preload.

The volume expelled and/or force of ejection during systole is proportional to the length of the muscle fibres or degree of cardiac filling at end diastole. Stretch-dependent calcium sensitivity of the myocardial cells forms the basis of the Frank–Starling mechanism.

Ventricular contractility

This can be described by three variables and their interrelationships:

The velocity of shortening;

The force of contraction;

The length of displacement.

Factors affecting the length of ventricular muscle fibres

Increased
    Stronger atrial contraction
    Increased total blood volume
    Increased venous tone
    Increased pumping action of the skeletal muscle
    Increased negative intrathoracic pressure

Decreased
    Standing
    Increased intrapericardial pressure
    Reduced ventricular compliance

Causes of displacement of ventricular function curve

Upward displacement (increased contractility)
    Sympathetic activation
    Positive inotropes

Downward displacement (decreased contractility)
    Hypoxia
    Acidosis
    Negative inotropes (beta-blockers, calcium antagonists)

Determinants of venous return to the heart

Pressure gradient for venous return: pressure at the end of capillaries.

Right atrial pressure.

Total blood volume.

Venous valves.

Skeletal muscle pump, which acts as a 'peripheral heart'.

Respiratory pump.

Abdominal pump.

Inotropic state of the heart, with the effect of ventricular contraction and relaxation. The ventricles exert a suction effect with diastolic relaxation. Blood is drawn into the atria during ventricular systole due to descent of atrio-ventricular fibrous rings.

Venomotor tone.

Central venous pressure is a measure of the filling pressure of the right ventricle. It can be used to estimate the intravascular volume, and as an estimator of left heart filling pressure in individuals with good LV function.

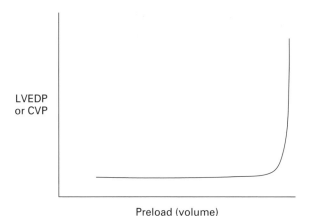

Figure 6.7 Compliance curve. LVEDP, left ventricular end-diastolic pressure; CVP, central venous pressure.

Pulmonary capillary wedge pressure(PCWP) and pulmonary artery diastolic pressure are estimators of left atrial pressure, which reflects LV end-diastolic pressure. Left ventricular end-diastolic pressure (LVEDP) is an indicator of LV preload in the form of LV end-diastolic volume. Pulmonary artery catheters are useful for assessing states where there is abnormal right or left ventricular compliance leading to disparities between left and right heart filling pressures.

The wedge pressure waveform is lower than that of the pulmonary artery, and demonstrates A and B waves in sinus rhythm.

Differences between pulmonary capillary wedge pressure and left ventricular end-diastolic pressure

These may occur under the following circumstances:

PCWP > LVEDP

Mitral valve disease

Increased pulmonary vascular resistance

Chronic obstructive pulmonary disease

Raised intrathoracic pressure

Positive pressure ventilation

Positive end-expiratory pressure

PCWP < LVEDP

Non-compliant left ventricle: ischaemia; hypertrophy

Aortic regurgitation

Systolic hypertension

LVEDP > 25 mm Hg

Jugular venous pressure

Positive deflections

a = right atrial contraction. It is absent in atrial fibrillation and increased by conditions impeding right atrial emptying, such as tricuspid or pulmonary stenosis.

c = right ventricular contraction, with bulging of the tricuspid valve into the right atrium during the initial isovolumic ventricular contraction.

v = filling of right atrium against a closed tricuspid valve in late ventricular systole causing a rise in atrial pressure. This occurs prior to the opening of the tricuspid valve in ventricular diastole. It is prominent in tricuspid regurgitation.

Negative deflections

x = atrial relaxation and downward movement of the leaflets of the tricuspid valve with ventricular contraction during the ejection phase.

x' = atrial relaxation, with return of tricuspid valve into position.

y = right atrial emptying through an open tricuspid valve.

The relationship of heart rate to contractility

This has been described in terms of the following effects:

- **Bowditch effect**: The contractile force of the isolated frog heart increases as a function of the frequency of contraction when the preload is kept constant.

- **Staircase or treppe phenomenon** in mammalian hearts: progressively higher plateaux of tension are reached following an incremental rise in stimulation frequency. At very high frequencies, beyond the physiological range, force generation diminishes.

The **Anrep effect** is a positive inotropic response to an abrupt and sustained increase in the pressure developed by the ventricle.

The LV pressure-volume plot provides a relatively load-independent method for the assessment of LV contractile function. The **ejection fraction**, which is the ratio of stroke volume to end-diastolic volume, is used in clinical practice as a measure of LV contractility, and hence systolic function. The reduction in ejection fraction that occurs with LV systolic dysfunction is brought about by a ventricular remodelling process, with a dilatation of the LV chamber and an increase in end-diastolic volume.

Heart failure

Heart failure can be due to either:

Systolic dysfunction:

Impaired ejection (forward failure), due to reduced inotropy (contractility)

Diastolic dysfunction:

Impaired filling (backward failure), due to reduced lusitropy (relaxation)

The term **hibernating myocardium** refers to reversible LV dysfunction due to chronic coronary artery disease which responds positively to inotropic stress. This is associated with reduced coronary blood flow reserve.

Adaptive mechanisms that allow maintenance of cardiac output in the presence of factors predisposing to congestive heart failure

These include:

The Frank–Starling mechanism;

The inotropic state of the cardiac muscle;

Increase in heart rate;

Myocardial dilatation (with chronic volume overload) or myocardial hypertrophy (with chronic pressure overload);

Increased sympathetic nervous system activity;

Humoral mechanisms, mediated via ANP.

Pathophysiology of the failing myocardium

Mechanical alterations

Reduction in force development per unit cross-sectional area;

Reduction in maximum rate of force development;

Reduced velocity of shortening;

Reduced relaxation (lusitropy).

Biochemical alterations

Catecholamines: reduced synthesis and myocardial content;

Reduced myofibrillar actomyosin-ATPase;

Increased hydroxyproline (hypertrophy);

Variable reduction in adenosine 5′-triphosphate (ATP);

Reduced calcium binding by sarcoplasmic reticulum, with myocardial calcium overload;

Reduced adenyl cyclase activity.

Exogenous changes

Increased cortisol, catecholamines and free fatty acids.

Factors that regulate cardiac myocyte hypertrophy

Positive: insulin growth factor-1; angiotensin II; endothelin 1; PGF2alpha; cardiotrophin 1.

Negative: vitamin A; ATP.

Inotropic mechanisms

These can be broadly classified as being:

Adenosine 3'-5'-monophosphate (cyclic AMP)-dependent mechanisms:

Beta-adrenoreceptor stimulation. These are G-protein-coupled cell membrane receptors that activate adenyl cyclase to produce cyclic AMP. Agonists at these receptors include noradrenaline, adrenaline, dopamine, dobutamine, isoprenaline and dopexamine.

Inhibition of phosphodiesterase isoenzyme in the myocardium. Inhibitors include bipyridine derivatives (amrinone, milrinone) and the imidazole derivatives (enoximone).

Cyclic AMP-independent mechanisms:

Inhibition of membrane bound Na^+/K^+-ATPase, causing an increase in intracellular sodium and intracellular calcium. This increases calcium stores in the sarcoplasmic reticulum and also increases the slow inward current responsible for the phase 2 plateau of the action potential in cardiac myocytes.

Partial agonists at the dihydropyridine receptor on the L-type calcium channel.

Calcium sensitisers, which promote prolonged actin and myosin interaction.

Alpha-1-adrenoreceptor agonists, such as phenylephrine and methoxamine.

■ Myocardial oxygen consumption

Determinants of myocardial oxygen consumption

Myocardial oxygen consumption involves a balance between oxygen demand and oxygen supply.

Myocardial oxygen supply depends on:

Oxygen content of the coronary arterial blood.

Coronary vessel calibre (concentration of myocardial metabolic products and the pCO_2).

Coronary perfusion pressure, which is diastolic and dependent on the LVEDP. It is equal to the difference between the aortic diastolic blood pressure (driving pressure) and the LVEDP or coronary pressure (back pressure), whichever is greater.

Coronary perfusion time, which equates to 1/heart rate. With faster heart rates diastole is shorter.

Myocardial oxygen demand depends on:

Basal oxygen requirements.

External work (mean arterial pressure × stroke volume), which is determined by LV preload, myocardial contractility or inotropic state (measured by the velocity of contraction), and LV afterload (dependent upon aortic contractility and arteriolar run-off).

Internal work (during isovolumetric contraction), which is pressure generated and dependent on the ventricular radius.

Myocardial mass.

Heart rate: tachycardia increases demand.

■ Coronary circulation

The **coronary circulation** consists of:

Arteries: The two coronary arteries arise from the coronary ostia just above the respective cusps of the aortic valve.

Left coronary artery, which gives off the following branches:

Left circumflex artery supplies posterior free wall of left ventricle

Left anterior descending artery supplies the anterior free wall of the left ventricle; a septal branch supplies the upper inter-ventricular septum

Right coronary artery supplies the free wall of the right ventricle and right atrium and the posterior free wall of the left ventricle.

Veins: epicardial veins; coronary sinus; Thebesian veins.

Features of coronary blood flow

The epicardial arteries give rise to small vessels that supply the outer third of the myocardium. They also give off penetrating vessels that anastomose with the subendocardial capillary plexus, which functions as an **end-arterial system**. There is no significant collateral circulation at the microcirculatory level, explaining the discrete nature of ischaemic lesions following myocardial infarction.

Flow is phasic, predominantly in diastole, owing to the aortic pressure wave and to intramural coronary vessel compression by cardiac muscle contraction in systole. During tachycardia, when myocardial oxygen demand is increased, the duration of diastole is reduced, thereby reducing coronary flow. The flow at rest in an adult with a cardiac output of 5 l/min is around 60–70 ml per 100 grams of myocardium per minute. The normal myocardium weight is 300 grams.

Maximal oxygen extraction takes place. Myocardial oxygen extraction ranges between 11 and 12 ml/100 ml per minute.

Coronary flow is subject to **autoregulation**. The difference between autoregulated flow and maximal flow constitutes the coronary vascular reserve. Flow is controlled by:

Myogenic response to change in luminal pressure (arterial smooth muscle contraction occurs in response to increased intraluminal pressure).

Metabolic vasodilatation (coronary arteriolar tone depends on the balance of myocardial oxygen supply and demand). Potential mediators for metabolic regulation include oxygen, carbon dioxide and adenosine. Adenosine is a product of ATP utilisation, and increased adenosine concentrations reflect an imbalance between energy demand and supply.

Autonomic innervation may play a role but the effects of sympathetic or parasympathetic activation on the coronary circulation may be difficult to isolate owing to concomitant changes in heart rate, blood pressure and contractility.

■ Cardiac cells

There are five functionally and anatomically separate types:
Sino-atrial node
Atrio-ventricular node
His-Purkinje system
Atrial muscle
Ventricular muscle

The properties of cardiac muscle

These are:
Automaticity (chronotropy): the ability to initiate an electrical impulse.
Conductivity (dromotropy): the ability to conduct an electrical impulse.
Contractility (inotropy): the ability to contract.
Lusitropy: the ability to relax and to fill.
Cardiac muscle cells form a structural and functional **syncytium** (a complex three-dimensional network), being linked by low-resistance intercalated disks. The cells measure 16–100 μm in length and 12–20 μm in diameter.

The **intercalated discs** serve the following functions:

The connection of adjacent cells via desmosomes.

The connection of actin filaments of adjacent cells.

Tight intercellular coupling through low-resistance gap junctions. Each gap junction consists of a cluster of several ion channels. Each channel comprises two hemi-channels or connexons. Each connexon is made up of six connexin molecules that traverse the lipid bilayer and form a central pore. Isoform-specific determinants of conductance, selectivity and gating are located in the cytoplasmic domains of the connexins.

■ Blood vessels

Types of blood vessels

- **Damping vessels**: arteries. The conduit and large distributing arteries offer little resistance to blood flow and help in the propagation of the arterial pulse. They have a windkessel or air cushion effect by virtue of partial accommodation of the stroke volume with ventricular systole. They offer dynamic resistance to the oscillatory components of pulsatile flow, constituting vascular impedance. This damps the pressure oscillations caused by intermittent ventricular ejection. With distal movement of the arterial pressure pulse, there is a rise in systolic pressure, a fall in diastolic pressure and a widening of the pulse pressure. The peak systolic pressure is amplified with passage down the lower limbs.

- **Resistance vessels**: small arteries; arterioles. These vessels are largely responsible for vascular resistance and the maintenance of blood pressure. A microcirculatory unit is a collection of vessels taking origin from an arteriole.

- **Exchange vessels**: capillaries, which are concerned with the transfer of nutrients and waste products between the blood and tissues. They are thin-walled, consisting of a single layer of endothelial cells (with no muscle or connective tissue) and have a large surface area. The endothelial cells are surrounded by a basement membrane and a fine network of reticular collagen fibres. Capillaries form branching networks and have a high density in metabolically active tissues such as glands, and cardiac and skeletal muscle. Capillary endothelial cells possess the property of forming new capillaries (angiogenesis).

  Capillaries may vary in structure according to functional needs as follows:

  Fenestrated or visceral capillaries (glomerulus, choroid plexus, intestinal epithelium, ciliary bodies of the eye) with fenestrations or pores, 60–80 nm in diameter, with or without a thin diaphragm.

Continuous or somatic capillaries (muscle; skin; lungs; brain; thymus; bone): with tight junctions and a continuous basal lamina.

Discontinuous capillaries (liver, bone marrow, spleen), with wide intercellular gaps.

- **Capacity vessels** (collecting and reservoir system): veins and venules, vena cavae, right atrium. Two thirds of the blood is contained within the venous system, which performs a reservoir function.

Arterio-venous shunts connect arterioles and venules and are common in the skin in certain parts of the body, including the fingertips and ear lobules. They are involved in thermoregulation.

Capillary exchange

The capillary acts as a selective filter. The movement of fluid across the capillary wall by filtration, between the capillary and the interstitial fluid, is governed by **Starling forces**. The Starling forces define water movement between the intravascular and extravascular spaces as the difference between hydrostatic forces forcing water out of the capillaries and osmotic forces drawing water into the intravascular space. The net fluid flux is directly proportional to the net driving pressure, which is outward at the arteriolar end and inward at the venous end of the capillary. This forms the basis of the plasma-interstitial fluid balance.

$$Qi = k((Pc - \pi i) - (Pi - \pi p))$$

Where

Qi = fluid movement across the capillary wall.

k = filtration constant for the capillary membrane (rate of filtration of fluid/ min per mm Hg per 100 grams of tissue). It is a measure of the leakiness of the capillary wall to water.

πp = plasma osmotic pressure.

πi = interstitial fluid osmotic pressure.

Pc = capillary hydrostatic pressure.

Pi = interstitial fluid hydrostatic pressure.

The **mechanisms of tissue oedema** can be considered in the light of the Starling forces as follows:

Increased capillary hydrostatic pressure, secondary to venous obstruction;

Reduced capillary plasma osmotic pressure, due to low plasma albumin levels as in liver disease or starvation;

Reduced interstitial hydrostatic pressure;

Increased interstitial fluid osmotic pressure, secondary to lymphatic vessel obstruction;

Alteration in the capillary filtration coefficient, i.e. increased capillary permeability due to local inflammation, hypoxia or local toxins as in anaphylaxis.

Light pressure on the skin can lead to a white response, caused by pre-capillary sphincter constriction. Harder pressure produces the **triple response**, which consists of a red reaction (dilatation of pre-capillary sphincters), a weal (raised capillary hydrostatic pressure and increased capillary permeability to proteins) and a flare (arteriolar dilatation).

Lymphatic vessels

These are thin-walled endothelial-lined vessels that aid in the return of tissue fluid to the venous system. They form a complex network of blind-ended permeable capillary vessels which are present in all organ systems except the CNS and the bone marrow. The volume of fluid transported through the lymphatics in 24 hours approximates the total plasma volume. The lymphatic vessels eventually drain into the great veins – the thoracic duct and right lymphatic duct draining into the junction of the internal jugular vein and the subclavian vein on the left and right sides respectively.

Flow of fluid through lymphatics is aided by:

The skeletal muscle pump: intermittent skeletal muscle activity;

Unidirectional valves;

Contractions of large lymphatic vessels;

The thoracic pump.

Functions of the lymphatic system

These include:

An in-line filter function of the lymph nodes;

Return of protein from the interstitial space to the venous system;

The transport of lipoproteins, long-chain fatty acids and cholesterol that has been absorbed in the small intestine;

Contributing to the maintenance of renal concentrating ability.

Factors determining smooth muscle tone

Intrinsic myogenic tone.

Locally produced vasoactive substances: metabolic products, including lactic acid, carbon dioxide, potassium, adenosine diphosphate (ADP), AMP and adenosine.

Circulating blood substances: adrenaline, vasopressin, angiotensin II, ANP.

Vascular endothelium

The endothelium is the confluent mono-cellular lining of blood vessels, which separates the blood from the extravascular tissues. It forms the structural and functional interface between the blood and the vessel wall. The endothelium constitutes the largest endocrine, paracrine and autocrine organ in the body, with a surface area of around 600 square metres in an average adult. It is responsible for the regulation of vasomotor tone (vasodilatation and vasoconstriction), vessel growth, platelet aggregation, monocyte adhesion and fibrinolysis. The endothelium plays a major role in the pathogenesis and progression of atherosclerosis and thrombotic disease.

Properties of endothelium

- Functions as a selective permeability barrier (permeability regulator: filter function).
  Large molecules: vesicular transport; passage through intercellular junctions
  Small molecules: vesicles; junctions; and through cytoplasm
- Forms a blood compatible container with a non-thrombogenic surface, which is achieved by the balance between the prothrombotic and the antithrombotic and fibrinolytic characteristics of the endothelial cell.
- Synthesis/metabolism/secretion of:
  Vasoactive (vasorelaxing and vasoconstricting) autacoids: prostacyclins; leukotrienes; nitric oxide; endothelin; angiotensin-converting enzyme.
  Connective tissue components: laminin, fibronectin, vitronectin.
  Chemokines: monocyte chemoattractant protein-1.
  Adhesion molecules: von Willebrand factor, E-selectin, intercellular adhesion molecule-1, vascular cell adhesion molecule-1.
- Binding and internalisation of lipoproteins: modify low density lipoproteins (LDLs)- LDL receptor; lipoprotein lipase.
- Synthesis of stimulating or inhibitory mitogens, with autocrine and paracrine effects.
- Regulator of vascular tone (regulation of smooth muscle contractility)
  Smooth muscle relaxation: nitric oxide.
  Smooth muscle contraction: endothelin; angiotensin II
- Regulator of haemostasis and inflammation: secretes procoagulant factors and inflammatory mediators:
  Platelet adhesion and activation: von Willebrand factor; P-selectin; E-selectin; platelet-activating factor
  Coagulation: thrombomodulin; heparin sulphate

Characteristics shared by all endothelial cells

Factor VIII/ von Willebrand factor staining;
Cell-specific surface lectins;
Uptake of acetylated LDL;
Response to angiogenic growth factors.

Vasoactive endothelial products

Endothelium-derived relaxing factors
Nitric oxide
Prostacyclin (PGI2)

Endothelium-mediated vasoconstrictors
Endothelin-I
Thromboxane
Prostaglandin H2
Oxygen free radicals

Fibrinolysis: tissue type plasminogen activator (t-PA); urinary (u)-PA;
  plasminogen activator inhibitor
Cytokines: interleukins -1, -6 and -8.
- Forms growth-regulating molecules: platelet derived growth factor; fibroblast growth factor; tissue growth factor beta.
- Forms connective tissue macromolecules (matrix factors): collagen; proteoglycans.

Endothelium-derived modulators of haemostasis

Anticoagulants
- Thrombin inhibition
  Antithrombin III (ATIII)
  Thrombomodulin
- Enhanced fibrinolysis
  Tissue plasminogen activator
- Platelet inhibition
  Prostacyclin (PGI2)

Procoagulants
- Coagulation factors:
  Tissue factor (thromboplastin)
  Factor VII

- Platelet aggregation:
  Von Willebrand factor
  Platelet activating factor
- Inhibition of fibrinolysis
  Plasminogen activator inhibitor

Endothelial secretion in acute inflammation

Vascular relaxation and inhibition of platelet aggregation: nitric oxide; prostacyclin

Vascular constriction: endothelin; thromboxane A2; ATIII

Promotion of inhibitors, e.g. heparin-like substances: growth factor platelet-derived growth factor(PDGF)

Chemokines

Endothelial role in haemostasis

Prothrombotic

Platelet function modulation: basement membrane collagen synthesis; von Willebrand factor synthesis.

Coagulation modulation: synthesis of basement membrane collagen; synthesis of factor V; synthesis and expression of tissue factor; binding site for thrombin.

Antithrombotic

Generates prostacyclin;

Binds thrombin, via thrombomodulin, which then activates protein C;

Adenosine;

Nitric oxide;

Synthesis of ATIII, protein S, plasminogen activator;

Binding site for plasmin;

Protein C activation.

Factors contributing to endothelial dysfunction

These include:
  Cytokines
  Bacterial products
  Viral infection
  Oxidised lipoproteins
  Homocysteine
  End products of advanced glycosylation
  Altered haemodynamic forces

Plasma markers

Those associated with endothelial cell damage or dysfunction may be predictive of cardiovascular complications, morbidity and mortality. They include:

Von Willebrand factor

Soluble thrombomodulin

Soluble E-selectin (CD62E)

Endothelin

Circulating endothelial cells

Normal artery wall

The arterial wall consists of the following layers:

The intima, which comprises a continuous monolayer of endothelial cells, and a subendothelial space comprising a proteoglycan layer and smooth muscle cells.

Internal elastic lamina.

Tunica media, which consists of interspersed layers of elastic tissue and concentrically arranged smooth muscle cells.

Adventitia or connective tissue sheath, which contains blood vessels, nerves and fibroblasts embedded in a network of collagen, elastic fibres, proteoglycans and glycoproteins. It helps in the maintenance of arterial shape. Vasa vasora feed into the capillary plexus in the adventitia and provide arterial wall nutrition.

Physiological functions of the components of the extracellular matrix

Arterial permeability; transfer of essential nutrients across the intima.

Structural integrity of intima.

Regulation of smooth muscle cell proliferation.

Vasopressors

Alpha 1-adrenergic receptor agonists

Ergot alkaloids

Vasopressin

Angiotensin II

Nitric oxide synthase antagonists

Nitric oxide

Nitric oxide is a diffusible, unstable or free radical gas. Having a low blood–gas partition coefficient, it readily enters the gas phase. Nitric oxide is synthesised by vascular endothelium from the terminal guanidine nitrogen of L-arginine in a single step reaction catalysed by nitric oxide synthase. It has a short half-life of under 5 seconds, undergoing rapid oxidation to stable metabolic end-products, nitrate and nitrite. Toxic metabolites include methaemoglobin, nitrogen dioxide and peroxynitrite.

The actions, which may be paracrine or autocrine, include:

Intracellular: stimulation of guanosine 3′–5′ monophosphate (cyclic GMP)-
dependent kinase ion channels or phosphodiesterase.

Extracellular:

- Neurally mediated vascular smooth muscle relaxation. This is responsible for vasodilator tone, which helps regulate systemic blood pressure.
- Anterograde and retrograde signalling between pre- and postsynaptic units, regulating smooth muscle function in the stomach, small intestine and uterus. It is the major mediator of relaxation regulated by the non-adrenergic, non-cholinergic system.
- Inhibition of platelet aggregation and adhesion, and of white blood cell aggregation.
- Regulation of cardiac contractility, via its negative inotropic effects.
- Neurotransmitter in the CNS and in the non-adrenergic non-cholinergic autonomic nervous system. In the CNS, it acts as a neurotransmitter at the presynaptic N-methyl-D-aspartate (glutamate) receptors which activate calcium channels.
- Modulation of immune cell defences, including stimulation of the formation of cytotoxic products by activated macrophages, thereby acting as an inflammatory mediator.
- Retinal phototransduction.
- Neuronal long-term potentiation and memory.
- Penile erection.
- Atherogenesis.

The synthesis of nitric oxide is catalysed by one of three isozymes of nitric oxide synthase, using nicotinamide adenine dinucleotide phosphate dehydrogenase (NADPH) as electron source and cofactors including tetrahydropterin and flavin nucleotides Flavine adenine mononucleotide (FMN), Flavine adenine dinucleotide (FAD). These enzymes are homodimeric cytochrome P450-like haemoproteins. The three types are neuronal, inducible and endothelial constitutive. Neuronal nitric oxide synthase is expressed by central and peripheral neurons. Inducible nitric oxide synthase is calmodulin-independent and cytokine-inducible. It is expressed by vascular smooth muscle cells, endothelial cells and inflammatory cells, including macrophages. Constitutive nitric oxide synthase is calcium/calmodulin and NADPH-dependent. It is expressed by endothelial cells and neurons.

Clinical uses of nitric oxide

These include:

Therapeutic role for inhaled nitric oxide: persistent pulmonary hypertension in neonates and adults; acute respiratory distress syndrome; high-altitude pulmonary oedema.

Nitric oxide donors, which include:

Organic nitrates, e.g. amyl nitrite, glyceryl trinitrate, isosorbide mononitrate

Sodium nitroprusside

Molsidomine and its metabolites

Diazeniumdiolites

S-nitrosothiols

Mesoimic oxatriazoles

Selective inhibitors of the synthesis of inducible nitric oxide.

■ Blood viscosity

Blood viscosity refers to the resistance to blood flow as a result of intermolecular attractions between its constituent fluid layers, leading to friction. Energy loss in the peripheral circulation occurs principally as a result of the need to overcome blood viscosity and to overcome inertia. The blood viscosity varies at different sites in the circulatory system, owing to differences in velocity gradient and vessel geometry.

The unit for measuring viscosity is the poise: 1 dyne s/sq.cm. The coefficient of viscosity is the ratio of the energy loss due to internal frictional resistance (shear stress) to the relative velocity of adjacent fluid layers (shear rate).

The relative viscosity or viscosity ratio relates the viscosity of a fluid to that of water.

Determinants of blood viscosity

Plasma proteins

Red blood cells

Haematocrit

Red cell aggregation: at low shear rates, rouleaux formation occurs

Red cell flexibility or rigidity

Platelet aggregation

Shear rate; blood behaves as a non-Newtonian fluid at low shear rates. At high shear rates, blood displays Newtonian behaviour, with the shear stress being directly proportional to the shear strain rate or velocity gradient.

Diameter of the blood vessel: Fahraeus–Lindqvist effect.

Hyperviscosity syndromes can be associated with polycythaemia, thrombocytosis, leukocytosis or elevated plasma protein levels (as in multiple myeloma or macroglobulinaemia).

Viscous properties of blood

Viscosity of blood changes with the rate of blood flow and shear rate. This anomalous viscosity can significantly increase resistance to flow when the perfusion pressure is low as in shock states, contributing to the resulting blood flow deficit. Blood is a non-Newtonian, thixotropic (demonstrating memory) fluid. In a Newtonian fluid viscosity is independent of shear rate and flow velocity.

Fahraeus–Lindqvist effect: viscosity is dependent on the diameter of the vessel it is flowing through. Viscosity appears to decrease as the vessel diameter decreases.

Plasma skimming: in vessels, red cells tend to accumulate in the centre of the flowing stream (axial streaming). Branches leaving a large vessel at right angles may receive a disproportionate amount of red cell-poor blood.

Laminar flow

This can be considered as being represented by a series of concentric layers or laminae sliding past each other, the outer ones nearly stationary, the inner ones moving faster. All motion is parallel to the walls of the tube. The maximal flow velocity is in the central axis of the vessel, resulting in a parabolic velocity profile. This difference creates a shearing effect greatest at the wall of the vessel. The shear rate is the rate of change of velocity of flow between concentric laminae of blood. The shear stress on the endothelial surface is directly proportional to the shear rate and inversely proportional to the viscosity of the fluid. Flow is directly proportional to pressure in laminar flow.

Turbulent flow

In **turbulent flow**, the velocity of flow varies rapidly with respect to space and time, and some of the fluid energy is dissipated as heat. Flow separation occurs, with the axial flow stream being separated from flow in areas more peripherally, as in aneurysms, and in segments just beyond arterial stenoses.

The tendency to turbulent flow is directly proportional to velocity of blood flow and to the diameter of the blood vessel, and inversely proportional to the viscosity of blood divided by its density. Turbulent flow is thus related to high flow rates, changes in vessel diameters, angles and branching points in the circulation.

Reynolds number $= v.d/(\eta/p)$

where $v =$ velocity of blood flow (cm/s)

$d =$ diameter of the vessel

$\eta =$ viscosity of blood in poises

$p =$ density of blood

Reynolds number

This describes the tendency for transition from laminar flow to turbulent flow. For blood the Reynolds number is around 1000. If the velocity of blood flow exceeds a critical value, or if there is an obstruction to blood flow, eddies start to form and turbulent flow may develop. When turbulent flow is fully developed, the velocity profile becomes rectangular in shape. Turbulent flow requires the expenditure of more energy than is required for laminar flow. Murmurs or bruits are audible over areas of turbulent flow.

Local flow disturbances leading to altered velocity profile and turbulent flow are related to curvature of vessels, branch points, bifurcations and the angle of branch take-off. A haemodynamically significant arterial stenosis is associated with cross-sectional area reduction by 75% and reduction in vessel diameter of at least 50%.

Poiseuille's equation

This is strictly applicable to steady (non-pulsatile) laminar (non-turbulent) flow of a Newtonian fluid (non-compressible fluid of uniform viscosity) within a straight, rigid, cylindrical tube. However, it can be used to derive the viscous energy losses associated with the flow of blood.

Blood flow is proportional to $\dfrac{\text{pressure difference} \times \text{radius}^4}{\text{viscosity} \times \text{length}}$

Poiseuille's formula is:

$$Flow = \frac{\text{pressure difference between the ends of a tube} \times \text{radius}^4}{8 \times \text{length of tube} \times \text{viscosity}}$$

$$Q = \frac{\Delta P \pi r^4}{8 l \eta}$$

Where Q = volume flow per unit time

ΔP = pressure head

r = radius

l = length of tube

η = viscosity of the fluid

The circulatory system uses blood pressure and radius of vessels for the short-term control of blood flow rate.

Laplace's law

This states that the wall tension required to withstand a given fluid pressure is directly proportional to the vessel radius. The intraluminal blood pressure exerts a distending and compressive force on the arterial wall, with a circumferential stretching force being applied tangentially to the arterial wall. The expansion of arterial walls is normally limited by collagen fibres, and weakening leads to aneurysm formation, progressing to rupture of the vessel.

Wall tension $T = Pr$, where P is the pressure and r is the radius of the lumen.

At a critical closing pressure, the vessel closes.

■ Phases of the cardiac cycle

Left ventricular contraction

Iso-volumetric (isometric) contraction: ventricles contract with aortic and pulmonary valves closed. The preload and afterload remain constant. The rate of pressure generation reflects the inotropic state of the myocardium.

Maximal ejection, with aortic valve opening.

Left ventricular relaxation (diastole)

Isometric ventricular relaxation, with both inlet and outlet valves closed. This ends with opening of the atrio-ventricular valves.

Passive ventricular filling.

Rapid phase, with ventricular suction;

Slow phase (diastasis);

Atrial systole or booster: it is debatable whether atrial systole actually boosts ventricular filling or merely prevents stagnation of venous blood in the atria.

The treatment of left ventricular diastolic dysfunction leading to failure involves the use of drugs that facilitate ventricular relaxation, such as diuretics, beta blockers, calcium channel blockers, ACE inhibitors and venodilators.

Cardiac contraction

This involves a sequence of:

- Cardiac **action potential** generation in the specialised conduction tissues.
- Propagation of the cardiac impulse by spread of current between adjacent cells at intercellular gap junctions or nexuses, which are formed by proteins known as connexins.
- The sarcolemmal excitation system is responsible for the spread of the action potential and for initiating intracellular events.
- The intracellular **excitation-contraction coupling** system amplifies the electrical excitation signal and converts it to a chemical signal. This comprises the sarcotubular system of transverse or T-tubules, and the sarcoplasmic reticulum. The T system represents invaginations of the sarcolemma, and the sarcoplasmic reticulum is a network of anastomosing, lipid bilayer membrane-limited intracellular tubules. The T system increases the cell membrane surface available for ion transport.
- The contractile system: The functional unit is the sarcomere, which is composed of two bundles of longitudinally oriented thick and thin filaments, separated by Z lines. The thin filaments are attached to each Z line and interdigitate with the thick filaments. The resting length of the sarcomere is between 1.6 and 2.4 μm.

Mechanism of cardiac muscle contraction and relaxation

Contraction is brought about by the following sequence:

Increased calcium influx into the cytosol increases calcium release from the sarcoplasmic reticulum by a positive feedback mechanism.

Calcium binds to troponin C.

Activated troponin C binds to troponin I.

Tropomyosin undergoes conformational change being consequently repositioned on the thin filament, removing its inhibitory effect on actin-myosin interaction.

Contractile regulatory proteins of the heart

Thick filament
Myosin: ATPase
Myosin binding protein C
Myomesin
M protein

Thin filament
Actin: activates myosin ATPase
Tropomyosin: modulates actin-myosin interaction
Troponin complex:
Troponin C: binds calcium
Troponin I: inhibits actin-myosin interaction
Troponin T: binds the troponin complex to tropomyosin

Titin filaments (third filament system)
Titin

Z discs
Alpha-actinin

The myosin heads interact with the actin filaments in cross-bridge cycling, with repetitive attachment and reattachment. The Z lines are drawn closer together, with shortening of the sarcomere.

The degree of shortening of the sarcomere is dependent on its initial length, providing an explanation for the Frank–Starling law, whereby the contractility of the heart increases with ventricular preload.

Relaxation is brought about by active reuptake of calcium from the cytosol into the sarcoplasmic reticulum. This is achieved by the sarcoplasmic reticulum calcium ATPase pump SERCA2a, which couples the hydrolysis of ATP to active transport of calcium. This cation pump cycles between a number of defined states, including calcium ion binding, ATP binding and phosphorylation, ion release, dephosphorylation and back to ion binding. It is a ten transmembrane-span helix with two cytoplasmic domains. Regulation of the calcium pump activity is modulated by an intrinsic sarcoplasmic reticulum protein, phospholamban. Myocardial energy consumption can be related to:

Myosin ATPase activity in cross-bridge cycling;
Active calcium reuptake by the sarcoplasmic reticulum;
Basal metabolism.

Role of calcium

Calcium plays a key role in modulating excitation-contraction coupling, acting at four major intracellular sites:

Sarcolemma

Sarcoplasmic reticulum

Myofilaments

Regulatory troponin-tropomyosin complex

■ Cardiac electrophysiology

Cardiac action potential

The cardiac action potential is generated independently of extrinsic innervation. Five phases are recognised:

Phase 0–**Initial rapid membrane depolarisation**

- This is represented by the upstroke of action potential.
- It is triggered by a decrease in the potential gradient across the membrane to the threshold potential of −70 to −60 mV.
- This leads to voltage-dependent opening of the fast Na^+ channels, resulting in the rapid influx of positively charged ions (the inward Na^+ current) and rapid reversal of membrane polarity. The transmembrane potential above 0 mV is referred to as the overshoot.

Phase 1–**Initial repolarisation**; rapid but limited depolarisation (spike)

- Activation of a transient outward K^+ current and rapid closure of fast inward Na^+ current.
- Most K^+ currents demonstrate rectification, i.e. decreased K^+ conductance with depolarisation.
- The K^+ currents include:

  Instantaneous inward rectifier K^+ current

  Outward (delayed) rectifier K^+ current

  Transient outward currents

  ATP-, Na^+, and acetylcholine-regulated K^+ currents
- The transient outward K^+ current has two components: one component is voltage-gated and the other is activated by a local rise in Ca2+.

Phase 2–**Plateau or prolonged depolarisation**, which is characteristic of the cardiac action potential and is the main determinant of the duration of the action potential.

- The net current is apparently small, as the flow of outward current and the inward flow of current are almost equal.
- The inward currents include: the slowly activating Na^+ current, a slow inward Ca^{2+} current through voltage sensitive L-type channels and an Na^+/Ca^{2+}-exchange current.

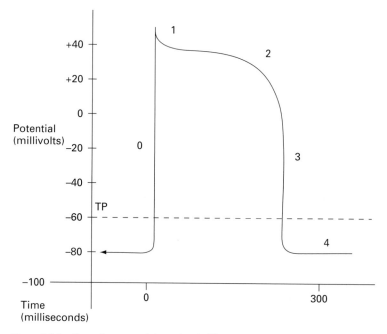

Figure 6.8 Cardiac action potential. TP, threshold potential; RP, resting potential.

- Outward currents include a slowly activating K^+ current, a Cl^- current, a more rapidly activating K^+ current and the Na^+/K^+-electrogenic pump.
- The cardiac cell cannot be excited by an electric stimulus, regardless of intensity–absolute refractory period.

Phase 3 – **Final rapid repolarisation**

- Net repolarisation of the membrane.
- Deactivation of inward Na^+ and Ca^{2+} currents occurs earlier than the K^+ currents.
- When the membrane is sufficiently repolarised, an inward K^+ rectifier current is progressively activated, resulting in a regenerative increase in outward currents and an increasing rate of repolarisation.
- Repolarisation is also achieved by the function of the Na^+/K^+-ATPase pump.
- The relative refractory period is when a greater stimulus intensity is required to generate an action potential than is required after full recovery of the resting membrane potential. This is also known as the relative refractory period.

Phase 4 – **Electrical diastole**

- This is represented by a stable resting membrane potential in atrial and ventricular muscle cells.

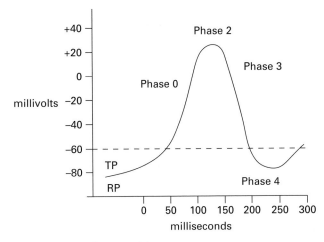

Figure 6.9 Pacemaker potential.

- Automaticity is the property of spontaneous initiation of an action potential in pacemaker cells. This is due to spontaneous steady diastolic depolarisation. The sino-atrial node normally has the fastest discharge rate and is hence the dominant cardiac pacemaker.
- Diastolic depolarisation is caused by a progressive reduction in membrane permeability to potassium ions and a gradual increase in permeability to calcium ions. At a critical threshold of $-40\,mV$ phase 0 depolarisation is triggered.

Pacemaker potential

The **pacemaker potential** is characterised by a less negative threshold potential and a less steep slope in phase 0. This is accompanied by the absence of a plateau phase (phase 2) and a negative phase 4 membrane potential. Spontaneous phase 4 depolarisation is characteristic.

Conduction system

The cardiac conduction system comprises:
- The sino-atrial node, located in the epicardial groove of the lateral part of the sulcus terminalis at the junction of the superior vena cava and the right atrium.
- The internodal tracts, sometimes described in three parts as the anterior (James), middle (Wenckebach) and posterior (Thorel) tracts.

Factors affecting the slope of phase 4 depolarisation

Increased slope
  Arterial hypoxia
  Hypercarbia
  Acute hypokalaemia
  Hyperthermia
  Catecholamines
  Sympathomimetic drugs

Reduced slope
  Vagal stimulation
  Acute hyperkalaemia
  Hypothermia
  Positive airway pressure

Classification of cardiovascular calcium channels

  L- type calcium channels
  T-type calcium channels
  Tetrodotoxin-sensitive calcium channels
  Sarcoplasmic calcium release channels
  Ryanodine receptor
  Inositol 1,4,5-triphosphate (IP3) receptors

- The atrio-ventricular node, which is located in the base of the atrial septum at the apex of a triangle formed by the tendon of Todaro, the tricuspid valve annulus and the coronary sinus.
- The bundle of His, which penetrates the central fibrous body beneath the non-coronary cusp of the aortic valve.
- The bundle branches.
- The Purkinje fibres.

The vagus nerve provides beat-to-beat control of the sino-atrial node. This is mediated by M2 type muscarinic cholinergic receptors coupled to G-protein-activated inward rectifying potassium channels. Respiratory sinus arrhythmia is completely abolished by muscarinic receptor blockade with atropine.

Electrocardiograph

The **electrocardiograph** is a record of the spread of cardiac electrical activity by surface electrodes. The body acts as a volume conductor. The recording electrodes depict the mean electrical vector, which is a sum of all individual vectors at a given instant in time. The magnitude of amplitude of the recorded potential is

Conduction velocities

Sino-atrial node: 0.05 m/s
Atrial muscle: 0.8–1.0 m/s
Atrio-ventricular node: 0.03–0.05 m/s
Bundle of His: 0.8–1.0 m/s
Ventricular muscle: 0.8–1.0 m/s

dependent on the mass of tissue involved and on the direction of the vector relative to the electrical axis (the angle between the lead and the cardiac dipole). The mean electrical axis is the mean electrical vector determined over time.

The electrocardiograph is essentially a record of impulse formation in the primary pacemaker (sino-atrial node), transmission through specialised conduction tissues, depolarisation of the myocardium and repolarisation of the myocardium.

Components of the electrocardiograph

P wave: atrial depolarisation.

QRS complex: ventricular depolarisation. Ventricular activation involves initially the septal area, followed by the apex and finally the bases.

T wave: ventricular repolarisation.

Electrophysiological mechanisms of cardiac arrhythmias

Impulse initiation

Enhancement of normal automaticity.

Abnormal automaticity, which is seen in partially depolarised muscle or Purkinje fibres.

Triggered activity from after-depolarisation of a preceding or triggering action potential. Early after-depolarisation is caused by membrane instability at the beginning of the repolarisation phase, and is associated with prolongation of the action potential. Delayed after-depolarisation occurs after completion of the repolarisation of the action potential.

Re-entry of the propagation wave, which can be either anatomical or functional requires:

A transient or permanent unidirectional conduction block;

A pathway (substrate) for impulse propagation;

Slow conduction within the re-entrant circuit, so that the cells are reactivated by the returning impulse being no longer refractory to further stimulation.

Classification of anti-arrhythmic agents

- Class I: sodium channel blockade (membrane stabilising agents) inhibit propagation of the action potential.

  a: increased refractory period: quinidine, procainamide, disopyramide

  b: reduced refractory period: lignocaine, mexiletine

  c: no effect on refractory period: flecainide, encainide
- Class II: beta-adrenoreceptor blockade.
- Class III: potassium channel blockade: prolong repolarisation: amiodarone, bretylium, ibutilide.
- Class IV: calcium channel blockade: verapamil, diltiazem.
- Miscellaneous: adenosine, digoxin.

Adenosine is an agonist at high-affinity A1 receptors in the atrio-ventricular node, increasing potassium conductance leading to hyperpolarisation of the cell membrane and reduction in or absence of spontaneous activity.

Digoxin inhibits the Na^+/K^+ pump and has agonist activity at muscarinic (M2 receptors), particularly in the atrio-ventricular node.

BIBLIOGRAPHY

Fahraeus, R. & Lindquist, T. The viscosity of the blood in narrow capillary tubes. *Am. J. Physiol.*, **96** (1931), 562–8.

Hallett, Jr, J. W., Mills, J. L., Earnshaw, J. J. & Reekens, J. A. *Comprehensive Vascular and Endovascular Surgery.* St Louis: Mosby, 2004

Klabunde, R. E. *Cardiovascular Physiology Concepts.* Baltimore: Lippincott, Williams & Wilkins, 2005

Mohrman, D. E. & Heller, L. J. *Cardiovascular Physiology.* New York: The McGraw-Hill Companies, Inc., 2003.

Moncada, S. & Higgs, A. The L-arginine-nitric oxide pathway. *New Engl. J. Med.*, **329** (1993), 2002–12.

Sperelakis, N., Kurachi, Y., Terzic, A. & Cohen, M. V. *Heart Physiology and Pathophysiology*, 4th edn. San Diego: Academic Press, 2001

Starling, E. H. On the absorption of fluids from the connective tissue spaces *J. Physiol.*, **19** (1896), 312–20.

Swan, H. J. C., Ganz, W., Forrester, J., *et al.* Catheterisation of the heart in man with the use of a flow-directed balloon tipped catheter. *New Engl. J. Med.*, **283** (1970), 447–51.

Vane, J. R., Anggard, E. E. & Botting, R. M. Regulatory functions of the vascular endothelium. *New Engl. J. Med.*, **323** (1990), 27–36.

Respiratory system

7

■ Introduction

The respiratory system allows oxygen delivery to, and carbon dioxide removal from, the bloodstream, which are mediated via the conducting airways and a gas-exchange region. The exchange of gases is termed respiration.

■ Functional components of the respiratory system

- The **pump** that drives ventilation: chest wall and pleura; respiratory muscles (intercostals and diaphragm). These can be supplemented by the accessory muscles of respiration (sternomastoids, scaleni, pectorals, latissimus dorsi) in situations where the work of breathing is increased. **Inspiration** is an active process, being brought about by negative intra-pleural pressure generated by contraction and descent of the diaphragm and rib cage elevation by the intercostal muscles. The contraction of the diaphragm expands the chest wall laterally (bucket handle effect) and antero-posteriorly (pump handle effect). The phasic action of the intercostal muscles helps in stabilisation of the chest wall. **Expiration** is mainly passive and dependent on the elastic recoil of the lungs and chest wall. Active expiration occurs during exercise and in hyperventilation states and primarily involves the anterior abdominal wall musculature, assisted by the internal intercostal muscles.
- The **distribution of ventilation**: upper respiratory tract, conducting airways, respiratory bronchioles. Apart from air conduction, these air passages are involved in the humidification and warming of inspired air.
- **Perfusion**: pulmonary arteries and veins, capillaries.
- **Bronchial clearance**: muco-ciliary escalator; macrophages.
- **Alveolar clearance and defence**: alveolar macrophages; pulmonary lymphatics; humoral mediators.

The process of **gas exchange** itself involves:

Ventilation of the lungs;

Capillary perfusion of ventilated alveoli;

Diffusion across the alveolar-capillary membrane.

The upper respiratory tract

This comprises:

- The **nose**, which serves the following functions:

  Air conduction.

  Particle and micro-organism clearance by the muco-ciliary mechanism, which comprises the pseudostratified ciliated epithelium, mucous blanket and the mucus-producing glands. The inspired air is thereby cleaned and filtered. In general, particle diameter requires to be greater than 10 μm to allow nasal filtration.

  Humidification and warming of inspired air by a counter-current heat and fluid exchange mechanism.

  Perception of smell, via the olfactory neuroepithelial receptors.

  Contributes to more than 50% of total airway resistance normally.

- The **pharynx**, which is involved in swallowing, while simultaneously preventing aspiration of food into the lungs.

- The **larynx**, which is involved with:

  The production of speech, which comprises the three components of phonation, resonance and articulation.

  Providing a sphincter for protection of the lower airway from soiling, especially during swallowing and vomiting.

  Acting as a sphincter in cough and expiration.

  Regulating airflow in and out of the lungs. When open, ventilation of the lungs is allowed.

  The Valsalva manoeuvre, of forced expiration against a closed glottis, which is involved in the control of venous return and also facilitates defaecation.

  Providing sensory input for respiratory control.

The **paranasal sinuses** are lined by ciliated stratified or pseudostratified columnar epithelium. They may subserve the following functions:

Humidification and warming of inspired air;

Regulation of intra-nasal pressure;

Provision of resonance to the voice;

Increase in the surface area of the olfactory mechanism;

Lessening the density and weight of the skull;

Providing an air buffer to the concussive effects of blunt trauma.

Nasal function testing

This can be carried out by:

- **Airflow measurements**

  Rhinomanometry: simultaneous trans-nasal pressure and airflow recording; which can be anterior, posterior or post-nasal;

  Peak nasal airflow;

  Acoustic rhinometry;

  Radiological imaging to assess the cross-sectional area of the nasal passages (computed tomography or magnetic resonance imaging).

- **Ciliary function testing**: saccharin taste test, which measures the time taken to taste saccharin in the back of the throat after application to the anterior tip of the inferior nasal turbinate. A time greater than 30 minutes is abnormal. Ciliated epithelium can be obtained by nasal brush biopsy of the inferior nasal turbinate and the sample is processed at 37 °C to determine ciliary beat frequency, and to assess the ciliary beat pattern by slow motion analysis. Ciliary ultrastructure can be assessed by transmission electron microscopy.

- **Tests of olfaction** using smell bottles.

Functional anatomy of the lower respiratory tract (Weibel)

The tracheo-bronchial tree can be described as a symmetrical dichotomous branching system of airways, comprising around 23 generations of airway from the trachea to the alveolar sacs. It comprises:

- Trachea: generation 0. This is 25 cm long in the adult and supported by 15–20 horseshoe-shaped cartilaginous rings that are joined posteriorly by smooth muscle.
- Main, lobar and segmental bronchi: generations 1–4. The major site of airways resistance to gas flow is at the level of the 3rd and 4th generation airways, contributing 60%–70% of total airways resistance.
- Small bronchi: generations 5–11. Bronchioles: generations 12–14. There is no cartilage in the wall at this level, and the air passages are held open not by structural rigidity but by elastic recoil.
- Respiratory bronchioles: generations 15–18.
- Alveolar ducts: generations 19–22.
- Alveolar sacs: generation 23. The 23rd generation airways possess a total cross-sectional airway diameter much greater than that of the trachea.

Airway calibre is determined by the coupling of airway wall elasticity and airway transmural pressure.

The topological unit of the lung is the **bronchopulmonary segment**, which is supplied by a principal branch of a lobar bronchus and its accompanying pulmonary artery.

Features of the pulmonary acinus (or terminal respiratory unit)

- The functional gas exchanging unit of the lung.
- The zone supplied by a first order respiratory bronchiole.
- Includes the respiratory bronchioles, alveolar ducts and alveolar sacs distal to a single terminal bronchiole, typically representing generations 15–23.
- A human lung contains between 30 000 and 50 000 acini, each with a diameter of about 3.5 mm and containing about 10 000 alveoli.
- This provides a total gas volume of 2500 ml and a surface area of between 50–80 square metres, through which gas exchange by diffusion can occur.
- The acini are connected by channels in the alveolar walls known as pores of Kohn, which act as portals for collateral ventilation and the transit of macrophages.

Respiratory epithelium

The **functions of respiratory epithelium** include:

Humidification of inspired air;

Chemical barrier and particle clearance;

Defence against infection.

Respiratory (bronchial) epithelium consists of the following cell types:

- Pseudostratified columnar ciliated epithelial cells, with 200–300 cilia per cell.
- Mucus-secreting (goblet) cells.
- Basal cells, which anchor the goblet and ciliated cells to the extracellular matrix.
- Mast cells, which secrete histamine, lysosomal enzymes, leukotrienes, platelet-activating factor, neutrophil and eosinophil chemotactic factors and serotonin.
- Non-ciliated bronchiolar epithelial (Clara) cells, which are specialised secretory cells in the terminal bronchioles. These cells synthesise, store, and secrete specialised lipids, proteins and glycoproteins.
- APUD (amine precursor uptake, decarboxylase) cells, which have a high content of amine and peptide hormones including serotonin, dopamine, noradrenaline and vasoactive intestinal peptide.
- Dense-core granulated cells (Kulschitzky cells)

Classification of alveolar cell types

Capillary endothelial cells with loose junctions.

Alveolar epithelial cells:

Type I: squamous lining cells, which comprise 90%–95% of the alveolar surface.

Type II: secretory cells: synthesise, secrete and store surfactant; cuboidal; microvilli; osmophilic inclusion bodies.

Alveolar macrophages, which are responsible for the phagocytosis of particles, viruses and bacteria.

Neutrophils.

Pulmonary defence mechanisms

These can be categorised as:

Mechanical

Filtration in the upper airways, especially the nose.

Humidification of the inspired air.

Epiglottic function.

A competent larynx allowing an effective cough reflex.

Ciliary action of respiratory epithelial cells, which allows upward clearance of mucus from the tracheo-bronchial tree – the muco-ciliary escalator. This characterises epithelial cells to the 17th generation of airways. There are over 200 cilia per cell.

Mucus blanket. Mucus is a mixture of water, electrolytes and macromolecules (lipids, mucins and enzymes) secreted by the goblet cells and mucosal glands.

Surfactant preventing alveolar atelectasis.

Glycoproteins (Fibronectin).

Immune defences

Immunoglobulins, especially IgA and IgG;

Complement factors, classical and alternative;

Cellular defence mechanisms (alveolar level): alveolar macrophages and T-lymphocytes; polymorphonuclear cells.

■ Diffusion

The **air–blood barrier** is about 2 μm thick and comprises:

The capillary endothelium;

The fused basement membranes of the endothelial and epithelial layers;

The epithelial type I and II pneumocytes.

The **pulmonary interstitium** separates the linings of the alveoli and of the capillaries. It comprises:

A fibrous scaffold of collagens and elastic fibres;

Extracellular matrix of vessel wall;

Fibroblasts, smooth muscle cells and macrophages;

Lymphatic vessels.

The rate-limiting steps for oxygen diffusion

These are:

The rate of passage of oxygen across the alveolo-capillary membrane;

The rate of combination of oxygen with haemoglobin in the red blood cells;

The driving pressure for diffusion, i.e. the differences in pressures between pO_2 in the alveolus and pO_2 in the red blood cell.

Diffusing capacity

This is measured using carbon monoxide as a tracer gas. The single breath-hold method involves the following steps:

- A single breath-hold for 10 seconds is followed by rapid inspiration from the residual volume to the total lung capacity of a gas mixture of 0.3%–0.4% carbon monoxide, helium, oxygen and nitrogen. This represents a vital capacity breath of gas from a reservoir bag.
- Slow even exhalation back to the residual volume follows. The first portion of the expired gas (750 ml) represents the anatomical and system dead space. The second portion (the last 75–100 ml) of the expired gas (the end-tidal gas) is collected and taken as representing alveolar gas.
- Carbon monoxide and helium concentrations are measured in alveolar gas.
- The carbon monoxide tension in pulmonary capillary blood is close to zero, owing to the long time required for the plasma to equilibrate with alveolar gas.
- The rate at which carbon monoxide leaves the alveoli depends on the rate of diffusion through the alveolar-capillary membrane.
- The diffusing capacity for carbon monoxide is equal to the volume of carbon monoxide transferred into the blood per minute per mm Hg of carbon monoxide partial pressure, i.e. the rate of uptake of carbon monoxide.

In the steady state method, the patient rebreathes the gas until equilibrium is reached.

Transport mechanisms for solute and water across the capillary endothelial cell

These include:

  Passive diffusion: transcellular or paracellular

  Pinocytosis

  Via endothelial channels

  Via inter-endothelial junctions

■ Dead space

Anatomical dead space

This refers to the volume of the conducting airways, and is around 130–180 ml (2 ml/kg throughout life) in the adult, i.e. about 1/3rd of the tidal volume (dead space ventilation (VD)/tidal volume (VT) ratio = 0.3). It can be measured by **Fowler's method**:

- A single breath of 100% oxygen is inhaled and followed by a single expiration.
- On expiration, nitrogen concentration is continuously measured at the mouth. Nitrogen is measured as it does not participate in gas exchange. A simultaneous measurement of expired gas volume is carried out.
- The nitrogen concentration in the expired gas gradually rises as 100% oxygen is washed out of the conducting airways by alveolar gas. It plateaus when only alveolar gas is being exhaled.
- The volume of the anatomical dead space is equal to the volume that occurs half-way to the plateau point.

Physiological dead space

This refers to the proportion of the tidal volume that does not participate directly in gas exchange. It consists of the anatomical dead space and the alveolar dead space (the volume of gas in alveoli that are ventilated but not perfused, and thereby not participating in gas exchange, i.e. wasted ventilation). It comprises 25%–35% of the normal tidal volume (the VD/VT ratio). It can be measured by **Bohr's method**, which is based on the following principles:

- Air ventilating perfused lungs will equilibrate with carbon dioxide in the blood. Alveolar pCO_2 is thus similar to arterial pCO_2.
- Inspired air contains virtually no carbon dioxide.

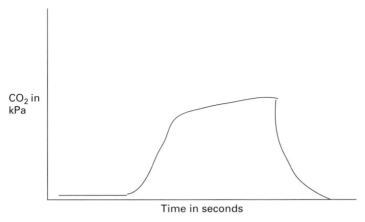

Figure 7.1 Expired CO_2 concentration during a normal breath.

- The product of the alveolar carbon dioxide concentration and the amount of inspired air reaching the alveoli equals the expired carbon dioxide concentration (multiplied by the tidal volume.

$$VD = \frac{(PaCO_2 - PECO_2)}{PaCO_2} \times VT$$

where

$PaCO_2 = $ arterial PCO_2

$PECO_2 = $ expired gas PCO_2

In general, alveolar dead space increases in disease and anatomical dead space increases with increasing age. Anaesthetic circuits and equipment will increase anatomical dead space.

■ Elastic properties

The **elastic behaviour of the lungs and chest wall** is due to:

The surface tension at the alveolar–air interface, which is determined by pulmonary surfactant.

Viscoelastic properties of the solid components of the lungs and chest wall, related to collagen and elastin fibre content.

Surfactant

Surfactant is synthesised by type II alveolar epithelial cells. It is comprised of about 90% lipids, predominantly the phospholipid dipalmitoylphosphatidylcholine and cholesterol, along with 5%–10% proteins. It is spread as a monolayer at the air–fluid interface.

It reduces the surface tension at the alveolar air–fluid interface. This stabilises the alveoli, preventing alveolar collapse during expiration, i.e. at low lung volumes. It changes surface tension characteristics as the surface is stretched. Surface tension increases as the alveoli distend and reduces as the alveoli contract. By Laplace's law, with a fall in alveolar pressure during expiration and reduction in alveolar radius, the pressure across the wall rises and would lead to alveolar collapse if surface tension were to remain constant. Reduction of surface tension increases lung compliance and reduces the work of breathing. Surfactant also reduces pulmonary capillary filtration and the transudation of fluid into the alveoli.

It is responsible for hysteresis in the lung, a phenomenon wherein the inflation and deflation volume–pressure curves of the lung are different. Surfactant may contribute to the lung defence mechanism.

Surfactant deficiency is a primary cause of neonatal respiratory distress syndrome, and exogenous surfactant therapy improves gas exchange and increases lung compliance in this condition.

■ Control of ventilation

Control of ventilation ensures delivery of oxygen, removal of carbon dioxide and the maintenance of pH. Central rhythm generation occurs in the medulla and the pons. Respiratory neurons possess inherent rhythmicity that is independent of higher influences. Rate and depth are adjusted by a combination of chemical and mechanical stimuli along with higher CNS inputs.

Components of the control system

The control of breathing comprises neural and chemical controls, which are closely interrelated. These include:

Sensors (afferent systems)
Chemoreceptors
- Central, in the ventral medulla oblongata in the floor of the fourth ventricle, responding to changes in cerebrospinal fluid (CSF) H^+ ion concentration. They are not stimulated by oxygen lack. Chronic increases in $paCO_2$ concentration causes the CSF pH to return to normal by virtue of altered bicarbonate

production by glial cells. Bicarbonate diffuses across the blood–brain barrier and raises the CSF pH.

- Peripheral: carotid and aortic bodies, which respond to reduced pO_2, reduced pH and raised $paCO_2$.

Mechanoreceptors

- Airways:

  Slowly adapting pulmonary stretch receptors in smooth muscle of bronchi and bronchioles, with vagal myelinated afferents, which respond to increase in lung volume, being activated by lung inflation. They are tonically active at the functional residual capacity, and are reponsible for the Hering Breuer inflation inhibitory reflex (stimulation of these receptors helps terminate inspiration). This reflex is a negative feedback control mechanism for ventilation.

  Rapidly adapting pulmonary stretch receptors, which are activated by rapid lung inflation. The rapidly adapting receptors in the trachea and large bronchi are responsible for the cough reflex, mucus production and bronchospasm.

- Juxta-pulmonary capillary C-fibre endings: type J receptors. These are unmyelinated vagus afferents that respond to increased pulmonary interstitial volume and mediate hyperventilation associated with increased left atrial pressure as in the presence of vascular congestion and pulmonary oedema.

- Musculoskeletal afferents stimulated by skeletal muscle stretch: muscle spindles and Golgi tendon organs. These form part of segmental spinal cord reflexes.

Pulmonary irritant receptors

Vagal myelinated afferents in airway epithelium.

Sensory nerves respond to inhaled chemical irritants and to endogenous chemical stimuli, e.g. histamine released by mast cells.

Stimulated by reduced lung compliance and deflation of the lung.

Control centre

Medulla oblongata

Pons

Cerebral cortex

Effectors (respiratory muscles)

Intercostals

Diaphragm

Accessory muscles

The rostro-caudal organisation of respiratory control is well recognised. The cortical areas, including the anterior hippocampal gyrus and the ventral and medial surfaces of the temporal lobe, are inhibitory. This effect is not clinically important. Rhythmic contraction of the respiratory muscles produces gas flow into and out of the lungs.

Brain stem respiratory neurons generate the basic respiratory rhythm and can drive the respiratory musculature rhythmically in the absence of any other input. They comprise three groups of neurons located bilaterally in the medulla and pons:

- The **pontine group**: the pneumotaxic centre in the upper pons, which transmits inhibitory signals to the inspiratory group.
- The **medullary group**:

    Dorsal respiratory group: ventro-lateral region of the nucleus of the tractus solitarius along the dorsal aspect of the medulla oblongata; the neurons are mainly found in the nucleus of the tractus solitarius and in the reticular formation. Contains mainly neurons that are active during inspiration and project to the contralateral spinal cord. They are driven by rhythm generated in the rostral ventro-medial medulla.

    Ventral respiratory group: in the nucleus ambiguus and nucleus retroambiguus of the medulla oblongata. Consist of both inspiratory and expiratory neurons, which project contralaterally to the spinal cord.

While breathing is primarily under involuntary control, a superimposed voluntary control system also operates. The latter allows speaking and voluntary breath-holding.

Peripheral chemoreceptors

These are fast-responding monitors of the arterial blood, responding to a fall in paO_2, a rise in $paCO_2$ or H^+ concentration, or a fall in their perfusion rate. Stimulation of peripheral chemoreceptors leads to an increase in ventilation.

The carotid bodies, which are located at the common carotid artery bifurcation, are almost exclusively responsible for the ventilatory response. The carotid bodies contain large sinusoids with a very high rate of perfusion. They have the highest blood flow per weight of any organ in the body. The arterial/venous pO_2 difference is small as the flow is high in relation to metabolism. The rapid response is within the range of 1–3 seconds.

The secretory glomus or type I cell is in synaptic contact with afferent nerve endings derived from an axon with its cell body in the petrosal ganglion of the glossopharyngeal nerve. Chemo-transduction following hypoxic stimulation is achieved via oxygen-dependent potassium channels.

In type I cells arterial hypoxia causes a reduction in the intracellular level of ATP, at levels of pO_2 which have little effect elsewhere in the body. The carotid bodies undergo hypertrophy and hyperplasia under conditions of chronic hypoxia. They are usually ablated in the operation of carotid endarterectomy.

■ Work of breathing

Breathing consists of rhythmic changes in lung volume brought about by the medullary respiratory neurons. The work of breathing, involved in the generation of a pressure gradient between the atmosphere and the alveoli, overcomes:

The non-elastic (mainly frictional) resistance to airflow in the airways;

The elastic recoil of the lungs and chest wall;

Inertial resistance of the tracheo-bronchial air column, the lungs and the chest wall.

Resistance

This is a measure of the change in pressure required for a unit change in flow. There are two components to resistance to airflow. Resistance during laminar airflow predominates in the small airways, while resistance during turbulent flow predominates in the larger central airways and is the major factor in determining resistance. With laminar flow, resistance is directly proportional to the length of airway and to the viscosity of the inhaled gas, and is inversely proportional to the fourth power of the radius of the airway.

Resistance to airflow is caused by:

Friction of air against the airway walls;

Turbulent flow, due to molecular interactions and velocity edges within the gas being breathed in.

Non-reversible molecular rearrangements within the tissue or the gas–liquid interface.

Airway resistance is equal to the pressure drop from the alveoli to the mouth, divided by airflow.

Turbulent gas flow

This is proportional to gas density and to the square root of the driving pressure. Turbulence is predicted by the Reynolds number, which is equal to vd/η, where v = velocity of gas flow, d = the diameter of the cylinder, and η = the kinematic viscosity of gas flow in a cylinder. When the number is under 2000, flow is usually laminar and gas flow is proportional to gas viscosity and to the driving pressure. When the number is greater than 4000, gas flow is turbulent. Intermediate values are associated with transitional flow.

Heliox

The inhalation of **Heliox** (a mixture of 20%–40% oxygen and 60%–80% helium) can reduce the work of breathing by:

Reducing the pressure gradient required to generate a given airflow rate by the fact that it is a low density gas, the density being lower than that of any other gas except hydrogen. The mixture has a density one third of that of air.

Reducing the Reynolds number favouring conversion of turbulent to laminar flow in the upper airways.

Pathophysiology of dyspnoea

Dyspnoea can be characterised as an abnormal and uncomfortable subjective awareness of the effort of breathing. The underlying causative factors include:
Increase in the mechanical work of breathing:

Increased airway resistance;

Chest wall muscle dysfunction;

Reduced pulmonary compliance: oedema, fibrosis, congestion.
Increase in ventilatory drive:

Chemical stimuli: hypoxia; metabolic acidosis;

Primary central nervous stimuli, which may be voluntary or involuntary;

Sensory stimuli, from the chest wall, arteries and veins, or lung interstitium.

■ Pulmonary circulation

The components of the pulmonary vasculature are:

Pulmonary arteries

Pulmonary arterioles

Pulmonary capillaries

Pulmonary venules and veins

Bronchial circulation

Pulmonary lymphatics

The pulmonary vessels are characterised by thin walls with relatively small amounts of vascular smooth muscle, a relatively sparse innervation and high distensibility.

Characteristics of the pulmonary circulation

The lungs together are the only organ to receive the total cardiac output, i.e. 5 l/min. The pulmonary circulation is in series with the systemic circulation. It is a low pressure, low resistance system with systolic/diastolic pressure of 25/10 mm Hg and a mean pressure of 15 mm Hg. Pulmonary vascular resistance is about 1/10 that of systemic vascular resistance.

The lungs contain 450 ml blood or 12% of the total blood volume, i.e. the pulmonary circulation has a high capacity. The lungs require 1%–2% of the total body consumption of oxygen for maintenance of activities. Ninety per cent of the cross-sectional area is located in the pre-capillary vessels of order 1. There are 17 orders of arterial vessels and 15 orders of veins in the pulmonary circulation.

The capillary network in the lungs is more dense than elsewhere in order to give a large interface for gas exchange. The capillaries form an extensive system of inter-connected parallel networks. The hydrostatic pressure in lung capillaries is much lower than the oncotic pressure of the plasma proteins, but the interstitial pressure is also lower than elsewhere due to lung factors, so net filtration is quite high.

The pulmonary arterioles constrict to a fall in pO_2 or a rise in pCO_2. Blood is preferentially distributed to dependent parts.

The bronchial circulation

This is a parallel circulation with the following functions:
Supplies the bronchial wall, from the carina down to respiratory bronchioles, with oxygenated blood;
Supplies the acinus if the pulmonary blood flow is interrupted;
Conditioning of inspired air, by providing water for humidification;
Clearance of locally produced mediators.
It is of systemic origin, arising from the thoracic aorta. The bronchial blood flow is around 40 ml/min, approximately 1% of pulmonary arterial flow.

Factors acting on the pulmonary vascular bed

These can be classified as:

Active influences on pulmonary vascular bed, which include:
Neurogenic stimuli
Humoral and chemical influences
Alveolar hypoxia and hypercapnia
Acidosis.

Functions of the pulmonary circulation

Respiratory gas exchange;

Metabolic conversion of circulating vasoactive amines and neurotransmitters by endothelium;

Metabolism of angiotensin I to angiotensin II;

Filtration of peripheral venous blood of clots;

Phospholipid synthesis, e.g. dipalmitoyl phosphatidyl choline, which is a component of surfactant;

Prostaglandin inactivation;

Leukotriene synthesis;

Immunoglobulin synthesis; IgA.

Factors influencing the pulmonary vascular resistance

Increase

Hypoxia

Hypercarbia

Acidosis

Increased pulmonary blood flow

Elevated airway pressure

Sympathetic stimulation

Pulmonary embolism

Hypothermia

Decrease

Oxygen

Hypocarbia

Alkalosis

Prostaglandin E1

Passive influences on pulmonary vascular bed, which include:

Left atrial pressure

Cardiac output

Changes in lung volume

Body position

Alveolar pressure

Factors involved in the production of pulmonary oedema

Increased pulmonary capillary permeability;

Increased pulmonary capillary hydrostatic pressure;

Reduced plasma protein colloid osmotic pressure;

Reduced lymphatic drainage.

The Starling equation can be used to predict the development of pulmonary oedema.

$$Qs = Kf(Pc - Pi) - (Op - Oi)$$

Where Qs = net fluid flow across the capillary membrane

Kf = fluid filtration and removal coefficient

Pc = pressure within capillaries

Pi = pressure within the interstitium

Op = plasma oncotic pressure

Oi = interstitial oncotic pressure

■ Ventilation–perfusion relationships

Alveolar perfusion and ventilation are non-uniform and change with posture.

West's three **zones of perfusion** provide a useful model for depicting the differential blood flow distribution in the lungs:

Zone 1: alveolar pressure > arterial pressure > venous pressure. No blood flow occurs.

Zone 2: arterial pressure > alveolar pressure > venous pressure.

Zone 3: arterial pressure > venous pressure > alveolar pressure.

■ Lung volumes and capacities

The right lung comprises 55% of the total lung volume and the left lung comprises 45% of total lung volume.

Specific functional lung volumes

Those that are determined by inspiratory and expiratory effort, include:

Types of alveolar-capillary unit
When considering ventilation (V) and perfusion (Q)
Normal ventilation and perfusion: normal unit
Ventilation without perfusion: dead space (high V/Q)
Perfusion without ventilation: right-to-left shunt (low V/Q)
No ventilation or perfusion: silent unit
Normal **venous–arterial admixture** is around 3%–5% of the cardiac output, and is due to drainage of bronchial venous deoxygenated blood into pulmonary venous oxygenated blood. Passage of blood from systemic venous to arterial system without going through gas-exchange areas of the lung constitutes a right-to-left shunt.

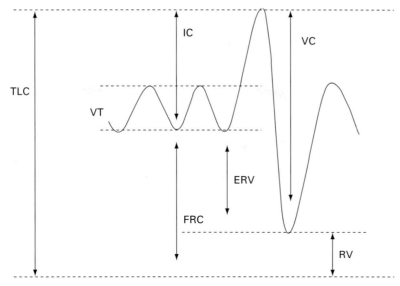

Figure 7.2 Lung volumes. TLC, total lung capacity; VT, tidal volume; IC, inspiratory capacity; VC, vital capacity; FRC, functional residual capacity; ERV, expiratory reserve volume; RV, residual volume.

- **Tidal volume (VT):** normal volume of gas inspired and expired with each normal breath. It is the volume of a normal breath beginning at the functional residual capacity. 400–600 ml (5–7 ml/kg).
- **Inspiratory reserve volume (IRV):** maximum volume of gas that can be inspired above the end of a normal spontaneous inspiration. 2500–3000 ml.
- **Expiratory reserve volume (ERV):** maximum volume of gas that can be forcibly exhaled after a normal expiration (i.e., below functional residual capacity). 900–1300 ml.
- **Vital capacity (VC):** maximum volume of gas that can be exhaled by forceful effort after a maximal inspiration. It is the sum of the VT, IRV, and ERV. 4000–5000 ml.
- **Residual volume (RV):** volume of gas in the lungs after a maximal expiratory effort. It normally comprises 20%–25% of the total lung capacity, or 25–30 ml/kg body weight, and increases with age. The RV is the smallest amount of gas possible in the lungs.

Lung capacities

These are determined by the size of the thorax and lungs, and consist of two or more volumes:

- **Functional residual capacity (FRC)**: volume of gas remaining in the lungs at the end of a normal expiration. This is around 3000–4000 ml and depends on the age, sex, height and weight of the subject. It is the sum of the RV and the ERV. Functional residual capacity represents the volume of gas remaining in the lungs that continues to take part in gas exchange, and is thus a measure of oxygen reserve.

  FRC = ERV + RV

- **Inspiratory capacity (IC)**: maximum volume of gas that can be inhaled after normal expiration. 3000–4000 ml.

- **Total lung capacity (TLC)** = IRV + ERV + VT + RV

  = volume of gas in the lungs after a maximal inspiration.

  The TLC is the largest possible volume of gas in the lungs.

- **Forced vital capacity (FVC)** is a vital capacity measurement taken as rapidly as possible. It evaluates the resistance properties of the airways and the strength of the expiratory muscles. The normal time required to exhale from a FVC to RV is less than 3 seconds. During a forced expiratory manoeuvre the volume of gas expired in the first second of expiration (FEV1) is usually 75% of the FVC (FEV1/FVC = 0.75). The peak expiratory flow rate occurs early in expiration, usually within the first 0.2 second, and is an index of both large airways resistance and of patient effort. It also depends on age, height and gender. The forced expiratory flow, defined as the slope of the expiratory flow between 25% and 75% of the FVC (FEV25–75), is effort independent and an index of small airways resistance. Forced vital capacity is equal to 50–60 ml/kg.

  Variability in the peak expiratory flow rate > 15%–20% daily or from day-to-day suggests obstruction. A fall in peak expiratory flow rate >15% following exercise is diagnostic of exercise-induced asthma. An increase in FEV1 > 20% with beta-adrenergic bronchodilator favours asthma over chronic obstructive airways disease.

  The values for lung volumes and capacities are generally expressed as percentages of the predicted value. For normally distributed values, 95% of the population values lie within two standard deviations of the mean.

Methods for the measurement of static lung volumes

- **Spirometry**: VC, VT, IC, ERV. A spirometer is a device for measuring the volume of air exhaled over time. It traditionally comprised an inverted air-filled bell with a water seal, connected to a pen writing on volume and time calibrated paper on a rotating drum. Flow transducer devices are currently used in spirometry. In these devices, the expired flow signal is electronically integrated with time to provide volume, and the expired volume signal is differentiated to provide flow. Hand-held models are now available.

Factors affecting the functional residual capacity

Body size
Sex
Age
Diaphragmatic muscle tone
Posture
Lung disease

- **Helium dilution**:
  Single breath hold: TLC
  Steady-state method: FRC
- **Constant-volume body plethysmograph** (body box): FRC. The body plethysmograph can measure the change in whole body volume during each respiratory cycle.

Methods for the measurement of functional residual capacity

Nitrogen wash-out by breathing 100% oxygen.
Wash-in of a tracer gas such as helium.
Body plethysmography, with seating of the subject within the box and recording of pressure changes in mouth and in the box of the plethysmograph while breathing against an occluded airway. The lung volume is proportional to the ratio of change of pressure within the box to the change of pressure within the lung (which is measured within the subject's mouth).

Flow–volume relationship

- This can be derived from spirometry. Spirometry is optimally performed in the standing or sitting position, with nasal clip occlusion to prevent air leaks. The performance of at least three tests with acceptable effort ensures the validity and reproducibility of the results obtained.
- Exhaled gas flow is plotted on the vertical or y-axis, and lung volume on the horizontal or x-axis. A continuous loop is formed, with inspiration below the line of zero flow and expiration above the line of zero flow.
- Gas flow is plotted as a function of lung volume during the performance of the FVC manoeuvre, i.e. maximal inspiration (from RV to TLC) followed by rapid forceful expiration back to RV. Forced vital capacity represents the volume between the RV and the TLC.

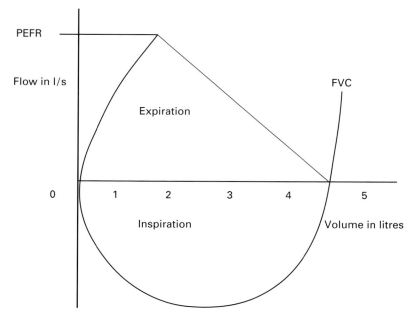

Figure 7.3 Flow–volume loop.

- The shape of the flow-volume loop depends on the properties of the airways, lung recoil and lung volume. The contours of the inspiratory and expiratory curves are different, demonstrating hysteresis (see p. 135).
- During forced expiration, there is an initial rapid increase of flow to a maximal or peak flow rate at a lung volume that is close to the TLC. Peak expiratory flow occurs at high lung volumes (about 70%–90% of the VC) and is effort dependent, with greater effort leading to greater flow. Peak expiratory flow records the greatest flow that can be sustained for 10 milliseconds on forced expiration, starting from full inflation of the lungs.
- With continued expiration, there is a reduction in lung volume, narrowing of the airways, increased resistance to flow and a progressive reduction in flow rate. The airflow rate is reduced linearly throughout this phase of expiration. This phase is effort independent, and depends on the elastic recoil of the lungs and the resistance of the airways distal to the point at which dynamic compression occurs. Air can be considered to be 'squeezed' out of the smaller airways in this phase.
- During forced expiration, the pleural pressure is greater than the intrathoracic tracheal pressure and the extrathoracic tracheal pressure is greater than atmospheric pressure.

- During forced inspiration, the extrathoracic tracheal pressure is less than atmospheric pressure and the pleural pressure is less than the intrathoracic tracheal pressure.
- The shape of the normal flow–volume loop can be likened to that of a triangle on a semicircle.
- Restrictive lung disease causes a proportionate reduction in flow rate and lung volume.
- Obstructive lung disease reduces flow rate but not lung volume. Extrathoracic airway obstruction reduces inspiratory flow, often causing the inspiratory limb of the flow–volume loop to become flat, while expiratory flow is unaltered. Intrathoracic airway obstruction reduces expiratory flow more than inspiratory flow.
- The flow–volume loop allows for the early detection of small airway disease. Oscillation of flow, giving a sawtooth pattern, can occur with irritability of the upper airway. This has been observed with upper airway stenosis, thermal injury to the airway, obstructive sleep apnoea and bulbar muscle weakness.

Flow–pressure relationship

- The term **compliance** refers to change in volume divided by change in pressure. It is a measure of the degree of distensibility of the lungs. It has a non-linear relationship with changing lung volume. Static compliance is determined from the ratio of the difference in lung volume at two different volume levels and the associated difference in intra-alveolar pressure. Dynamic compliance relates VT to intrathoracic pressures at the instants of zero airflow that occur at the end inspiratory and expiratory levels with each breath.
- The lung volume/pressure relationship forms characteristic counter-clockwise loops demonstrating **hysteresis**, i.e. the shape is different during inspiration and expiration. The term hysteresis denotes failure of a system to respond identically to the application and the withdrawal of a force. The presence of hysteresis denotes a proportionate energy loss for the system due to the resistive behaviour of the lungs.
- The width of the loop can be used as a quantitative measure of resistive behaviour. When divided by the rate of gas flow, it yields resistance.
- At low end-expiratory lung volumes hysteresis is mainly due to the opening and closing of airways. At high lung volumes, the primary source of hysteresis is surfactant, reducing the surface tension at the gas–liquid interface in the alveoli.
- Lung volume can be expressed as a proportion of the VC and pressure that the respiratory muscles must generate.

The static pressure–volume curve of the lung is obtained by the simultaneous measurement of airway opening pressure, lung volume and pleural pressure as estimated by a balloon in the lower one third of the oesophagus.

■ Lung function testing

- **Tests of ventilatory capacity**: FEV, forced expiratory flow (FEF); expiratory flow–volume curve; peak expiratory flow rate (PEFR).
- **Tests of gas exchange**: arterial blood gases; diffusing capacity for carbon monoxide (single breath; re-breathing; steady state or continuous breathing).
- **Static lung volumes**: VC; VT; IC; ERV; FRC; RV.
- **Lung elasticity: pressure–volume curve**. A stiffer lung has a more horizontal curve, as greater pressure is required to achieve the same inflation volume compared with normal lung.
- **Tests of uneven ventilation**: single breath nitrogen test; closing volume; multi-breath nitrogen washout; radioactive xenon scan.
  In patients with uneven ventilation, the nitrogen concentration rises in the alveolar plateau phase as poorly ventilated regions with relatively high nitrogen concentrations empty last. Normally the nitrogen concentration is almost flat in this phase.
- Airway resistance.
- Exercise tests.
- **Distribution of pulmonary blood flow**: perfusion scan; catheterisation.

Features of an obstructive pattern on lung function testing
Reduced FVC, FEV1, maximum voluntary ventilation (MVV), PEFR, FEF at 25%–75% lung volume
Reduced FEV1/FVC ratio ($< 80\%$)
TLC normal or increased
FRC normal or increased
Normal or increased residual volume and RV/TLC ratio (normally 20%)

Features of a restrictive pattern on lung function testing
Reduced FVC, FEV1
Normal or increased FEV1/FVC ratio
Reduced TLC
Normal or reduced RV
Normal or reduced FRC
Reduced compliance

- **Small airway function**: frequency dependence of dynamic compliance; closing volume.

Causes of arterial hypoxia

Reduced alveolar pO_2

Low inspired pO_2: e.g. high altitude or low administered oxygen concentrations.
Reduced ventilation (associated with raised $paCO_2$).

Increased alveolar-arterial pO_2 difference

Right to left intracardiac or intrapulmonary shunt.

Alveolar-capillary diffusion block: alveolar space filling with fluid, or alveolar collapse.

Ventilation-perfusion mismatch, brought about by some perfusion of non-ventilated alveoli (insufficient gas exchange) or by the ventilation of non-perfused alveoli (wasted ventilation).

Increasing the ambient oxygen concentration corrects hypoxia due to reduced alveolar ventilation, or due to impaired alveolar-capillary diffusion, but has no effect in the presence of right-to-left shunting.

Normally there is an **alveolar-arterial pO_2 difference** of about 10–15 mm Hg. This is produced, under physiological circumstances, by:

- Venous admixture, produced by the drainage of desaturated blood from the bronchial circulation into the pulmonary veins, and the drainage of coronary venous blood into the left ventricle by the thebesian veins. This represents blood that has bypassed the gas exchange zone.
- Ventilation/perfusion gradients from the bases to the apices of the lungs, leading to the admixture of relatively less oxygenated blood from the bases with better oxygenated blood from the apices.

The alveolar-arterial pO_2 difference $= PAO_2 - PaO_2$

where, by the alveolar gas equation, $PAO_2 = FiO_2 - (PaCO_2/0.8)$

Rectangular hyperbolas relating alveolar gas concentrations to alveolar ventilation all obey the following general rules:

The vertical asymptote is zero alveolar ventilation;

The horizontal asymptote is the inspired concentration of the gas under consideration;

The curve is concave upwards for gases being eliminated from the body and concave downwards for gas being taken up into the body;

The curves move away from the intersection of the asymptotes as the volume of the gas being exchanged increases.

Causes of falsely low saturation readings

Poor peripheral perfusion
Skin pigmentation
Nail polish
Intravascular dye, e.g. methylene blue
Hyperlipidaemia

Causes of falsely high saturation readings
Hypothermia
Carbon monoxide poisoning
Hyperbilirubinaemia

Pulse oximetry

This is based on:

The presence of an arterial pulsatile signal;

The different absorption spectra of oxyhaemoglobin and reduced haemoglobin;

Oxyhaemoglobin absorbs more infrared light and less red light than reduced haemoglobin.

Method

Two light emitting diodes emit light at 660 nm (red) and 940 nm (infrared) wavelengths. The no-light waveform is subtracted from the red and infrared waveforms to correct for the presence of background light. The red and infrared light absorption waveforms are normalised by division of their pulsatile components by their constant components.

The relative amplitudes of the normalised pulsatile components is compared with an empirically derived calibration curve to estimate the arterial oxygen saturation. The saturation obtained is a time-weighted average of the calculated saturation.

A co-oximeter is required in the presence of dyshaemoglobins, e.g. carboxy-haemoglobin, which has a similar absorption spectrum to oxyhaemoglobin.

Saturation is of little value in the differentiation of high but safe oxygen tensions from those that are associated with a risk of oxygen toxicity.

BIBLIOGRAPHY

Haefeli-Bleuer, B. & Weibel, E. R. Morphology of the human pulmonary acinus. *Anat. Rec.*, **220** (1988), 410–14.

Levitzky, M. G. *Pulmonary Physiology*, 6th edn. New York: The McGraw-Hill Companies, Inc., 2003.

West, J. B. Regional differences in gas exchange in the lung of erect man. *J. Appl. Physiol.*, **17** (1963), 893–8.

   Respiratory Physiology. The Essentials. Baltimore: Lippincott, Williams & Wilkins, 2005.

Woolcock, A. J., Vincent, N. J. & Macklem, P. T. Frequency dependence of compliance as a test for obstruction in the small airways. *J. Clin. Invest.*, **48** (1969), 1097–106.

8

Blood

■ Introduction

Blood is a suspension of cellular elements in an aqueous solution. Forty-five per cent of this volume comprises cellular elements (the haematocrit), the remainder being plasma. About 8% of the plasma volume consists of solutes, the remainder being water.

■ Plasma proteins

Most plasma proteins are synthesised in the liver. They are generally synthesised as pre-protein on membrane-bound polyribosomes and initially contain amino-terminal signal peptides. Almost all are glycoproteins. Many exhibit polymorphism. They are mainly anions. Each plasma protein has a characteristic half-life in the circulation.

Functions of plasma proteins

- Maintenance of colloid osmotic pressure, of about 25 mm Hg across capillary wall, and thereby control of extracellular fluid volume. This is mainly due to

Cellular composition of human blood		
Red blood cells	4 500 000–5 000 000/cu mm	
Platelets	150 000–400 000/cu mm	
White blood cells	5000–10 000/cu mm	
Neutrophils	63.5%	
Lymphocytes	30.0%	
Monocytes	4.0%	
Eosinophils	2.0%	
Basophils	0.5%	

albumin. Human albumin is a single chain polypeptide of 584 amino acids, with 17 disulphide bonds. The plasma half-life is around 20 days.

- Carrier proteins for lipids, hormones, drugs and excretory products (transport functions). Albumin, in particular, binds a range of physiologically important ligands, including various hydrophobic molecules and metal ions.
- Defence reactions: immunoglobulins, complement system.
- Buffering of hydrogen ions. Plasma proteins provide about 15% of the total buffering capacity of the blood.
- Coagulation (haemostasis) and fibrinolysis.
- Specialised functions: protease inhibitors, haemoglobin binding, renin–angiotensin system, lipoprotein metabolism.

The plasma proteins can be considered to include five **interactive systems**:

Coagulation proteins
Fibrinolytic enzymes
The complement system
The kinins
Inhibitors to the preceding four systems

Electrophoresis

Electrophoretic separation of plasma proteins yields the following fractions:

Albumin
Alpha 1-globulins   alpha 1-antitrypsin
                     alpha 1-acid glycoprotein
Alpha 2-globulins   alpha 2-macroglobulin

Functions of transport proteins

Pre-albumin	Retinol, thyroxine (T4), triiodothyronine (T3)
Albumin	Inorganic plasma constituents (e.g. calcium)
	Free fatty acids
	Hormones
	Excretory products
	Drugs
Hormone-binding proteins	Corticosteroids: cortisol-binding globulin
	Sex hormones: sex-hormone-binding globulin
	Thyroid hormones: thyroxine-binding globulin
Metal-binding proteins	Copper (caeruloplasmin)
	Iron (transferrin)
Apolipoproteins	Lipids

Protease inhibitors of human plasma

Antithrombin III (ATIII) (heparin cofactor)
Heparin cofactor II
Alpha 2-macroglobulin
Alpha 1-antitrypsin
Alpha 2-antiplasmin (alpha 2-plasmin inhibitor)
C1-inactivator (C1-esterase inhibitor)
Extrinsic pathway (tissue factor pathway) inhibitor
Activated protein C inhibitor

	haptoglobin
	caeruloplasmin
Beta globulins	transferrin
	low density lipoprotein
	C3 fraction of complement
Gamma globulins	immunoglobulins

Acute phase reactants

The levels of certain plasma proteins increase during acute inflammatory states or secondary to certain types of tissue damage. Acute phase reactants are serum proteins that are produced by hepatocytes in the liver in response to pro-inflammatory cytokines (tumour necrosis factor-alpha, interleukin-1 and interleukin-6). Their synthesis constitutes a normal response to tissue inflammation or injury. These reactants help in minimising local tissue damage and participate in tissue repair, as well as aiding microbial killing. They include:

C-reactive protein: binds bacterial, fungal and parasitic polysaccharides and peptidopolysaccharides; activates complement; acts as opsonin to facilitate phagocytosis

Anti-protease inhibitors: alpha 1-antitrypsin

Caeruloplasmin

Alpha 1-acid glycoprotein

Fibrinogen

Haptoglobin

Serum amyloid A

Complement proteins

Metallothionein.

The acute phase response allows the detection, diagnosis and therapeutic monitoring of diseases that involve tissue damage and inflammation.

Causes of an acute phase response

These include:

Bacterial infections

Rheumatic diseases: rheumatoid arthritis; seronegative spondarthritis

Vasculitis

Crohn's disease

Trauma including burns and surgery

Malignancy

Cytokines

Cytokines are a group of soluble, low molecular weight glycoproteins, which are involved in cell proliferation, immunity and inflammation. They regulate both the amplitude and duration of the systemic inflammatory response, and may be either pro-inflammatory or anti-inflammatory. They may act on cells in a paracrine and autocrine manner. The systemic inflammatory response syndrome appears to result from excessive, inappropriate and/or prolonged release of cytokines into the systemic circulation. They are synthesised *de novo* and released in response to tissue damage.

Classification of cytokines

Interleukins: IL-1 to IL-13;

Interferons: alpha-interferon, beta-interferon, gamma-interferon;

Colony-stimulating factors: macrophage-colony stimulating factor (M-CSF), granulocyte-macrophage-colony stimulating factor (GM-CSF), granulocyte-colony stimulating factor (G-CTF).

Plasma lipoproteins

These include:

Chylomicrons: dietary triglyceride transport.

Very low density lipoproteins (VLDL): endogenous triglyceride transport to adipose tissue.

Intermediate density lipoproteins (VLDL remnants).

Low density lipoproteins (LDL): contain a high concentration of cholesterol and cholesterol esters and are involved in the transport of dietary and endogenous cholesterol. Cholesterol is delivered from the liver to peripheral tissues, especially adipose tissue and the adrenal glands, and also returned to the liver.

High density lipoproteins (HDL): HDL2 and HDL3: involved in the return of cholesterol from peripheral tissues to the liver (reverse transport).

Enzymes involved in lipid transport

Lecithin cholesterol acyltransferase (LCAT)
Lipoprotein lipase
Hepatic lipase
Mobilising lipase

Lipoproteins consist of a core of hydrophobic non-polar triacylglycerol, surrounded by a shell of polar lipids (phospholipids and cholesterol), in turn surrounded by a shell of protein, which together constitute a hydrophilic complex. Apolipoproteins, the protein components of the lipoproteins, are named ApoA, ApoB, ApoC and ApoE. The density of lipoproteins is inversely proportional to their lipid/protein ratio.

The low density lipoprotein supergene family of receptors

These possess four major structural characteristics:

Cysteine-rich C-type repeats;

Epidermal growth factor precursor-like repeats;

A cytoplasmic domain;

A transmembrane domain.

The low density lipoprotein receptor is an 839 amino acid transmembrane protein. It includes an N-terminal extracellular domain which binds apoB-100, and a C-terminal cytosolic domain that binds adapter proteins involved in modulation of clathrin coat formation (receptor-mediated endocytosis).

Normal lipoprotein metabolism

This involves three major pathways mediating:

The transport of exogenous dietary triglyceride and cholesterol;

The transport of endogenous triglyceride and cholesterol synthesised in the liver;

Reverse cholesterol transport, i.e. transfer back from peripheral tissues to the liver, in which HDL plays a major role.

■ Haemoglobin

Structure of haemoglobin

Haemoglobin consists of four polypeptide chains, two alpha chains of 141 amino acid residues each and two beta chains of 146 amino acid residues each. Each chain harbours one haem, a cyclic tetrapyrrole. A single polypeptide chain combined with a single haem is called a subunit of haemoglobin or monomer of the molecule. In the complete molecule the four subunits are closely joined by hydrogen bonding to form a tetramer. Functions of haem proteins include oxygen binding, oxygen transport and electron transport.

Each polypeptide chain is divided into helical and non-helical areas. The helical areas are designated A to H. Amino acids can be designated by number or according to helical region. Each haem consists of protoporphyrin IX, with four nitrogen atoms co-ordinated to a ferrous ion, Fe^{2+}. The Fe^{2+} is also co-ordinated to a nitrogen atom in a histidine residue of the globin part of the molecule. Oxygen binding causes alterations in the plane of the Fe^{2+}, triggering a sequence of intermolecular rearrangements that are transmitted to the other subunits.

Haemoglobin is structurally adapted to bind strongly to oxygen in the lungs and to release it in oxygen depleted tissues. It can also transport some carbon dioxide back to the lungs for release.

Determinants of oxygen-carrying capacity of blood

Partial pressure (kPa) of oxygen: pO_2.
Haemoglobin concentration. Each gram of haemoglobin can combine with 1.34 ml of oxygen. One millimole of haemoglobin (64.5 grams) can carry up to 4 milllimole of oxygen if all binding sites are occupied, i.e. if haemoglobin is fully saturated.
Oxygen saturation of haemoglobin present: p50.
Tissue oxygen delivery depends on:
   Blood oxygen content, which is determined by:
      PO_2
      Haemoglobin level
      Haemoglobin function
   Blood flow, which is determined by:
      Cardiac output
      Peripheral perfusion

Oxyhaemoglobin dissociation curve

The curve consists of an X axis representing the percentage saturation of haemo-globin and a Y axis representing pO_2. The sigmoid shape of the curve comprises:
   The **loading region**: oxygen-free molecules (deoxyhaemoglobin) are reluctant to take up the first oxygen molecule but their appetite for oxygen grows with the eating (Perutz).

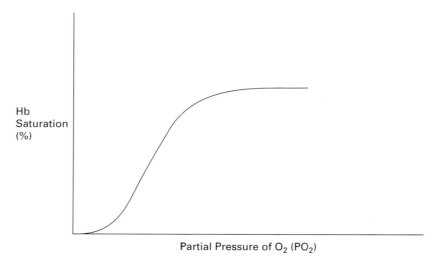

Figure 8.1 Oxyhaemoglobin dissociation curve. (Hb, haemoglobin.)

The **flat region** or plateau is observed above pO_2 of about 10 kPa.

The non-linearity of the dissociation curve allows optimisation of maximum oxygen diffusion in the lungs. Maximum arterial oxygen saturation is associated with maintenance of a nearly constant paO_2 despite fluctuations in alveolar O_2 tension. This provides a margin of safety as a fall in paO_2 does not result in profound desaturation.

The unloading region.

The steep portion of the curve below a pO_2 of about 10 kPa. Small falls in pO_2 cause a large transfer of O_2 to the tissues. This allows ready release of oxygen if the tissue oxygen consumption increases.

The more pronounced the sigmoid shape of the equilibrium curve the greater the fraction of oxygen in the red cells that can be unloaded to the tissues. The sigmoid curve favours oxygen transport, allowing the saturation of haemoglobin in the lungs and deoxygenation in the capillaries.

Characteristics of oxygen binding by haemoglobin

- It is determined primarily by local oxygen tension (paO_2).
- It is affected by local tissue conditions (pH, temperature) and local concentrations of substances (2,3-diphosphoglycerate; 2,3-DPG).
- It produces an allosteric change in haemoglobin structure to a 'relaxed' form. In the absence of an allosteric effect a hyperbolic binding curve would result.

- It is 'co-operative', i.e. binding oxygen at each site promotes binding at the remaining sites due to allosteric changes. An allosteric protein is one in which binding of a ligand to one site affects the binding properties of another site on the same protein. Haem–haem interaction and the interplay between oxygen and the other four ligands are known collectively as the co-operative effects of haemoglobin.
- Deoxygenation of haemoglobin increases affinity of several proton-binding sites on its molecule.

Co-operativity

This implies that:

Binding sites exist for more than one ligand.

Binding of each ligand facilitates binding of successive ligands.

With partial saturation of haemoglobin with oxygen, the affinity of the remaining haems on the tetramer for oxygen increases markedly. This is because alpha 1 beta 2 interface destabilisation causes the transition of the quaternary structure from the T (tense or taut form) to the R (relaxed) state.

Oxygen has significantly higher affinity for haemoglobin in the R state.

Oxygen binding stabilises the T state.

Oxyhaemoglobin and deoxyhaemoglobin differ markedly in quaternary structure. The **Perutz mechanism** is a description of the dynamic behaviour of haemoglobin based largely on the static structure of its R and T end states. The quaternary structure of deoxyhaemoglobin is the T form, with low affinity for oxygen; that of oxyhaemoglobin the R form, with high affinity. Changes in conformation of Fe^{2+} trigger a sequence of intermolecular rearrangements. The contacts between the haemoglobin subunits are described as the $\alpha 1\beta 2$ and the $\alpha 1\beta 1$ regions. The $\alpha 1\beta 1$ contact change is slight. The $\alpha 1\beta 2$ contact region is designed to act as a switch between two alternative structures. When oxygen is absent experimentally, the T state is more stable and is thus the predominant configuration of deoxyhaemoglobin.

The T to R transition is triggered by changes in the positions of key amino acid side chains surrounding the haem. The T state is stabilised by a network of C-terminal salt bridges that must break to form the R state.

The allosteric properties of haemoglobin arise from interactions between its subunits. Allosteric theory explains haem–haem interaction without postulating any direct communication between the haem groups. The functional unit of haemoglobin is a tetramer consisting of two kinds of polypeptide chains. A structural change (oxygenation) within a subunit is translated into structural changes at the interfaces between subunits. Binding of oxygen at one haem site is thereby communicated to parts of the molecule that are far away.

Shift of the HbO$_2$ dissociation curve to the right implies increased tissue oxygen delivery, reduced oxygen affinity of haemoglobin (fall in P50) and a more sigmoid shape. P50 is the pCO$_2$ at which haemoglobin is 50% saturated with oxygen under standard conditions of temperature and pH.

Causes of shift to the right:

Carbon dioxide with increase in H$^+$

Hydrogen ions-protons (Bohr shift), associated with a fall in pH (acute acidosis). Haemoglobin binds one H$^+$ for every two oxygen molecules released. This favours the conversion of carbon dioxide into the bicarbonate ion promoting its transport back to the lungs.

2,3-Diphosphoglycerate (depletion of intracellular 2,3-DPG in stored blood may impair tissue oxygen delivery with transfusion).

Rise in intracellular pH.

Increased temperature.

Causes of shift to the left (increased P50):

Reduction in temperature.

Increased oxygen tension: Haldane effect.

Reduced H$^+$ and paCO$_2$: rise in pH and fall in paCO$_2$.

Increased CO tension: carbon monoxide has 150 times the affinity of oxygen for the haem iron.

Fetal haemoglobin: binds oxygen more strongly than maternal haemoglobin. The difficulty in oxygen release is compensated for by higher haemoglobin concentrations in the fetus.

Carboxyhaemoglobin.

Methaemoglobin.

Fall in 2,3-DPG.

Fall in intracellular adenosine triphosphate (ATP).

2,3-Diphosphoglycerate

2,3-Diphosphoglycerate is a negative allosteric heterotropic effector of oxygen binding to haemoglobin. It modulates the oxygen affinity of haemoglobin, binding tightly to the deoxygenated form (T state) of the molecule, but poorly to the oxygenated or other ligand-bound forms. Binding occurs stereo-specifically within the central cavity of the haemoglobin tetramer. It stabilises deoxyhaemoglobin, favouring oxygen release. Each red blood cell contains 15 μmol/g 2,3-DPG (molar ratio of 1:1 with haemoglobin). A polyanion, it forms 15% of the anionic content of red blood cell. One mole of 2,3-DPG binds to one mole of deoxyhaemoglobin. It is bound between the two beta subunits by ionic salt bridges.

The rate of synthesis is controlled by the concentrations of unbound 1,3-DPG and 2,3-DPG (**Rapoport–Luebering shuttle**)

Chronic hypoxia

Prolonged exercise

Enzyme abnormalities of the red cells

Molecular pathology of haemoglobin

Sickle syndromes, due to single amino acid mutations in the beta chain;

Thalassaemias, due to defects in synthesis of one or more globin polypeptide chain(s) leading to absent synthesis of the chain(s);

High oxygen affinity haemoglobins associated with erythrocytosis;

Low oxygen affinity haemoglobins associated with cyanosis;

M haemoglobins associated with pseudo-cyanosis;

Unstable haemoglobins associated with haemolytic anaemia;

Dyshaemoglobins: sulphaemoglobinaemia and methaemoglobinaemia;

Compound haemoglobinopathies.

Red blood cell defences against excess methaemoglobin formation

Reducing substances in the red cells: ascorbic acid; glutathione.

Binding of haem to the apoprotein creates a protective environment for the iron.

Enzyme methaemoglobin reductase reduces methaemoglobin back to normal haemoglobin, using nicotinamide adenine dinucleotide (NAD) H as a reductant.

Erythropoietin

Erythropoietin is a 165 amino acid polypeptide with a molecular weight of 34 kDa. Heavy glycosylation leads to a 40% carbohydrate content. Ninety per cent is synthesised in the adult by peritubular capillary endothelial cells in the kidneys, and the remainder by centrilobular hepatocytes. In infants the hepatocyte is the primary site of synthesis. The kidneys become the primary site of synthesis shortly after birth. The normal serum level ranges from 5 to 25 μg/ml. The plasma half-life is around 3 to 8 hours.

Erythropoietin is produced by the action of an enzyme secreted by the kidney, erythrogenin, on a plasma alpha-globulin produced in the liver. Production is

Mechanisms of carbon dioxide transport in blood

Dissolved carbon dioxide: 5%

Carbonic acid

Bicarbonate ions

Carbamino compounds: 5% (CO_2 combined with terminal NH_3 groups on protein side chains)

Effects of altitude acclimatisation

Hyperventilation, initiated by the stimulation of peripheral chemoreceptors;

Polycythaemia;

Shift to right of oxygen dissociation curve with better unloading of oxygen in venous blood at a given pO_2 (increased 2,3-DPG concentration);

Increased peripheral muscle capillary concentration;

Increased maximum breathing capacity;

Pulmonary vasoconstriction (pulmonary hypertension; high altitude pulmonary oedema);

Exercise tolerance.

stimulated by a reduced oxygen content in the renal arterial circulation. Increased serum levels are seen in states of chronic tissue hypoxia, including anaemia, cyanotic heart disease and lung disease. Deficiency of erythropoietin is the principal cause of anaemia associated with chronic renal failure, and recombinant human erythropoietin is used for the treatment of anaemia in this situation.

Erythropoietin acts mainly on the early phases of cell division in the bone marrow. Circulating erythropoietin binds to high affinity erythropoietin receptors on the surface of erythroid progenitors resulting in replication and maturation to functional red blood cells.

■ Iron metabolism

Iron metabolism involves a balance between dietary intake, absorption, transportation, storage, recycling and excretion. The total body iron content in an adult ranges between 4 and 5 grams, mainly in haemoglobin of red blood cells. The liver is the major site of storage. Three milligrams of the total body iron circulates in the plasma in an exchangeable pool, bound to transferrin. The average losses, mainly from epithelial desquamation, amount to about 1 mg per day in the adult, with around 1.5–2 mg per day in the menstruating female.

Enzymes containing iron

Cytochromes a,b,c, P450
Cytochrome c oxidase
Succinate dehydrogenase
Catalase
Myeloperoxidase
Monoamine oxidase
Xanthine oxidase
NADH dehydrogenase
Ribonucleotide reductase
Tryptophan pyrrolase

Functions of iron

It is a component of several enzymes involved in critically important cellular reactions;

It constitutes the functional group for oxygen binding by haemoglobin and myoglobin;

It is a carrier for electrons;

The ability to reversibly cycle between the ferrous and ferric states makes it important in oxidation reactions;

In excess, ionic iron contributes to toxic free radical generation.

Iron absorption

This occurs in the duodenum and proximal jejunum and depends on:

The dietary iron content;

Bioavailability of the dietary iron;

Absorption by mucosal cells, which depends on the extent of the body iron stores and the erythropoietic activity of the bone marrow.

About 10% of the normal dietary intake of 10–20 mg of dietary iron is absorbed daily. Ferric iron is converted in the presence of gastric acid by ferric reductase in the duodenal brush border to ferrous iron. Absorption is facilitated by the divalent metal transporter 1 protein, which transports ferrous iron from the gut lumen over the apical border of the enterocyte. After an oral iron load, down-regulation of iron absorption (**mucosal block**) by the enterocytes ensues. This is presumably created by intracellular iron accumulation in the enterocyte, and operates even in the presence of systemic iron deficiency states.

Factors affecting the **bioavailability** of iron include:

Evaluation for iron deficiency anaemia

- Peripheral blood smear, which shows microcytic hypochromic red cells;
- Reduced serum ferritin;
- Reduced serum iron;
- Increased serum iron-binding capacity;
- Reduced serum iron saturation;
- Serum transferrin receptor levels;
- Raised red cell protoporphyrin;
- Therapeutic response to oral iron;
- Bone marrow aspiration showing reduced or absent stainable iron and delayed cytoplasmic maturation.

Evaluation of body iron stores

Lowered stores
Serum ferritin
Serum iron-binding capacity

Increased stores
Serum ferritin
Liver biopsy
Dual energy computed tomography; magnetic resonance imaging
Urine iron excretion after administration of chelating agents

The intra-luminal pH of the duodenum;

Chelation with ascorbate or citrate, which facilitates absorption;

The presence of plant phytates and tannins, which reduce the availability of iron.

Iron distribution is achieved by **transferrin**, the major iron transporting protein in the serum and the extracellular fluid. Transferrin is a single chain glycoprotein with two similar iron-binding sites. It is predominantly synthesised in the liver and has a half-life of 8 days. The high iron affinity of transferrin protects the body from free iron. The iron–transferrin complex is attached to high affinity cell surface transferrin receptors in the liver and in developing red blood cells in the bone marrow. The ensuing complex is internalised into clathrin-coated endosomes. An ATP-dependent proton pump lowers the endosomal pH to less than 6, when transferrin divests itself of its attached iron and exits the endosomal membrane in a process mediated by divalent metal transporter 1 and an endosomal oxido-reductase. The transferrin molecule is recycled to the cell surface and released back into the circulation.

Iron is stored as ferritin and haemosiderin.

■ Blood cells

Stem cells

Stem cells are the precursor of all blood cells as well as of further stem cells. They comprise about 1 in 10 000 of cells in the bone marrow. They possess the properties of lacking specialised function yet being able to transform to specialised cells, self-renewal over long periods of time and pluripotentiality (the ability to develop into many different cell types).

Pluripotential haematopoietic stem cells maintain haematopoiesis by clonal proliferation. Stem cells express CD34, a surface protein.

Red blood cells

Features

Each red cell is a non-nucleated biconcave disc $7.5 \times 2 \, \mu m$. This shape maximises the surface area/volume ratio, allowing more effective gas exchange. The discs are also deformable, allowing passage through small blood vessels such as capillaries.

There are a total of about 3×10^{13} cells in the body, containing 1 kg of haemoglobin. The average lifespan of a red blood cell is 120 days. Normal development takes 7–10 days. It comprises 90% haemoglobin by dry weight. Red cells are derived from reticulocytes, which are also non-nucleated, but possess ribosomes for globin synthesis, and mitochondria to allow oxidative metabolism and haem synthesis. They mature in 24–48 hours to red cells.

The red cell uses anaerobic metabolism as an energy source. It does not possess any mitochondria or ribosomes. Glucose is metabolised anaerobically primarily by glycolysis (Embden–Meyerhof pathway) and secondarily by the pentose phosphate pathway (hexose monophosphate shunt). The glycolytic pathway converts 90%–95% of the glucose metabolised in red cells to lactate. This generates one mole of ATP per mole of glucose metabolised. Five per cent to ten per cent of glucose is metabolised by the pentose phosphate pathway, generating one mole of nicotinamide adenine dinucleotide phosphate dehydrogenase (NADPH) for each mole of glucose metabolised. This is a cofactor for glutathione reductase, which maintains glutathione in the reduced state to protect against the toxic effects of free oxygen radicals, which are generated by intracellular haem oxidation.

The functions of red cells consist of oxygen transport, carbon dioxide transport and regulation of extracellular fluid pH.

ATP is used by the red cell for:

The provision of energy for Na^+/K^+ -ATPase (sodium pump) and Ca^{2+}-ATPase (calcium pump);

Protein phosphorylation;

The maintenance of cell shape;

Reduction of the oxygen affinity of haemoglobin.

Red cell membrane

The **red cell membrane** is composed of:

Lipids:

Phospholipids: phosphatidylcholine; phosphatidylethanolamine; sphingo-myelin; phosphatidylserine)

Cholesterol

Proteins:

Integral membrane proteins:

Band 3 or anion exchange protein

Glucose transporter GLUT 1

Glycophorins, which have a high sialic acid content

Cytoskeletal proteins (which form a dense two-dimensional fibrous network):

Spectrin protein family: alpha and beta spectrins; spectrin deficiency is a hallmark of red cells in hereditary spherocytosis

Ankyrin

Short filaments of F-actin

Proteins 4.1, 4.2 and 4.9

p55

Adducins

White blood cells

White blood cells can be classified as:

Granulocytes:

Neutrophils: 12–15 μm in diameter; nucleus with clumped chromatin and 2–5 lobes; drumstick in normal females; acidophilic cytoplasm. A right shift refers to an increase in lobe count.

Eosinophils: 12–17 μm in diameter; nucleus with 2–3 lobes; spherical granules; weakly basophilic cytoplasm. They are phagocytic cells with a special affinity for antigen–antibody complexes. The granules contain four cationic proteins: eosinophilic cationic protein, major basic protein, eosinophil derived neurotoxin and eosinophil peroxidase.

Basophils: 10–14 µm in diameter; purple black granules.

Mononuclear cells:

Lymphocytes: small: 10–12 µm in diameter; large: 12–16 µm in diameter.

Monocytes.

Functions of white blood cells

These depend on the cell type:

- Neutrophils phagocytose bacteria, fungi, protozoa, viruses, foreign cells, tumour cells and toxins. Chemotaxis occurs in response to activated complement proteins, cytokines and microbial products.
- Eosinophils phagocytose antigen–antibody complexes and larval forms of helminthic parasites. They inactivate mediators of anaphylaxis.
- Basophils possess IgE receptors and release mediators from granules in inflammatory and allergic reactions.
- Lymphocytes.

  B lymphocytes synthesise antibodies (immunoglobulins), contributing to humoral immunity. In response to a specific antigen they give rise to a monoclonal proliferation of plasma cells, which produce specific antibodies. T lymphocytes, which comprise 65%–80% of circulating lymphocytes, are responsible for cell-mediated immunity. They mediate the cell-mediated response to intracellular parasites, viruses, bacteria and fungi; delayed hypersensitivity; graft-versus-host reactions; and organ transplant rejection. They include subpopulations, which can be distinguished by cell surface markers.

  Helper (CD4 marker): enhance antibody production by B cells and stimulate the activity of other T cells.

  Cytotoxic (CD8 marker): kill virus infected and tumour cells, based on previous experience.

  Suppressor: block helper T cells.

- Monocytes are phagocytic and become macrophages in the tissues.

Macrophages occur in the following locations:

Connective tissues: histiocytes

Liver: Kupffer cells

Lungs: alveolar macrophages

Lymph nodes: free and fixed macrophages

Spleen: free and fixed macrophages

Bone marrow: fixed macrophages

Skin: Langerhans cells; histiocytes

Serous fluids: pleural and peritoneal macrophages

Blood groups

Blood group antigens are polymorphic, genetically inherited, structural characteristics of the outer surface of the red cell membrane.

The red cell phenotype depends on two classes of antigens:

- Carbohydrate moieties attached to membrane proteins or lipids (glycoproteins or glycolipids): e.g., ABO, Lewis and P systems. The A and B antigens are defined by a terminal sugar attached to a carbohydrate chain in membrane glycolipids and glycoproteins. A, B and H antigens may also be found in secretions such as saliva in secretors.
- Membrane proteins, e.g. Rhesus(Rh), Duffy, Kell, Kidd, MNSs systems. The Rh blood group system comprises 45 antigens, of which 5 are routinely identified, D, C, c, E and e.

The clinical importance of antigens depends on the degree of antigenicity, the frequency of occurrence of the antigen in the population and the activity of antibodies to the antigen at $37°$ C.

Blood transfusion principles

The recipient plasma must not contain antibodies corresponding to donor A and/or B antigens.

Rhesus D positive individuals may receive either RhD positive or RhD negative red cells.

Rhesus D negative individuals should only receive RhD negative red cells.

Table 8.1 ABO blood groups

Blood type	Genotype	Antigens (agglutinogens)	Antibodies (agglutinins)
O	OO	none	anti-A, anti-B
A	OA, AA	A	anti-B
B	OB, BB	B	anti-A
AB	AB	A, B	none

Blood components used for transfusion

Whole blood
Packed red blood cells
  Leukocyte added
  Adenine-saline added
Fresh frozen plasma
Cryoprecipitate: the portion of plasma remaining insoluble after thawing
Cryosupernatant
Platelet concentrates
Granulocytes
Platelet-rich plasma
Platelet-poor plasma

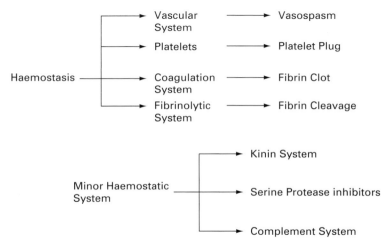

Figure 8.2 Components of haemostasis.

■ Haemostasis

Normal haemostasis is a balance between the simultaneous, opposing processes of clot formation and fibrinolysis. For a clot to form normally, there must be functioning vascular endothelium, platelets with adequate number and function, and sufficient plasma coagulation factors. Primary haemostasis refers to the formation of the platelet plug, a process that occurs within 1–3 minutes of injury. This involves platelet activation, platelet–vessel wall and platelet–platelet interaction. Secondary haemostasis refers to the action of the coagulation cascade to form clot. Normally haemostasis involves a sequence of vasoconstriction, platelet aggregation (adhesion, activation and aggregation) and blood coagulation.

Pathophysiology of haemostatic defects

Thrombocytopenia
Functional platelet abnormalities
Blood vessel defect
Coagulation factor(s) defect
Excessive fibrinolysis
Combined defect

Screening tests for bleeding tendency

Platelet disorders
Bleeding time (Ivy technique; Duke technique)
Platelet count (150–300 000/cu.mm)
Fresh blood film inspection

Vascular disorders
Bleeding time
Tourniquet test (Hess)

Coagulation disorders
Prothrombin time and international normalised ratio: extrinsic pathway
Activated partial thromboplastin time: intrinsic pathway
Thrombin time
Fibrinogen assay

Viscoelastic devices
Thromboelastography
Sonoclot

■ Platelets

Features

Platelets are derived from megakaryocytes in the bone marrow.

Thrombopoietin is the major regulatory protein for platelet production. They are discoid anucleate cells 2–3 μm in diameter. The surface is flat, with numerous pit-like openings that lead to an internal anastomosing system of membrane-bound tubes (canalicular system) continuous with the plasma membrane. The canalicular system serves as a reservoir of plasma membrane and membrane receptors, and as a conduit for the release of the contents of intracellular cytoplasmic granules after activation.

Platelet microanatomy

The following zones are recognised:

Peripheral zone
  Exterior coat or glycocalyx
  Unit plasma membrane
  System of filaments
  Open canalicular system

Sol-gel zone
  Submembrane fibres
  Dense tubular system
  Microtubules
  Microfilaments

Organelle zone
  Mitochondria
  Lysosomes
  Peroxisomes
  Alpha-granules
  Dense bodies

Membrane zone
  Surface-connected open canalicular system
  Dense tubular system
The contractile apparatus of the platelet is responsible for filopodium and lamellipodium formation, secretion and clot retraction.

The circulating blood level ranges from 150 000–400 000/cu.mm. About 2/3rds of the platelet mass circulates in the plasma and the other 1/3rd is sequestered within the spleen. The circulating platelet is inactive. Under normal circumstances it does not interact with other cells during its normal survival of 9–10 days. The turnover rate is around 10% per day.

Normal platelet function comprises adherence and aggregation, release of procoagulant factors and provision of phospholipid surface for the assembly of enzyme complexes.

Platelet granule types

There are three types of granules in platelets, which are listed below along with their constituents:

Alpha
  Coagulation proteins: factor V; fibrinogen; von Willebrand factor
  Growth factors: platelet-derived growth factor

Platelet modulators: platelet factors 1–7; beta-thromboglobulin

Adhesive proteins: thrombospondin; fibronectin; P-selectin

Dense body granules

Divalent cations: Ca^{2+}; Mg^{2+}

Adenine nucleotides: ADP; ATP

Platelet modulators: bioactive amines; serotonin

Lysosomes

Acid hydrolases

Platelet glycoprotein receptors

Receptor	Ligand
Ia/ IIa	Collagen
Ib	Thrombin
Ib/Ix/ V	von Willebrand factor
IIb/IIIa	Fibrinogen, von Willebrand factor
IV	Thrombospondin

Platelet factors

Coagulation factor V

Thromboplastic material

Platelet thromboplastin

Anti-heparin factor

Fibrinogen coagulant factor

Anti-fibrinolytic factor

Platelet co-thromboplastin

Physiological agents acting on platelets

Platelet activating agents can be classified as:

Indirect: collagen

Direct: thrombin; adrenaline; ADP; thromboxane A2

Physiological inhibitors of platelet activation include:

PGI2-prostacyclin

Nitric oxide

Endothelial cell ecto-ADPase(s)

Adenosine

Inhibitors of thrombin generation and thrombin action

Haemostatic role of platelets

The role of platelets in haemostasis involves the following steps:

- Adherence: platelets adhere to the exposed subendothelial matrix (the components of which include collagen, fibronectin and von Willebrand factor) through an interaction between the glycoprotein Ib-IX-V complex on their surface and von Willebrand factor in the subendothelium. This is aided by high fluid shear stresses within the lumen secondary to vascular constriction.
- Other adhesive reactions ensue and involve platelet integrins such as the platelet glycoprotein IIb-IIIa complex which bind subendothelial matrix components such as fibrinogen, von Willebrand factor, collagen and fibronectin. This brings about platelet-to-platelet aggregation.
- The adherence of platelets is followed by their activation.
- Platelets are activated by specific agonists, of which thrombin is probably the most important. These agonists bind to their specific receptors, G-protein-coupled receptors, in the platelet cell membrane, and trigger a cascade of intracellular signals, mediated by the sequential activation of several enzymes, including phospholipase C (which produces inositol 1,4,5-triphosphate and 1, 2-diacylglycerol) and protein kinase C.
- Activation of protein kinase C and the generation of thromboxane A2 are crucial for the activation of the fibrinogen receptor – the IIb-IIIa complex (glycoprotein(GP)IIb/IIIa).
- Fibrinogen binds to the GPIIb/IIIa complex of adjacent platelets, mediating linkage of platelets and thereby causing them to aggregate.

Platelet plug formation thus entails the steps of surface adhesion, change in shape, degranulation and release of granule contents, aggregation, and consolidation.

Inhibition of platelet function

Inhibitors of platelet prostaglandin synthesis
Cyclo-oxygenase (COX-1) inhibitors: aspirin; indomethacin; sulphinpyrazone; indobufen; ibuprofen
Thromboxane synthase inhibitors: Dazoxiben
Thromboxane A2 receptor antagonist: Ridogrel
Prostacyclin mimetics
Platelet calcium channel inhibitor: Suloctidil
Phosphodiesterase inhibitors: Dipyridamole; Cilostazol
ADP receptor inhibitors: thienopyridine derivatives
    Ticlodipine
    Clopidogrel

Classification of inhibitors of platelet GP IIb/IIIa receptor

Monoclonal antibody to Gp IIb/IIIa receptor: abciximab-Fab fragment of monoclonal antibody

Intravenous peptide and non-peptide (peptidomimetic) small molecule inhibition: eptifibatide; tirofiban

Oral inhibition: sibrafiban

Prothrombin time

- A crude preparation of tissue factor (usually an extract of brain) is added to citrate-anticoagulated plasma. The plasma is recalcified and clotting time is measured.
- Usually both the thromboplastin and calcium chloride are added in a single step.
- The thromboplastins are calibrated against an international reference preparation to derive an international sensitivity index (ISI). Once the ISI of the thromboplastin is assigned, the results can be reported as the international normalised ratio (INR).
- A prolonged prothrombin time is due to deficiencies of factors II, V, VII or IX, or to the presence of a factor inhibitor.

International normalised ratio

The INR is the prothrombin time of patient/mean prothrombin time of a normal plasma pool.

The ISI is determined for each batch of the thromboplastin reagent by comparison to an international reference on a specific instrument utilised in the testing.

The INR was adopted as a way to eliminate inter-laboratory variations in test results caused by the use of thromboplastins with different sensitivities.

Causes of prolonged prothrombin time

Inherited
Quantitative deficiency
Functional abnormality

Acquired
Consumption, e.g. disseminated intravascular coagulation
Production failure, e.g. liver disease
Massive transfusion
Anticoagulation with coumarin derivatives
Presence of inhibitors (high levels of heparin)
Very low levels of fibrinogen

Vitamin K

Vitamin K acts as a cofactor for carboxylase, which causes post-translational modification of coagulation factors II (prothrombin), VII, IX, and X, and of plasma regulatory proteins, proteins C and S.

Vitamin K-dependent coagulation factors or zymogens are a group of calcium-binding proteins. They are characterised by a $-NH_2$ terminal Gla domain that contains 10–12 gamma-carboxyglutamate residues. Vitamin K acts as a cofactor for the carboxylase involved in the conversion of NH_2-terminal glutamic acid residues to the gamma-carboxyglutamate residues in these proteins.

The primary site of synthesis of vitamin K-dependent proteins of the blood is in the liver. They are synthesised in a non-functional precursor form (pre-proenzymes), reduced vitamin K being required for activation.

Activated partial thromboplastin time

A surface-activating agent, e.g. kaolin or ellagic acid and phospholipid, is added to citrate-anticoagulated plasma. After a standardised incubation time to allow optimal activation of the contact factors, the plasma is recalcified and the clotting time recorded. A prolonged activated partial thromboplastin time is due to deficiencies of factors II, V, VIII, X, XI, XII, kallikrein, high molecular weight kininogen and fibrinogen.

Coagulation cascade

The cascade is a multi-component enzyme system of circulating inactive pro-enzymes, cofactors and inhibitors, forming a sequential self-amplification process. This involves serial activation of zymogens by serine proteases, with cleavage of a vulnerable arginine site. This releases a small peptide, alters the three-dimensional configuration of the protein and exposes an active serine for the subsequent reactions. This leads to:

A sequence of reactions resulting in generation of a prothrombin activator, via activated factor X (the formation of which represents the convergence of the intrinsic and extrinsic pathways).

Cleavage of prothrombin by the prothrombin activator to form thrombin. This is associated with a positive feedback loop, whereby thrombin activates substrate pro-coagulant proteins.

The reaction of thrombin with fibrinogen and factor XIII leads to deposition of cross-linked polymers of fibrin.

The extrinsic pathway is initiated by tissue factor (factor III) and the intrinsic pathway by collagen exposure. Tissue factor is a transmembrane glycoprotein with a large extracellular domain (responsible for haemostatic activity), a transmembrane segment, and a cytoplasmic tail. The distinction between extrinsic and intrinsic pathways is somewhat artificial, but is useful for a conceptual understanding of the coagulation process. It is more than likely that a network model of coagulation can be invoked, which involves a linkage between the two pathways, regulated by a series of positive and negative feedback loops.

FLOW CHART

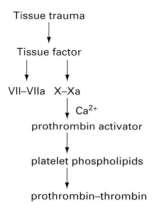

Figure 8.3 Extrinsic pathway (contact-activation pathway).

FLOW CHART

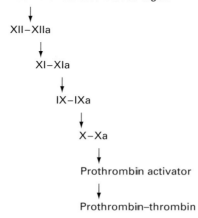

Figure 8.4 Intrinsic pathway.

Factor XII activation

This can be brought about by:
  Glass
  Kaolin
  Cartilage
  Kallikrein
  Bacterial endotoxins
  Collagen
  Basement membrane
  Trypsin
  Factor XI
  Sodium urate crystals

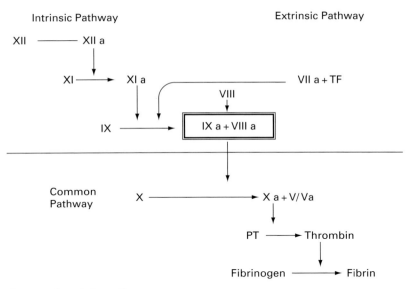

Figure 8.5 Coagulation pathways.

Control mechanisms of coagulation cascade

Anti-proteases (specific serine protease inhibitors), e.g. ATIII, thrombin, protein C and S;
Proteolytic feedback inhibition;
Protein C activation;
Fibrinolytic system.

Coagulation factors

These can be categorised as:

Vitamin K-dependent factors: II, VII, IX, X

Contact factors: XII, XI

Thrombin-sensitive factors: I, V, VIII, XIII

The factors were numbered according to the sequence of their discovery.

Factor	Other names
I	Fibrinogen
II	Prothrombin
IV	Labile factor; proaccelerin
VII	Stable factor; proconvertin
VIII	Antihaemophilic globulin
IX	Christmas factor
X	Stuart–Prower factor
XI	Plasma thromboplastin antecedent
XII	Hageman factor
XIII	Fibrin-stabilising factor

Thrombin actions

Thrombin has both procoagulant and anticoagulant actions.

Procoagulant

Cleaves fibrinogen to fibrin

Activates XI, VIII, V, XIII

Stimulates platelet activation

Anticoagulant

Activates protein C, which inactivates VIIIa, and Va

Heparin

Heparin is a mucopolysaccharide with unbranched chains of alternating sulphated hexosamine (N-sulphated-D-glucosamine) and uronic acid (L-iduronic acid) residues. It is found in the lungs, liver and intestinal mucosa of mammals. Heparin has a half-life of 30 minutes. The mean molecular weight of heparin ranges from 12 to 15 kDa. The mean number of saccharide units is from 40 to 50.

The anticoagulant activity has been localised to a unique pentasaccharide sequence, the third residue of which contains a 3–O sulphated glucosamine that is required for binding to a lysine-binding site in ATIII. This accelerates the binding of the arginine reactive centre of ATIII to activated serine proteases over 2000 fold, with the formation of inactive ATIII-serine protease complexes. Once binding of ATIII to the serine protease occurs, heparin dissociates and binds to a new ATIII molecule. The ATIII-protease molecules are removed by the reticulo-endothelial system. The anticoagulant activity of heparin is also mediated by heparin cofactor II, which only inhibits thrombin. Activity is monitored by the activated partial thromboplastin time.

The actions of unfractionated heparin include:

Enhanced action (cofactor) of ATIII on serine protease coagulation factors (IIa, Xa, XIIa, IXa and XIa): prevents fibrin aggregation.

Reduced platelet aggregation.

Increased vascular permeability.

Release of lipoprotein lipases into plasma.

Characteristics of low molecular weight heparins

They are derived from unfractionated heparin by either enzymatic or chemical depolymerisation. Their mean molecular weight is between 4 and 6.5 kDa, with a range of 2 to 8 kDa. The mean number of saccharide units is between 13 and 22.

Low molecular weight heparins do not prolong the activated partial thromboplastin time. They possess higher anti-Xa than antithrombin effect, i.e. reduced anti-IIa activity relative to anti-Xa activity. Activity is measured by anti-Xa assay. The target range for anti-Xa activity in blood samples drawn 4–6 hours after a dose should be between 0.5 and 1.0 unit/ml.

Advantages:

Predictable anticoagulant dose–response relationship.

High bioavailability; less non-specific binding to cationic plasma proteins and to cell surfaces as a result of less negative charge density.

Longer plasma half-life (greater than 30 minutes).

Therapeutic anticoagulant effect with once or twice daily subcutaneous injections at fixed, weight-adjusted doses.

Reduced binding to platelet factor IV (reduced risk of heparin-induced thrombocytopenia).

Less interference with the physiological activation of protein C.

Reduced binding to osteoclasts (reduced risk of heparin-induced osteoporosis).

Disadvantages:

More difficult to reverse with protamine.

Too small to inactivate IIa well.

Mechanisms preventing intravascular coagulation in the normal human

Blood flow.

Naturally occurring plasma inhibitors, i.e. the circulating antiproteases.

Heparin sulphate-ATIII mechanism.

Protein C-thrombomodulin-protein S mechanism.

The fibrinolytic system: plasmin.

Endothelial activity: prostacyclin production; ADPase activity; nitric oxide production; tissue type plasminogen activator (tPA) release.

Hepatic and phagocytic clearance of activated coagulation factors.

Clearance by the liver.

Inactivation by ATIII (proteases except VIIa), tissue factor pathway inhibitor (VIIa), protein C (factors V and VIII).

Elimination of clotting factors from blood.

Protein C

The zymogen (inactive form) of a serine protease with plasma concentration of 3–5 mg/l. It is synthesised in the liver as a 461 amino acid single chain precursor that contains a signal peptide and a propeptide. It consists of two polypeptide chains, a 150 amino acid light chain and a 260 amino acid heavy chain, linked by a single disulphide bridge. The molecular weight is 62 000.

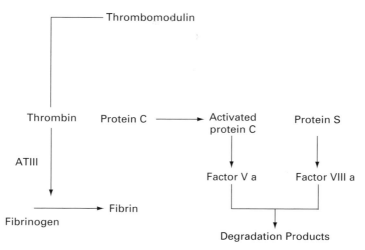

Figure 8.6 Antithrombotic mechanisms. ATIII, antithrombin III.

Classification of therapeutic anticoagulants

Heparins: standard unfractionated; low molecular weight
Coumarins: coumarin; 4-hydroxycoumarin; warfarin; bishydroxycoumarin (dicoumarol)
1, 3-indanediones: anisidione; 1, 3-indanedione

Effects of aspirin

Cyclo-oxygenase inhibitor: reduced thromboxane A2; reduced platelet aggregation.
Low dose aspirin:
   Reduced platelet cyclo-oxygenase activity.
   Prostaglandin synthesis is not impaired as there is no reduction of endothelial cell
cyclo-oxygenase activity.

Protein S

It consists of a single chain polypeptide with a molecular weight of 71 000 that is
synthesised in the liver, endothelium and megakaryocytes. The polypeptide
chain consists of 635 amino acids, with ten gamma-carboxyglutamic acid residues. It serves as cofactor for activated protein C.

■ Thrombosis

Thrombosis refers to the formation of solid intravascular clot. It can be consid-
ered as a pathological extension of normal haemostasis. The steps in thrombus
formation include:
   Endothelial cell damage with the exposure of subendothelial collagen
   Platelet plug formation;
   Activation of the intrinsic coagulation cascade;
   Formation of fibrin;
   Entrapment of blood cells;
   This is followed by granulation tissue formation, recanalisation and scar
      formation.
   Virchow's triad enumerates the pathogenetic mechanisms in thrombus for-
mation. The triad comprises:
Changes in blood flow pattern
   Reduced speed of flow: General: (e.g., congestive heart failure)
      Local: prolonged limb dependence
                reduced muscle pump activity
                proximal occlusion of venous drainage

Turbulence:
>   Arterial branch points
>   Narrowed arterial segments

Changes in vessel wall intimal surface
>   Atheroma
>   Injury to endothelium: mechanical/chemical
>   Inflammation
>   Neoplastic invasion

Changes in blood constituents
>   Increase in circulating platelets

Disseminated intravascular coagulation

This is characterised by systemic activation of coagulation with the formation of fibrin–platelet thrombi throughout the vascular tree. This is triggered by increased tissue factor activity in the circulation, which can be produced by a variety of stimuli including bacterial endotoxin and lipopolysaccharide. Thrombotic occlusion of small to medium sized vessels by fibrin clot can lead to multiple organ failure. Continual depletion of platelets and coagulation factors creates a consumption coagulopathy. Secondary activation of the fibrinolytic system ensues. The clinical manifestations represent a combination of those due to thrombosis and those due to bleeding, either of which may predominate. Treatment is essentially directed towards management of the underlying disorder. Acute disseminated intravascular coagulation is usually haemorrhagic, and chronic disseminated intravascular coagulation usually presents as a prothrombotic state.

A screen for thrombophilic states

This includes the measurement of:
>   Antithrombin III antigen level and activity assay;
>   Protein C antigen level and activity assay;
>   Activated protein C resistance;
>   Protein S antigen level;
>   Activated protein C resistance assay and factor V Leiden genetic analysis;
>   Prothrombin 20201A gene analysis;
>   Homocysteine level;
>   Anti-phospholipid and anti-cardiolipin antibody screen.

Diagnostic tests for disseminated intravascular coagulation

Laboratory markers of thrombin generation
D-dimer
Protamine procoagulation assay for fibrin monomer
Ethanol gel assay for fibrin monomer
Fibrinopeptide A
Prothrombin fragment 1–2
Thrombin–antithrombin complex

Screening assays for factor and platelet consumption
Prothrombin time
Partial thromboplastin time
Thrombin time
Quantitative fibrinogen
Platelet count

Ancillary tests
Fibrin/fibrinogen degradation products
Euglobulin or dilute whole-blood clot lysis
ATIII level
Alpha 2-antithrombin level
Factor V level

Causes of thrombophilic states

Activated protein C resistance: factor V Leiden, which may manifest in heterozygous
  and homozygous states
Prothrombin gene mutation: G20201A mutation
Protein C deficiency
Protein S deficiency
ATIII deficiency
Plasminogen deficiency
Dysfibrinogenaemia
Homocystinuria

■ Fibrinolytic system

Fibrinolysis is the plasmin-mediated enzymatic breakdown of fibrin. The fibrinolytic system is usually activated in concert with the coagulation system. The procoagulant, anticoagulant and fibrinolytic systems are tightly inter-regulated in order to maintain the fluidity of blood, while allowing controlled clot formation for haemostatic purposes followed by clot dissolution.

Table 8.2 Factors affecting fibrinolysis

Activation		Inhibition
Tissue activator		
Vascular wall activator	PLASMINOGEN	Anti-activators
Urokinase	(beta globulin)	Plasminogen activation inhibitor
	PLASMIN	Antiplasmins
		• Alpha 2-antiplasmin
		• Alpha 2-macroglobulin
		• Alpha 1-antitrypsin
		• C1 inactivator
		• Interalpha-trypsin
		• ATIII
	FIBRIN	
	Fibrin degradation products	

Plasminogen activators can be intrinsic (or blood-borne) such as factor XII, pre-kallikrein, high molecular weight kininogen and pro-urokinase; or may be extrinsic, such as tissue plasminogen activator, urokinase and streptokinase.

Endogenous extrinsic plasminogen activators are of two distinct structural, immunological and functional types: tissue-type plasminogen activator and urokinase-like plasminogen activator. They are serine proteases, which convert the inactive zymogen plasminogen to plasmin. Tissue type plasminogen activator is the major activator in the intravascular space and is released from stimulated endothelial cells. Urokinase is the major activator in the extravascular space and is synthesised by a range of cell types.

Plasminogen is a 790 amino acid with a 77 amino acid pre-activation peptide sequence, 5 homologous triple-loop structures called kringle domains, an activation cleavage site and a catalytic domain. Thrombolytic agents act by the hydrolysis of the arginine 560–valine 561 peptide bond in plasminogen to form plasmin.

Plasmin, a non-specific serine protease, brings about enzymatic degradation of fibrinogen, cross-linked fibrin and other plasma procoagulant proteins including factors V, VIII and XII. D-dimer is a degradation product of cross-linked fibrin. Fibrin degradation products result from the breakdown of cross-linked fibrin, fibrin monomers and uncross-linked polymers, and hence are less reliable markers of active thrombosis.

Resistance to thrombolysis may arise from selective lysis of fibrin, leaving activated platelets as a source of re-thrombosis. Platelets can release plasminogen activation inhibitor-1 and thromboxane A2. Clot-bound thrombin remains catalytically active, promoting thrombolysis.

Inhibitors of fibrinolysis

Aprotinin (trasylol): non-competitive inhibition of plasmin; 58 amino acid residue polypeptide

Synthetic lysine analogues:
  Epsilon-aminocaproic acid: complex formation with heavy chain of plasmin
  Cyclic aminocarboxylic acids: transexamic acid (AMCA)
Natural plasma inhibitors of tissue plasminogen activator (PAI-1) and plasmin (alpha 2-antiplasmin)

Tests for fibrinolysis

- Direct measurement of the clot lysis time, by manual or viscoelastic tests. The changes in viscosity of blood as it clots can be measured using thrombo-elastography, or by the Sonoclot test, which measures the changing impedance on an ultrasonic probe that is immersed in a coagulating blood sample.
- Measurement of the end-products of fibrin degradation. Fibrin degradation products, resulting from the cleavage of fibrin monomers and polymers, using a latex agglutination assay. Cleavage of cross-linked fibrin by plasmin yields dimeric units comprising one D-domain from each of two adjacent fibrin units (D-dimers), which are measured either by enzyme-linked immunosorbent assays or latex agglutination techniques.

■ Spleen

Structural features

- Weight: 75–250 grams. This depends on age, sex, race and blood content in the venous sinuses of the red pulp.
- Cranial to caudal axis: 15 cm; elliptical axis: 8 cm; thickness: 2–3 cm.
- The normal adult spleen contains 20–40 ml of blood.
- It receives about 5% of the cardiac output in the adult.
- The **white pulp** includes periarteriolar lymphoid sheaths containing T lymphocytes and antigen-presenting cells, and lymphoid nodules with germinal centres (secondary lymphoid follicles).
- The **red pulp** comprises vascular sinusoids lined by fixed and free phagocytes, and large numbers of interdigitating macrophages with long dendritic processes forming the splenic cords of Billroth.

Post-splenectomy blood picture

Red blood cell inclusions:
  Howell-Jolly bodies
  Heinz bodies
  Pappenheimer bodies

Poikilocytosis:
  Target cells (thinner than normal red cells; greater surface area–volume ratio)
  Acanthocytes or spur cells (multiple irregular surface projections)
  Nucleated red blood cells (rarely)
  Red cell fragments
Thrombocytosis (usually transient), which may be associated with thrombotic complications and necessitate temporary therapeutic anticoagulation.

Leukocytosis:
  Lymphocytosis (may persist)
  Monocytosis (may persist)
  Eosinophilia

Splenic function

The **functions of the spleen** include:
Filtration:
  Culling: Red blood cell (or other blood cell) destruction
    Physiological (aging)
    Pathological
  Pitting ('facelifting' of red blood cells)
    Removal of cytoplasmic inclusions:
        Howell-Jolly bodies (remnants of nuclear material);
        Heinz bodies (denatured haemoglobin);
        Siderotic granules (iron deposits): Pappenheimer bodies;
        Intracellular parasites (e.g. malarial parasites).
  Remodelling of cell membranes;
  Erythroclasis: destruction of abnormal red cells with liberation into circulation
    of red cell fragments;
  Removal of other particulate material, e.g. bacteria, colloidal particles.
Immunological function:
  Trapping and processing of cytoplasmic antigens in the marginal zone promotes the interaction of antigens with cells of monocytic and lymphocytic cells;
    'Homing' of lymphocytes;
    Lymphocyte transformation and proliferation;

Causes of hyposplenism

Congenital
- Asplenia
- Hypoplasia
- Immunodeficiency disorders

Acquired
- Splenectomy
- Acute atrophy and/or infarction:
  - Sickle cell disease
  - Radiotherapy
  - Autoimmune disorders
  - Essential thrombocythaemia
  - Chronic alcoholism
  - Hypopituitarism
  - Malabsorption syndromes

Functional asplenia with normal-sized or enlarged spleen
- Infiltration by leukaemia, lymphoma, multiple myeloma, mastocytosis
- Early sickle cell disease
- Amyloidosis
- Sarcoidosis
- Benign and malignant vascular tumours
- Malabsorption syndromes

Reduced immune function
- AIDS
- Endocrine: hypopituitarism, hypothyroidism, diabetes mellitus
- Chronic alcoholism
- Post chemotherapy/radiation therapy

Antibody (IgM) and lymphokine production in lymphoid follicles (B cells).
Macrophage activation;
Production of opsonins: tuftsin, properdin.
Reservoir:
Storage or normal sequestration of platelets, granulocytes;
Recycling of iron;
Red blood cell storage-blood reservoir (minor in humans).
Haematopoietic function:
Erythropoiesis, granulopoiesis, megakaryopoiesis;
Lymphocyte and macrophage production;
The haematopoietic role is primarily seen during fetal life and in situations of bone marrow destruction or dysfunction.

Greer, J. P., Foerster, J., Lukens, J. N., Rodgers, G. M., Paraskeva, F. & Glader, B. *Wintrobe's Clinical Haematology*, 11th edn. vols. 1 and 2. Philadelphia: Lippincott, Williams & Wilkins, 2004.

Hoffbrand, A. V., Pettit, J. E. & Moss, P. A. H. *Essential Haematology*, 4th edn. Oxford: Blackwell Science, 2001.

Schiffmann, F. J. *Haematologic Pathophysiology*. Philadelphia: Lippincott-Raven Publishers, 1998.

Neurophysiology

9

■ Introduction

The nervous system is broadly divided into the central nervous system (CNS) and the peripheral nervous system. The CNS consists of the brain and spinal cord, which are enclosed by the meninges and enclosed within bone of the skull and the spinal column, respectively. The brain is composed of the cerebrum, the cerebellum and the brain stem. The cerebrum includes the cerebral hemispheres, basal ganglia and thalamus, while the brain stem consists of the midbrain, pons and medulla oblongata. The spinal cord carries sensory information from the peripheral nervous system to the brain, and motor information from the brain to the muscles and glands.

The brain processes and integrates sensory inputs and controls and co-ordinates motor output. The brain and spinal cord are both broadly comprised of white matter, representing myelinated axons within a matrix of glial cells, and grey matter, representing cell bodies and dendrites with connecting axons and synapses.

The peripheral nervous system, lying outside the dura mater, comprises the somatic or spinal nerves and the visceral or autonomic nerves. The 12 paired cranial nerves may be either part of the central or the peripheral nervous system. There is a close relation between structure and function in the nervous system.

■ Cells of the nervous system

- **Neurons** are the fundamental structural and functional units of the nervous system. They are specialised for the reception, integration and transmission of information. Neurons can be broadly classed as afferent, efferent and inter-neurons (integrators and signal changers). There are about 10^{10} neurons in the body. Neurons act on other neurons, muscle cells and glandular cells via neurotransmitters. The signalling functions of neurons allow the processing of sensory information, and the programming of motor and emotional responses, learning and memory.

- **Neuroglial cells** are the supporting cells of the nervous system, occupying the spaces between the neurons. They are not excitable (not generating action potentials) and do not possess axons or form synapses, thereby not being involved in the transmission of information. They retain the capability to undergo mitosis, and secrete growth promoting molecules. Glial cells form myelin sheaths, provide nutrition to the neurons, contribute to the formation of the blood–brain barrier and are involved in the reuptake of neurotransmitters. The glial cells outnumber neurons 10:1.

Neurons

A neuron consists of:

- A **cell body** or soma. This contains the nucleus, cytosol and organelles including the rough and smooth endoplasmic reticulum.
- **Dendritic processes** (afferent or receptive zone), which are responsible for synaptic contacts with other nerve cells. Neurons can be morphologically classified as either unipolar, bipolar or multipolar, based on the number of processes arising from the cell body. **Synapses** form a functional communication between neurons. There are broadly three types of synapses, axo-dendritic, axo-somatic and axo-axonic. In the CNS, the presynaptic elements are axon terminals, whilst the postsynaptic elements are predominantly dendrites.
- **Axon** (transmission zone), involved in signal conduction. This consists of an initial segment, the axon proper and the terminal synaptic bouton:

The neuroglial cells

These can be subdivided into:
  Macroglial cells:
  Central nervous system:
    Astrocytes (star cells)
    Oligodendrocytes
  Peripheral nervous system:
    Schwann cells
  Microglial cells, which are involved in the phagocytosis of cellular debris produced
    as a result of pathological processes in the CNS.

The cytoplasm of the axons, or axoplasm, contains mitochondria, microtubules, neurofilaments and smooth endoplasmic reticulum. There are no free ribosomes and no rough endoplasmic reticulum, hence no protein synthesis is possible.

Axonal transport is carried out by microtubules and microtubule-associated proteins, which convey subcellular organelles and matrix proteins. This transport can be either antegrade or orthograde, from the neuron to the axon terminal, or retrograde, in the reverse direction. Kinesin is responsible for anterograde flow and dynein for retrograde flow. The axon terminal contains abundant mitochondria but does not possess microtubules.

Glial cell functions

Functions of astrocytes

- Provide structural support for nerve cells.
- Contact both capillaries and neurons and form the blood–brain barrier, thereby regulating the chemical composition of the extracellular space.
- Proliferation and repair following injury to nerves. They are responsible for reactive gliosis in response to injury to the CNS.
- Astrocytes produce a large number of growth factors, which act singly or in combination to selectively regulate the morphology, proliferation, differentiation and/or survival of distinct neuronal subpopulations.
- Isolation and grouping of nerve fibres and terminals.
- Participate in metabolic pathways which modulate ions, transmitters, and metabolites involved in the function of neurons and their synapses.

Functions of oligodendrocytes

Formation of myelin sheaths of axons in the CNS.

Neuronal inclusions

Nissl bodies or tigroid substance: rough endoplasmic reticulum
Golgi apparatus
Mitochondria
Microfilaments
Microtubules
Lysosomes
Lipofuscin; melanin
Glycogen; lipid

■ Peripheral nerve fibres

Peripheral nerve fibres were classified by Erlanger and Gasser on the basis of fibre diameter, conduction rate and the degree of myelination. Myelin is a dense, laminated structure of lipids and membrane proteins, consisting of 70% lipids. The proteins include myelin basic protein, proteolipid protein and protein zero.

Membrane potentials

There are two kinds of membrane potential change, local graded potentials and propagated action potentials. **Graded potentials** vary continuously in amplitude, and may produce an action potential if a threshold potential is exceeded. Graded potentials rapidly decrease in amplitude with propagation distance.

Action potential

An action potential is a cycle of membrane depolarisation, hyperpolarisation, and return to the resting value, and lasts one to two milliseconds. It is generated by voltage-gated cation (sodium and potassium) channels.

Table 9.1 Nerve fibre types

Group	Fibre diameter(μm)	Conduction velocity(m/s)
A		
Alpha	12–20	70–120
Beta	5–12	30–70
Gamma	3–6	15–30
Delta	2–5	12–30
B	1.5–3	3–15
C		
Dorsal root	0.4–1.2	0.5–2
Sympathetic postganglionic	0.3–1.3	0.7–2.3

Group A alpha: somatic motor to extrafusal muscle fibres; proprioception (somatic nervous system)

    Beta: touch, pressure (preganglionic autonomic nervous system)

    Gamma: motor to muscle spindle

    Delta: pain, cold, touch

B: sympathetic preganglionic

C: dorsal root; sympathetic postganglionic

Julius Bernstein in 1902 proposed the first satisfactory hypothesis for the genesis of the resting potential. He used the Nernst equation as a theoretical framework on which to develop the hypothesis that the resting potential of neurons is based on the selective permeability of the membrane to K^+. He also proposed that the membrane became permeable to all ions in the process of generation of the nerve action potential.

Bernstein's hypothesis was tested primarily by Hodgkin and Huxley and their colleagues, who provided the first complete description of ionic mechanisms underlying the action potential:

The membrane potential is equal to the potassium (K^+) equilibrium potential.

One can predict the resting potential by applying the Nernst equilibrium equation for potassium.

The resting potential is maintained by the influence of the Na-K ATPase. Most of the sodium channel gates are in a closed position. Slow facilitated diffusion of K^+ ions through leaky or semi-open potassium channels takes place.

Kenneth Cole and Howard Curtis in 1938 using giant squid axon recordings showed that membrane conductance to ions increases during the action potential. Cole designed the voltage clamp in 1949, which interrupts the interaction between the opening and closing of voltage-gated channels and the membrane potential. It was used by Hodgkin and Huxley in the early 1950s in a series of experiments revealing ionic mechanisms underlying the action potential to show the existence of separate channels for Na^+ and K^+. The action potential in the squid giant axon is generated by rapid opening and subsequent voltage inactivation of voltage-dependent Na^+ channels and delayed opening and closing of voltage-dependent K channels.

The **voltage clamp** allows direct measurement of permeability changes. It comprises three components:

A circuit to measure membrane potential;

A command amplifier, under the control of the experimenter;

A circuit to measure current flow across the cell membrane.

This forms an electronic negative feedback device. The output of the command amplifier is directly proportional to the differences in inputs. The voltage clamp maintains a constant membrane potential or voltage at any desired level.

The technique involves the insertion of two electrodes into the squid giant axon. One records the voltage difference across the membrane, i.e. the membrane potential. The other is used for the intracellular injection of current. The electrodes are connected to a feedback circuit that compares the measured voltage across the membrane with the voltage desired by the experimenter. If these two values differ, current is injected into the axon to compensate for this difference. This continuous feedback cycle keeps the voltage across the membrane constant so that the amplitude and time course of the ionic currents can be measured.

The membrane potential is clamped to the predetermined command potential. The current injected into the axon to keep the membrane potential clamped is equal to the current flowing through the ionic channels in the membrane. Ionic currents are both voltage and time dependent. Keeping voltage constant allows these two variables to be separated. Voltage dependence and kinetics of ionic currents flowing through the plasma membrane can be directly measured.

Patch clamping techniques, which permit measurement of ion movement through single open ion channels, are used to determine the potential at which a channel opens, its ion conductivity and the rate of channel inactivation and closing. The patch clamp represents a method of voltage clamping a small patch of membrane.

The principles involved are:

Electrical isolation of a small patch of cell membrane containing a few ion channels, by placement of a glass micropipette in close contact with the membrane. The heat-polished end of the micropipette is sealed onto the surface of the cell by the application of negative pressure through the pipette.

The ion current through the open channel completes its circuit through the current sensing amplifier connected to the interior of the micropipette. This is due to the high electrical resistance produced by the micropipette.

Sequence of events in generation of an action potential

- Depolarisation to threshold: a stimulus depolarises the membrane, i.e. makes less negative, from its resting potential to its threshold potential, around −55 mV. Threshold depolarisation is the level of depolarisation that results in an action potential 50% of the time. Subthreshold stimuli produce local graded potentials, which rapidly decrease in amplitude with propagation distance.
- Activation of Na^+ channels, with increased sodium permeability, leads to rapid depolarisation, with a voltage change from −70 mV to +30 mV: the upstroke.
- Activation is associated with conformational change leading to opening of the channel. Sodium channels can be either ligand-gated, opening in response to binding of ligand to channel, or voltage-gated, opening in response to cell membrane depolarisation. Local anaesthetics prevent opening of voltage-gated sodium channels and stop action potential initiation

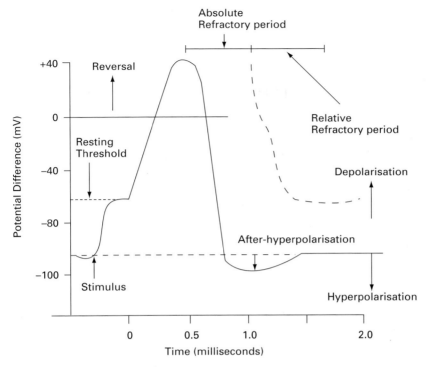

Figure 9.1 Nerve action potential.

and conductance along nerves. They delay recovery of these channels from inactivated state and prolong the absolute refractory period. Activity is enhanced at alkaline pH.

- Inward Na^+ flow further depolarises the membrane, opening more Na^+ channels by a positive feedback mechanism. This increases membrane Na^+ conductance by a factor of up to 5000, leading to an overshoot of the membrane potential.
- The overshoot is associated with a positive membrane potential, the peak of the action potential.
- Inactivation of Na^+ channels and activation of K channels leads to repolarisation. Slow opening of K channels is associated with increased K permeability.
- There is an undershoot, of hyperpolarisation, when the membrane potential becomes more negative than its resting value. The interior of the cell becomes briefly electropositive.
- This is followed by a return to normal permeability.
- The inactivation of Na^+ channels is associated with the absolute refractory period, and the transitory hyperpolarisation of the membrane with the relative

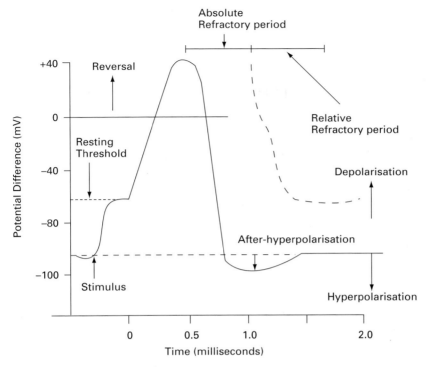

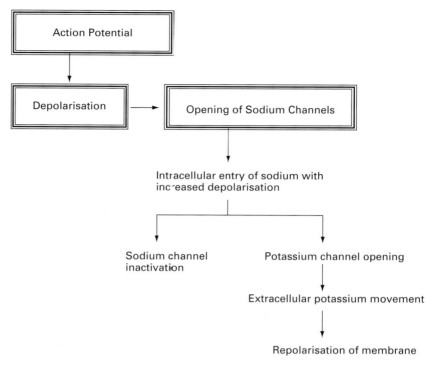

Figure 9.2 Nerve excitation.

refractory period. During the absolute refractory period, no generation of a further action potential is possible. During the relative refractory period, a greater than threshold depolarisation is required to trigger an action potential.

Properties of the action potential

- It depends on voltage-gated ion channels, representing a diffusion potential set up by a sequential change in membrane conductance for sodium and potassium, namely:

  A rapid increase in membrane conductance to Na;

  A slower increase in membrane conductance to K with peak in repolarisation phase.

- It is an **all or none response** to a stimulus. The action potential is triggered at a threshold level of depolarisation, about 15 mV depolarised relative to the resting potential. This causes complete depolarisation of the membrane, i.e. reduction in membrane potential.

- It has the same amplitude in all nerves, from –70 mV to +40 mV.

- Action potentials cannot be summed.

- The cell is refractory during the action potential.
- It is self-propagating and unidirectional, without decrement (maintains constant amplitude). Unidirectional transmission is due to the presence of synapses.
- The velocity is proportional to the diameter and myelination of the nerve fibre.
- The action potential is regenerative.

Physiological effects of action potentials
These include:
   Transmission of impulses along nerve fibres;
   Release of neurosecretions or chemical transmitters in synapses;
   Muscle contraction;
   Activation or inhibition of glandular secretion.

Myelin

The myelin sheath increases the velocity of action potential conduction by increasing the length constant of the axon, reducing capacitance of the axon, and restricting generation of action potentials to the nodes of Ranvier, where the sodium channels are concentrated.

An action potential over the myelinated internodes is conducted with little decrement and at great speed from one active node of Ranvier to the next. The process is called **saltatory conduction**. This is achieved because time is not lost in bringing the internodes to threshold potential.

Sodium pump

The **sodium pump**, or Na-K ATPase, is found in all cells. It is an integral membrane protein, formed by a tetrameric complex of two polypeptides: two transmembrane catalytic alpha subunits and two glycoprotein regulatory beta subunits.

The catalytic subunits form the gated channel and possess binding sites for Na^+ and adenosine S'-triphosphate (ATP) on the intracellular surface, and for K^+ and ouabain on the extracellular surface. They have phosphorylation sites and span the plasma membrane ten times. The beta subunit comprises a single membrane-spanning domain and has three extracellular glycosylation sites.

It requires oxygen for the provision of the substrate, ATP. It is electrogenic, extruding 3 Na^+ ions for every 2 K^+ ions (coupling ratio of 3:2). The pump is an antiport, transporting two different ions in opposite directions across the membrane. Sodium Na^+ ion pumped out of the cell is used to drive active co-transport systems.

Ion translocation by Na-K ATPase

This involves:

Intracellular binding of ATP and 3 Na^+ ions;

Phosphorylation of the pump by ATP;

Conformational change and Na^+ release to the extracellular fluid;

External binding of 2 K^+ ions and dephosphorylation of the pump;

Conformational change and release of K^+ to intracellular fluid.

Functions of the sodium pump

Maintenance of intracellular sodium concentration at a low level;

Regulation of intracellular potassium concentration controls cell volume and osmolality;

Provision of a sodium gradient as an energy source for co-transport;

Generation and maintenance of the transmembrane potential.

Role of potassium channels

They contribute to the resting membrane potential;

They shorten the duration of the action potential;

The relative refractory period for action potential generation is produced by prolongation of the after-hyperpolarisation following an action potential;

Termination of burst firing by neurons;

Mediation of some forms of inhibitory postsynaptic potentials.

Nernst equation

This can be used to find the equilibrium potential – the membrane potential at which ions are in equilibrium – of any ion present on both sides of a membrane permeable to that ion. The Nernst potential is the potential difference at which

Measurement of membrane potential

Intracellular electrode inserted into nerve cell: glass pipette filled with a concentrated salt solution (salt bridge) connected to a metal electrode. A glass capillary tube is drawn in heat to a tip size of 0.5–1.0 μm.

A second extracellular electrode using a concentrated salt solution of similar ionic composition connected to a metal electrode.

The two metal electrodes are connected to a voltage amplifier.

The amplifier is connected to an oscilloscope.

The amplitude of the membrane potential is displayed as the vertical deflection of a spot of light on the screen.

there is no ionic flow in spite of the presence of a concentration difference. It describes the potential difference between two compartments as a consequence of the activity difference at equilibrium.

The Nernst equation calculates the membrane potential at which net flux of an ion across the membrane is zero. The electrical potential across a cell-surface membrane is given by a more complex version of the Nernst equation in which the concentrations of the ions are weighted in proportion to the relative magnitudes of their permeability constants.

ENa = (RT/ZF) In ((Na)1/(Na)2)

ENa is the voltage difference between side 1 and side 2 of the membrane at equilibrium

R is the gas constant

T is the absolute temperature

Z is the valence of the sodium ion

F is Faraday's constant

In is the symbol for the natural, or base e, logarithm

(Na)1 and (Na)2 are the sodium concentrations on sides 1 and 2 of the membrane.

The **Goldman–Hodgkin–Katz equation** can be used to predict the equilibrium voltage or resting potential. It can be used to determine the potential developed across a membrane permeable to Na^+ and K^+. It relates the membrane potential to alterations in permeability or concentration of all permeable ions.

The Gibbs–Donnan equilibrium

If a large impermeable organic ion is present on one side of a membrane, the permeable ions distribute themselves unequally on either side of the membrane. The product of the permeable ions outside the membrane are thus equal to the product of the permeable ions inside the membrane. This allows preservation of chemical equilibrium and electrical neutrality. The system is, however, not in osmotic equilibrium, as the total number of particles in the solution with the non-permeable anions is greater than the total number of particles in the other solution. This situation arises from the accumulation of excess protein with anionic charge on one side of a membrane.

With a Gibbs–Donnan equilibrium:

● The concentrations of ions on either side of the membrane do not match each other.

● Within each solution, the concentrations of anions and cations are equal to each other, maintaining electroneutrality.

● The concentration of diffusible cations is greater in the solution containing the non-permeable, negatively charged particles.

- The concentration of diffusible anions is greater in the solution without the non-permeable particles.

Nerve conduction velocity can be measured in sensory, mixed and motor nerves. Measurement entails recording of evoked response potentials caused by supra-maximal stimulation with skin electrodes.

■ Neurotransmission

The **neuromuscular junction** comprises the triad of:
  Motor nerve terminus: synaptic boutons or terminals on the presynaptic terminals;
  Neurotransmitter: acetylcholine;
  Postsynaptic muscle end-plate.

Sequence of transmission at the neuromuscular junction

- The neuronal action potential arrives at the synaptic terminal of the motor neuron nerve fibre. Depolarisation of the synaptic terminal occurs. Opening of voltage-gated calcium channels leads to an increase in intracellular calcium concentration.
- Acetylcholine is released by a process of vesicular exocytosis from membrane-bound synaptic vesicles in axon terminals into the junctional cleft (10–20 nm width). Each vesicle contains about 10 000 molecules of the neurotransmitter – accounting for quantal release in multi-molecular packets or quanta in the absence of presynaptic electrical activity. This coupling of depolarisation and neurotransmitter release is caused by the influx of calcium ions.
- Diffusion of acetylcholine occurs down a concentration gradient towards the motor end-plate, which contains ligand-gated, nicotinic acetylcholine receptors.
- Acetylcholine interacts with postsynaptic or postjunctional acetylcholine receptors. The chemical signal (binding of two acetylcholine molecules) is converted into electric signals (i.e. a transient permeability change and depolarisation in the postsynaptic membrane). Denervation hypersensitivity in skeletal muscle is due to the increased expression of nicotinic cholinergic receptors and their spread to regions away from the motor end-plate.
- Depolarisation of the motor end-plate produces an end-plate potential. When the end-plate potential exceeds a threshold potential of excitability, an action potential is triggered.
- The action potential passes into the T-tubules and causes depolarisation with opening of voltage-gated calcium channels of the sarcoplasmic reticulum.

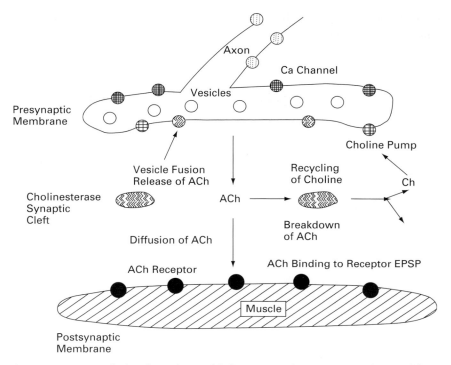

Figure 9.3 Neuromuscular junction. Ach, acetylcholine; EPSP, excitatory postsynaptic potential.

- Dissociation of the acetylcholine/receptor complex occurs.
- Acetylcholine is hydrolysed by acetylcholinesterase. Reuptake of choline back into the nerve terminal ensues. Re-synthesis of acetylcholine follows, with storage in the synaptic vesicles.

The synaptic potential at the neuromuscular synapse was first studied in detail in the 1950s by Paul Fatt and Bernard Katz. Using curare they reduced the amplitude of the synaptic potential below the threshold for the action potential, thus isolating the synaptic potential in intracellular voltage recordings.

Miniature end-plate potentials

At the neuromuscular junctional cleft small packets (quanta) of acetylcholine are constantly being released in the absence of nerve activity, probably due to the random release of single vesicles from the nerve endings, giving rise to miniature end-plate potentials.

These potentials arise due to an increase in the ratio of 'open' to 'closed' time of the acetylcholine-sensitive channels, so that there is an increase in the number of ions crossing the membrane per unit of time.

Classification of neuromuscular blocking agents

Non-depolarising, which produce competitive inhibition of nicotinic acetylcholine
receptors on the motor end-plate.

Isoquinoline:
  D-Tubocurarine
  Metocurine
  Doxacurium
  Atracurium
  Cisatracurium
  Mivacurium
Steroid:
  Pancuronium
  Pipecuronium
  Rocuronium
  Rapacuronium
  Vecuronium
Depolarising, which produce prolonged depolarisation of neuromuscular junction.
  Decamethonium
  Succinylcholine

Agents used for reversal and antimuscarinic effects with non-depolarising blocking agents

Reversal agent
  Edrophonium
  Pyridostigmine
  Neostigmine

Antimuscarinic agent
  Atropine
  Glycopyrrolate

They are spontaneous, random, of constant and small amplitude (0.4 millivolts)
and are abolished by curare. They are increased in frequency and amplitude by
acetylcholinesterase inhibitors.

Characteristics of the perfect neuromuscular blocking agent

  Non-depolarising blockade;
  A rapid onset of action;
  A predictable and controllable duration of action;

Table 9.2 Differentiation of the type of neuromuscular blockade

	Depolarising	Non-depolarising
Fasciculation	yes	no
Tetany	no fade	fade
Post-tetanic potentiation	no	yes
Anticholinesterases	increase block	reduce block
Additional non-depolariser	antagonism	potentiation

Haemodynamic stability at all levels of block and rate of administration;

Predictable kinetics, independent of age or gender;

No active metabolites or toxicity;

Elimination independent of hepatic or renal function;

Inexpensive.

Uses of neuromuscular blocking agents

To facilitate endotracheal intubation;

As an adjuvant to anaesthesia to provide muscle relaxation during surgery;

To enhance carbon dioxide removal in patients who are difficult to ventilate;

  Life-threatening asthma

  Status epilepticus

  Neuromuscular toxins: strychnine, methaquolone poisoning

  Tetanus

Reduction of intracranial pressure in intubated patients;

Prevention of injury during the administration of electroconvulsive therapy.

Acetylcholine receptors

Characteristics of the nicotinic receptor

Each nicotinic acetylcholine receptor is a pentameric glycoprotein complex composed of five subunits, alpha, beta, delta and epsilon in a ratio of 2:1:1:1. These subunits are integral membrane proteins, spannning the cell membrane. Each of the two alpha subunits acts as a high-affinity acetylcholine-binding site. When stimulated, the channel undergoes conformational change and opens for one millisecond, allowing non-selective passage of small positively charged ions, mainly sodium, potassium and calcium. The Na^+ influx depolarises nearby muscle membrane, triggering local voltage-gated Na^+ channels, thereby creating a self-propagating depolarisation.

Characteristics of the muscarinic receptor

The muscarinic receptor acts indirectly on ion channels or second messengers via G-proteins. It comprises G-protein-coupled receptors, which activate phospholipase C, inhibit adenyl cyclase, or open K ion channels. There are five subtypes: M1, M2, M3, M4 and M5.

Criteria for identification of a chemical messenger as a neurotransmitter

Presence at the synapse in the neurons from which it is released;

Storage in the presynaptic terminal;

Processes for synthesis present in the presynaptic neurone;

Release on presynaptic nerve stimulation;

Postsynaptic membrane application of exogenous postulated neurotransmitter mimics the action of endogenously released transmitter;

Specific mechanisms for inactivation are present at the synapse;

Agents that block the response to presynaptic stimulation also block the response to exogenously applied neurotransmitter.

Techniques for study to confirm the above criteria involve:

Microelectrodes for recording from or stimulating neurons;

Micropipettes for application of putative neurotransmitters and probes for removal of extracellular fluid for analysis;

Biochemical and isotopic techniques for detection of neurotransmitters or precursors and metabolites;

Ligand binding, immunological and molecular (e.g. *in situ* hybridisation) techniques to map distribution of a receptor and its subtypes in the CNS;

Histochemical fluorescence techniques for localisation of putative monoamine neurotransmitters;

Immunological techniques for localisation of enzymes involved in neurotransmitter synthesis and breakdown, or for identification of putative peptide neurotransmitters;

Lesion making, and neuroanatomical tracing.

Known or postulated neurotransmitters

Acetylcholine

Biogenic monoamines

Catecholamines

Dopamine

Noradrenaline

Adrenaline

Indoleamines: Serotonin(5-hydroxytryptamine)

Histamine

Amino acids

Excitatory: L-glutamate (α-amino-3-hydroxy-5-methyl-isoxazole AMPA) and N-methyl-D-aspartate (NMDA receptors); L-aspartate

Inhibitory: gamma-amino-butyric acid (GABA) (GABA A and GABA B receptors) (increases Cl⁻ permeability at postsynaptic membrane); glycine

Neuropeptides (neuroactive peptides)

Endogenous opioid peptides: enkephalins; endorphins; dynorphins

Substance P: undecapeptide of the tachykinin family

Substance K

Neuropeptide Y: 36 amino acid peptide

Somatostatin

Angiotensin II

Nucleosides and nucleotides

ATP

Adenosine

Miscellaneous

Gases: nitric oxide

Purines: adenosine/ATP

Excitatory amino acid receptor activation may cause neuronal death (excitotoxicity). There may be a role for glutamate release blockers or excitatory amino acid antagonists (which modulate NMDA receptors) in the prevention of neuronal damage.

Neuropeptide Y

This is a 36 amino acid peptide, which plays a role as an inhibitory neuromodulator in appetite, thirst and blood pressure control. It is found mainly in brain interneurons and is also found in noradrenaline-containing neurons in the hypothalamus, ventro-lateral medulla and locus coeruleus, as well as in sympathetic ganglia.

Classification of opioid receptors	
Mu	Mu-1
	Mu-2
Kappa	Kappa-1
	Kappa-2
	Kappa-3
Sigma	Delta

■ Synapses

A synapse is a specialised contact zone that acts as the site for functional inter-neuronal communication or information transfer. It can represent either the site of functional contact between two neurons, or between a neuron and a target organ (gland or muscle). A synapse consists of a presynaptic ending containing the synaptic vesicles, a synaptic cleft, or intersynaptic space, and a postsynaptic membrane, where neurotransmitter receptors are located.

Synapses can be classified as one-to-one (neuromuscular junction), one-to-many (axon collaterals of motor neurons on Renshaw cells in spinal cord) and many-to-one: spinal motor neurons.

Properties of synapses

One-way conduction
Synaptic fatigue: with repetitive stimulation of the presynaptic neuron at a rapid rate there is progressive decrease in the number of impulses from the post-synaptic neuron. This is due to exhaustion of neurotransmitter stores in synaptic knobs and progressive inactivation of postsynaptic receptors.

Post-tetanic facilitation: increased excitability of the postsynaptic neuron that follows repetitive stimulation of an excitatory synapse, following on a period of synaptic delay. This is due to accumulation of Ca^{2+} in the presynaptic terminals.

Synaptic delay: minimum time required for transmission across one synapse (0.5 ms).

Modes of transmission

Synaptic transmission can be electrical or chemical.

Electrical synapses possess symmetrical morphology. They can allow either unidirectional or bidirectional transfer of information. Ionic currents are used as the mode of transmission. Transmission is generated by voltage-gated channels in the presynaptic neuron. Electrical transmission allows for rapid and synchro-nous firing of interconnected cells. The pre- and postsynaptic elements are in close apposition, being bridged by gap junctions.

Chemical synapses possess asymmetrical morphology, with differences in the structure of the pre- and postsynaptic elements. Pre- and postsynaptic elements are separated by a synaptic cleft, a gap of 200–300 nm. Chemicals are used as the mode of transmission. The transfer of information is unidirectional. Chemical transmitter receptors are membrane-spanning proteins and carry out an effector

Modulation of synaptic transmission

Presynaptic
Receptor activation of a presynaptic neuron;
Direct effect of a pharmacological agent on neurotransmitter release, on either vesicular apposition to the synaptic terminal, or on fusion or fission of synaptic vesicles.

Postsynaptic
Changes in ligand affinity for the receptor;
An effect on ion conductances;
Long-term changes in receptor numbers, either down-regulation or up-regulation, mediated by pharmacological manipulation.

function within the target cell, either gating an ion channel directly or indirectly, or initiating a second messenger cascade via activation of G-proteins. The depolarisation signal in the presynaptic membrane is destroyed by diffusion of neurotransmitter from the synaptic cleft, reuptake of neurotransmitter and/or enzymatic breakdown of neurotransmitter.

The synaptic vesicle exo-endocytic cycle comprises transmitter uptake from cytoplasm, cytoskeletal and intervesicular anchoring, plasma membrane docking, membrane fusion (exocytosis) with liberation of neurotransmitter into synaptic cleft, endocytosis and recycling.

Features of synaptic transmission in the CNS (neuron-to-neuron)

There is poly-synaptic input into neurons;
Synapses can be excitatory or inhibitory;
Single presynaptic action potentials lead to small depolarisation of the postsynaptic cell;
Synaptic potentials undergo spatial (spatially distinct simultaneous inputs on a single postsynaptic cell) or temporal (series of sequential action potentials) summation to produce threshold depolarisation.

This differs from synaptic transmission at the neuromuscular junction (neuron-to-muscle), which has the following characteristics:

Excitatory synaptic transmission;
A one-to-one synapse, with one action potential in the input cell leading to one action potential in the output cell;
A single presynaptic action potential triggers a postsynaptic action potential.

Generation of postsynaptic potentials

Stimulation of the presynaptic nerve fibre at an excitatory synapse results in the depolarisation of the postsynaptic membrane: an excitatory postsynaptic

Synaptic vesicle proteins

Synapsin: Ia; Ib; IIa; IIb
Synaptophysin
Synaptotagmin
Syntaxin
Synaptobrevin/VAMP (vesicle-associated membrane protein)
Rab3 and rabphilin
SV-2 : large glycoprotein with 12 transmembrane domains
Vacuolar proton pump: membrane ATPase

potential (epsp). A single epsp normally produces insufficient depolarisation to reach threshold for generation of an action potential. Generation of a postsynaptic impulse requires summation of several epsps. An epsp is associated with simultaneous increase in membrane permeability to potassium and sodium.

Stimulation of the presynaptic nerve fibre at an inhibitory synapse results in a hyperpolarisation of the postsynaptic membrane: an inhibitory postsynaptic potential (ipsp). The effect of ipsps is to move the membrane potential away from the threshold for excitation, thus opposing the effect of epsps.

Types of postsynaptic potentials in the CNS

Ionotropic: direct binding of transmitter molecule(s) with a receptor-channel complex, with opening of either excitatory or inhibitory ion channels. Ionotropic glutamate receptors are divided into two broad classes based on sensitivity to the agonist NMDA: NMDA-receptors and non-NMDA receptors.

Metabotropic: indirect effect of transmitter molecule(s) binding with a receptor via stimulation of second messengers. Most act through protein phosphorylation, regulated by G-proteins

Genotropic: a specific compound translocated into the nucleus activates ribonucleic acid (RNA) polymerase activity.

■ Reflexes

A reflex is a stereotyped specific involuntary response to an adequate sensory stimulus. The pathway for a reflex includes an afferent (sensory)signal that evokes an efferent (motor) response.

The **reflex arc** is composed of five components:
A peripheral receptor (sensory organ);

An afferent or sensory limb, from the receptor to the spinal cord or brain stem;

Integrative centre: one or more inter-nuncial neurons which link the afferent and efferent limbs;

The efferent or motor limb;

A terminal effector organ (muscle or glands).

The neural components responsible for the tendon jerk or stretch reflex, or myotactic unit

The afferent primary ending in the muscle spindle, which is a stretch receptor, responding to sudden passive muscle stretch.

The afferent Ia fibre.

Cell body in the dorsal root ganglion.

Collateral branch at the root entry zone to the anterior horn cell, via the central grey matter. An excitatory synapse with the anterior horn cell.

The efferent limb is through group I fibres to the motor units (extrafusal muscle fibres of the muscle).

The tendon reflex has a latency (stimulus–response interval) of 15–25 milliseconds.

The alpha motor neuron can be stimulated by Ia afferents of muscle spindles, the corticospinal, lateral vestibulospinal, or reticulospinal tracts.

General properties of reflexes

An adequate stimulus is necessary.

Local sign: pattern of response depends on the afferent nerve fibre stimulated.

Irradiation of the stimulus: the more intense a stimulus is, the greater is the spread of activity in the spinal cord, involving more and more motor neurons.

Summation: several synaptic inputs from different sources may have a cumulative effect (spatial summation) or repeated stimuli in a brief time can also have a cumulative effect (temporal summation).

Occlusion.

Recruitment and after-discharge.

Reciprocal innervation (or reciprocal inhibition).

Final common path: the motor neuron is the common efferent path for several reflexes.

Response time is an indicator of the number of synapses in the reflex arc.

Rebound phenomenon: the exaggeration of a reflex after a temporary period of inhibition.

■ Cerebral blood flow

The cerebral blood flow is carried by the paired internal carotid arteries and the basilar artery. These vessels provide input to the anastomotic circle of Willis at the base of the brain, which gives rise to the paired anterior, middle and posterior cerebral arteries. Variability in the development of anterior and posterior communicating arteries is associated with variability in functional adequacy of the circle. The circle of Willis is anatomically incomplete in 50% of cases.

The brain comprises 2% of the body mass and accounts for 15% of the resting metabolic rate. The cerebral blood flow comprises 15% of the total resting cardiac output. This is equal to 50–55 ml/100 g brain tissue per minute. Grey matter blood flow equals 70–80 ml/100 g per minute. White matter blood flow equals 15–20 ml/100 g per minute. Grey matter blood flow relative to white matter blood flow = 3–4:1. A fall in cerebral blood flow to less than 10 ml/100 g per minute is associated with irreversible neuronal damage secondary to failure of the Na-K ATPase pump mechanism.

The **Fick principle** for measuring cerebral blood flow involves the use of a metabolically inert, freely diffusible tracer with a known partition coefficient between the blood and the brain. Providing that full saturation is achieved, the brain concentration of the tracer can be estimated from the cerebral venous blood.

Techniques for measuring cerebral blood flow

Indirect
> Carotid duplex scanning.
> Transcranial Doppler to measure blood flow velocities in basal cerebral arteries.

Direct
> Intermittent:
>> Inert gas inhalation (Fick principle): nitrous oxide, argon, krypton 85, xenon 133. This requires arterial and jugular venous bulb sampling.
>> Single photon emission computed tomography.
>> Intra-arterial injection of inert gas: Xenon 133.
>> Stable xenon computed tomography.
>> Positron emission tomography.
> Continuous:
>> Laser Doppler flowmetry.
>> Thermal diffusion.

Cerebral metabolism

Cerebral metabolic rate of oxygen:

Consumption = Cerebral blood flow × arterio-venous oxygen content difference
= 3–6 ml oxygen/100 g per minute

Oxygen consumption is higher in the cortex than in the white matter. Under physiological conditions, cerebral metabolic consumption of oxygen is relatively stable, irrespective of whether the subject is asleep or engaged in intense mental activity.

D-glucose is the sole energy substrate of the brain, except in states of ketosis, when ketone bodies derived from the catabolism of non-esterified fatty acids in the liver can be utilised. Ketone body uptake into the brain is mediated by the monocarboxylic acid transporter-1. The brain consumes about 100–120g of glucose per day, equivalent to 60% of total hepatic production. Glucose oxidation in the CNS accounts for 20% of whole-body oxygen consumption.

D-glucose is transported into the brain by facilitated diffusion across the blood–brain barrier, involving membrane-based carrier mechanisms specific for D-glucose. Glucose uptake is mediated by glucose transporter-1, expressed at high density in the capillary endothelium, in an insulin-independent action. The glucose transporter-3 is responsible for glucose uptake into the neurons, and is also insulin-independent. There is a tight coupling between cerebral metabolic demand and cerebral substrate supply, which is in turn regulated by cerebral blood flow. Functional imaging demonstrates regionally specific increases in metabolism with cognitive, motor or visual activation. As glycogen stores in the brain are negligible, acute lowering of glucose causes the rapid onset of severe compromise of brain function.

The metabolic rate is reduced in sleep, coma, general anaesthesia and hypothermia.

The metabolic rate is increased with sensory stimulation, epileptiform activity, mental concentration, ketamine anaesthesia and hyperthermia.

Cerebral energy consumption

The high energy consumption of the brain is used for:

Maintenance of transmembrane ionic gradients (Na^+-K^+ ATPase) by the continuous activity of ionic pumps. These are necessary for neuronal transmission.

Neurotransmitter synthesis, release and reuptake. These substances are necessary for synaptic transmission.

Macromolecular synthesis and distribution: proteins, amines, lipids, carbohydrates.

Cerebrospinal fluid (CSF) formation.

Fast axoplasmic transport, which is bidirectional.

The structural and metabolic functions of the glial cells.

At the regional level, glucose and oxygen utilisation, as well as enzyme distribution, is heterogeneous.

Cerebral ischaemia

Cerebral ischaemia is associated with a number of events, which potentiate each other. These include:

Neuronal changes

Depletion of ATP;

Disruption of ion and amino acid transporters;

Influx of sodium;

Efflux of potassium;

Intracellular acidosis;

Increased intracellular calcium concentrations;

Activation of proteases, phospholipase and caspase;

Formation and breakdown of arachidonic acid;

Production of free radicals;

Release of excitatory amino acids (excited to death).

Vascular changes

Vasospasm;

Red cell sludging;

Hypoperfusion.

The ischaemic penumbra at the periphery of an ischaemic lesion is functionally silent but may be capable of recovery under favourable circumstances, such as the opening of collateral vessels or the resolution of cerebral oedema.

Regulation of cerebral blood flow

The cerebral blood flow is regulated by:

Cerebral perfusion pressure, which is equal to mean arterial pressure − (venous pressure + intracranial pressure).

Arterial oxygen tension.

Arterial carbon dioxide tension, which is the most potent physiological determinant of cerebral blood flow. The response to arterial carbon dioxide

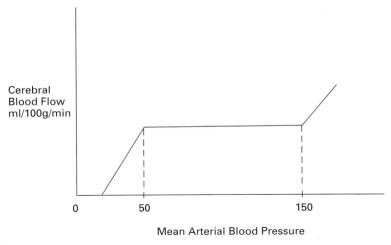

Figure 9.4 Cerebral blood flow–perfusion pressure relationship.

tension is mediated by the hydrogen ion concentration in the extracellular fluid of the vascular smooth muscle.

Cerebral metabolic demands (flow-metabolic coupling). Loss of the normal tight coupling between cerebral blood flow and cerebral metabolic rate may lead to zones of luxury perfusion (with cerebral blood flow exceeding metabolic demands) or penumbral zones (regions of potentially viable tissue with marginal cerebral blood flow).

The cerebral circulation demonstrates **autoregulation**, maintaining a constant blood flow, over a mean arterial pressure range of 50–160 mm Hg. This is evident in the cerebral cortex, basal ganglia and the white matter. Autoregulation can be considered as the intrinsic capability of the cerebral blood flow to regulate itself in accordance with the metabolic needs of the brain. Myogenic and metabolic control mechanisms are involved, which affect the smooth muscle in the arterial and arteriolar segments. Autoregulation is primarily mediated by alterations in the vascular tone of the precapillary resistance vessels or arterioles, which constrict in response to elevations in transmural pressure. With reduction in blood flow, vasodilator mediators accumulate. Within the physiological range, autoregulation protects the brain against hypoxic damage with a reduction in cerebral perfusion pressure, and against hyperaemia, capillary damage and cerebral oedema with increased perfusion pressure.

With loss of autoregulation, cerebral blood flow and blood volume change passively with changes in systemic arterial blood pressure – leading to a linear relationship.

Causes of increased cerebral blood flow

Hypoxia
Hypercapnia
Hyperthermia
Rapid eye movement sleep

Causes of reduced cerebral blood flow

Hypocapnia
Hyperoxia
Hypothermia

Unique features of cerebral capillaries

Lack of fenestrations;

Tight junctions between adjacent cells (zonulae occludens), which create high electrical resistance;

ATPase pumps on luminal surfaces form interstitial fluid;

Increased numbers of mitochondria for high energy needs;

Glucose transporters and amino acid carriers;

Basal lamina, pericytes and astrocytes. The astrocytic foot processes are closely invested around the vessels.

Autoregulation is lost with arterial hypotension or hypertension outside the specified limits, raised intracranial pressure, hyperviscosity and raised arterial pCO_2.

■ Blood–brain barrier

The blood–brain barrier is a dynamic interface between blood and the brain, maintaining homeostasis in the cerebral interstitial fluid. Structurally it consists of the pericapillary astrocyte end-feet and the tight quintuple-layered junctions between the non-fenestrated capillary endothelial cells. The endothelial cells rest on a continuous basement membrane. The barrier is further augmented by the extracellular matrix. This arrangement reduces transcellular and paracellular solute movement across the capillaries. The tight junctions represent a barrier to passive diffusion of drugs with low lipid solubility, protein macromolecules and smaller hydrophilic molecules such as glucose. In general, the threshold

Blood–brain interfaces

	Tight junction localisation
Blood–CSF	Choroid plexus epithelial cell
CSF–blood	Arachnoid membrane in arachnoid villi
Blood–brain	Capillary endothelial cell
CSF–brain	Ventricular ependyma

These barriers help maintain a stable microenvironment for neurons, axons and glia of the CNS.

Causes of disruption of blood–brain barrier function

Infection
Inflammation
Neoplastic infiltration
Circulating toxins
Cerebral ischaemia and reperfusion
Malignant hypertension
Osmotic injury
Seizure activity

molecular weight for allowing free diffusion is below 400–600 daltons. Pinocytotic vesicles transport plasma and interstitial fluid bidirectionally across the endothelium. The capillary endothelial cells have a high mitochondrial content to supply energy for the transport of water-soluble substances. P-glycoprotein, a unique membrane glycoprotein with a molecular weight of 170–180 kDa , is expressed at the luminal membrane of the endothelial cells and at the astrocytic foot processes.

The blood–brain barrier can be bypassed by intrathecal administration of drugs into the CSF and by drug modification (increased lipid solubility; carrier transport). Disruption of barrier function can be recognised radiologically on computed tomographic scanning by the phenomenon of contrast enhancement, and is associated with vasogenic cerebral oedema. Disruption is associated with acute increases in CSF protein levels. Loss of integrity of the barrier function is related to partial and reversible relaxation of endothelial tight junctions, and to increased vesicular transport across the endothelial cells.

Mechanisms of transport across the blood–brain barrier

Electrolyte transport: simple diffusion through capillary endothelial cells; diffusion through pores within and between cells; and carrier mediated active and/or passive transport.

Micronutrient transport (of vitamins, nucleotides, purine bases): facilitated diffusion at the capillary endothelial cell; active transport at the choroid plexus epithelium.

Carrier mediated transport systems in the CNS:

Monosaccharides: D-glucose

Monocarboxylic acids: L-lactate

Neutral amino acids: L-leucine

Basic amino acids: L-arginine

Dicarboxylic acids: L-glutamate

Amines: choline

Nucleosides: adenosine

Purines

Brain areas outside the blood–brain barrier

'Windows of the brain' are characterised by higher capillary densities and by the presence of fenestrated capillaries. They help form a functional interface between the CNS and the endocrine system, sensing hormonal changes. They are essentially midline structures located adjacent to the ventricular spaces and arising from the ependymal lining of the ventricular system. The **circumventricular organs,** which abut on the third and fourth ventricles can be classified as either:

Secretory:

Posterior lobe of the pituitary gland: neurohypophysis.

The area of the median eminence of the hypothalamus: releasing or inhibiting hormones from the hypothalamus are released into capillaries of the hypothalamic–pituitary portal system.

Pineal gland.

Subcommissural organ.

Receptor:

The organum vasculosum of the lamina terminalis, which monitors cytokines in the blood.

The area postrema at the inferior border of the fourth ventricle: drugs stimulate the chemoreceptor trigger area in the floor of the fourth ventricle; monitors cholecystokinin.

Subfornical organ: monitors angiotensin II levels.

Immunological privilege

The brain is a relatively **immunologically privileged site.** This is due to:

The blood–brain barrier preventing the entry of circulating antibodies and lymphocytes into the brain;

A low level of antigenicity of neurons, which express very low levels of surface histocompatibility molecules;

A paucity of lymphatic drainage.

■ Intracranial pressure and cerebrospinal fluid

The cranium becomes an almost rigid container following closure of the fontanelles and sutures, with three minimally compressible components contained within:

The brain parenchyma: 80%–85%

The circulating CSF: 10%

The cerebral vascular bed: 5%–10%

The cranium is in direct communication with the vertebral canal, which forms part of the cranio-spinal axis. According to the **Monro–Kellie doctrine** (Alexander Monro, 1783 and George Kellie, 1824) of constant intracranial contents, any increase in either brain, blood or CSF occurs at the expense of the other components.

The slope of the intracranial pressure–volume curve dP/dV defines the elastance of the system and reflects the resistance to deformation exerted by the intracranial contents in the face of rising intracranial volume.

The brain is contained within the meninges, which comprise, from outside inwards:

The vascular pia mater;

The subarachnoid space;

The arachnoid membrane;

The subdural space;

The dura mater, which contains the dural venous sinuses.

The cranial dura forms two sheets, the falx cerebri and the tentorium cerebelli, which divide the cranial cavity into compartments. Rises in intracranial pressure result in pressure gradients between these compartments and a shift of brain structures.

Cerebrospinal fluid

The CSF represents a plasma ultrafiltrate, supplemented by products of active endothelial secretion. It is a clear aqueous solution that circulates through

Functions of the cerebrospinal fluid

Mechanical protection for the brain and spinal cord, similar to that provided by a water jacket, against the effects of external acceleration and gravity.

Removal of waste products of cerebral metabolism, including carbon dioxide, lactate, hydrogen ions. This affects the acid–base status of the CSF, which contributes to the control of pulmonary ventilation.

Maintenance of a stable chemical environment for neurons and their medullated fibres.

A medium for nutrient exchange between the blood and the extracellular fluid compartment of the brain.

macroscopic and interstitial spaces that are in continuity. The macroscopic spaces include the ventricles, aqueduct, central canal of the spinal cord and the subarachnoid space. The interstitial space surrounds the neurons and glial cells of the CNS.

The average intracranial volume of CSF in adults equals 150–170 ml, with around 75 ml in the cisterns, 50 ml in the subarachnoid space and 25 ml in the ventricles. The formation rate is about 0.5 ml/min, or 400–500 ml per day. Over 75% is produced by the choroid plexus in the lateral, third and fourth ventricles. The flow occurs successively through the lateral ventricle, third ventricle, aqueduct, fourth ventricle and the subarachnoid space. The total CSF pool is replaced three to four times a day.

Reabsorption is a passive process via the macroscopic arachnoid granulations of the superior sagittal sinus (85%–90%) and the microscopic arachnoid villi of the venous drainage of the spinal nerve root sleeves (10%–15%). The rate of absorption increases with increasing CSF pressure.

Intracranial pressure

This represents the summation of the volumes of the brain (1200–1600 ml), blood (100–150 ml) and CSF (100–150 ml). It increases exponentially in the presence of an expanding intracranial mass lesion once a critical point is reached when compensatory mechanisms are overwhelmed. Compensation can be achieved by a reduction in intracranial blood volume, displacement of CSF into the spinal subarachnoid space and by increased absorption of CSF. Rapid development of a mass lesion is associated with earlier decompensation.

The elastance of the cranio-spinal axis is determined by the rigidity of the skull; the elasticity of the intracranial and spinal dura; and displacement of the mobile neuraxis contents, blood and CSF, within the cranio-spinal axis.

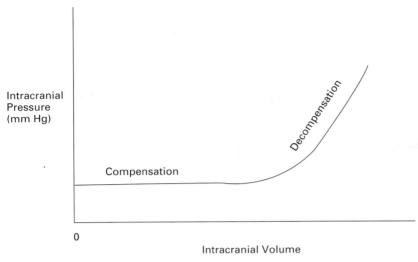

Figure 9.5 Intracranial volume–pressure relationships.

Intracranial pressure range

Normal: 0–15 mm Hg (0–2.0 kpa)
Equivocal: 15–20 mm Hg (2.0–2.7 kpa)
Moderately increased: 20–40 mm Hg (2.7–5.3 kpa)
Severely increased: > 40 mm Hg (5.3 kpa)
The pressure is identical in the lumbar subarachnoid space, the cisterna magna, the
    lateral ventricles and the cerebral subarachnoid space.

The clinical effects of raised intracranial pressure

These can be broadly considered as being due to hydrocephalus, brain ischaemia
and brain shifts.

The **brain shift** sequence associated with rising intracranial pressure involves:

Subarachnoid space compression;

Midbrain and basal cisterns compression;

Ipsilateral ventricle compression;

Herniation of the cingulate gyrus;

Dilatation of the contralateral ventricle;

Uncus of medial temporal lobe herniates between the free edge of the tentorium
    and the midbrain;

Foramen magnum cone.

Measurement of intracranial pressure

Intracranial pressure can be measured with systems incorporating the following components:

  Placement in either the intraventricular, subarachnoid, subdural, epidural or intraparenchymal space. A lateral ventricular catheter placed via a burr hole is the gold standard for intracranial pressure measurement. Subdural bolts or parenchymal silicone strain gauge monitors can be used alternatively.

  A deformable membrane.

  An optico-electric mechanical device to convert the pressure signal to an electrical signal.

  An amplifier.

  A display device.

The **normal intracranial pressure waveform** consists of three arterial components superimposed on the respiratory rhythm: a percussion wave, a tidal wave and a dicrotic wave.

Lundberg waves are categorised as large plateau-like A waves, smaller sharper B waves and small rhythmic oscillatory C waves.

  A waves are characterised by a steep rise from a near normal value to 50 mm Hg or greater and persist for 5–20 minutes.

Methods of reduction of raised intracranial pressure

  Hyperventilation, which can also reduce cerebral blood flow leading to secondary brain injury. The primary mechanism of action is by blowing out carbon dioxide. This produces extracellular alkalosis and cerebral vasoconstriction.

  Osmotic diuretics, e.g. mannitol, which acts by creating an osmotic gradient across the intact blood–brain barrier.

  Cerebrospinal Fluid drainage: ventricular drain; lumbar drain.

  Loop diuretics.

  Glucocorticoids: dexamethasone; methylprednisolone.

  Removal of space-occupying lesion.

Types of cerebral oedema

  Cytotoxic: cell membrane damage due to ischaemic hypoxia and failure of the Na-K ATPase pump.

  Vasogenic: extravasation of protein-rich fluid from the intravascular to the extracellular space, caused by capillary endothelial damage, i.e. disruption of the blood–brain barrier. This responds to high dose glucocorticoids.

  Interstitial: shift of fluid from the ventricles into the periventricular interstitium.

B waves are rhythmic oscillations every 1–2 minutes.

C waves are oscillations at a frequency of 4–8 per minute.

■ Cerebral hemispheres

- These comprise the cerebral cortex or pallium, a mantle of grey matter, and the underlying white matter. The white matter consists of multiple inter-and intra-hemispheric tracts connecting the cortical and subcortical structures of grey matter.
- Each hemisphere comprises four lobes: frontal, parietal, temporal and occipital.
- The neocortex comprises six layers: molecular or plexiform, external granular, external pyramidal, internal granular, internal pyramidal or ganglionic, and multiform or fusiform.
- The six-layered isocortex displays two patterns of cellular arrangement: the homotypical cortex with the six layers easily recognisable, and the hetero-typical cortex with a predominance of certain cell types.
- The surface of the cortex demonstrates convolutions and folds, the sulci and gyri respectively, which serve to significantly increase its surface area.
- The cortex is divided into cytoarchitectural areas based on the types, amounts and arrangement of neurons in each area. Brodmann's system of numbering cerebral surface areas (52 areas in each hemisphere), which is based on micro-scopically identified variations in neuronal architecture, is still widely used in spite of its imperfections. Along with regional variations in cytoarchitecture, there are variations in neurochemical activity and in physiological function.
- The lobes are connected by fibres of white matter, which can be classified as:

Association fibres

Ipsilateral: short; long (cingulum; uncinate fasciculus; arcuate or short long-itudinal fasciculus)

Commissural: anterior commissure; corpus callosum; posterior commissure

Projection fibres

Afferent: corticopetal

Efferent: corticofugal

Cerebral function

The cerebral hemispheres demonstrate functional asymmetry with respect to language production, praxis or skilled movements, mechanisms of attention, visuospatial abilities, and perception and expression of emotion.

Projection fibres

The internal capsule
Thalamic radiations: anterior; middle; posterior
Motor projection fibres:
  Pyramidal motor system
  Corticobulbar(corticonuclear)
  Corticospinal: ventral; lateral
Other fibres:
  Corticorubral
  Corticoreticular
  Cortico-olivary

Methods for the study of localisation of cortical function

Neuroanatomical studies;
Stimulation studies;
Regional cerebral blood flow;
Positron emission tomographic scanning;
Evoked potentials.

Frontal lobes

They lie anterior to the central or Rolandic sulcus and superior to the Sylvian fissure. Functional areas include:

The primary motor cortex: area 4: precentral gyrus, in the anterior bank of the central sulcus. This forms a homunculus, a cortical map of the body. The area directly controls all voluntary movement.

The premotor (supplemental motor) cortex: area 6: the superior and middle frontal gyri of the precentral gyrus.

The frontal eye field: area 8: posterior part of the middle frontal gyrus

The prefrontal areas: areas 9–12, 32 and 45–47. These are concerned with personality and insight.

Motor speech area (Broca's area): areas 44, 45: the opercular and triangular parts of the inferior frontal gyrus. This area is concerned with the production of written and spoken language.

Areas 4 and 6 comprise the frontal agranular cortex.

Corticofugal pathways from the frontal lobe include corticospinal; cortico-reticular; and corticostriate, corticothalamic and corticopontine pathways.

Frontal lobe lesions

These may be associated with:

Personality changes, such as disinhibition, impaired judgement, lack of initiative, irritability and jocularity.

Expressive aphasia: involvement of the posterior part of the left inferior frontal gyrus.

Hemiparesis: projection fibres in the posterior frontal lobe traversing the white matter to the corona radiata and internal capsule.

Gaze preference.

Primitive reflexes, such as forced grasping and the snout reflex.

Frequency and urgency of micturition.

Unilateral anosmia: pressure on the olfactory nerve.

Parietal lobes

Functional areas

The somatic sensory cortex: postcentral gyrus: areas 3, 1, 2: in the banks of the calcarine sulcus. This region receives somato-sensory pathways from the thalamus that mediate skin sensation and the discriminative senses (such as position sense, stereognosis). Somatic sensory input is integrated with visual and auditory input in the region.

Superior parietal lobule: areas 5, 7: the somato-sensory association area.

Supramarginal gyrus: area 40: inferior parietal lobule.

Angular gyrus: area 39: inferior parietal lobule.

Parietal operculum of postcentral gyrus: area 43: taste.

Deep pathways

Superior longitudinal fasciculus;

Optic radiation.

Temporal lobes

Functions

Integration of sensations, emotions, memory, learning and behaviour.

Involved in the processing of auditory and visual information

Functional areas

Primary auditory receptive area: transverse gyri of Heschl within the Sylvian fissure: areas 41 and 42. The region receives the auditory pathway from the medial geniculate body of the thalamus.

Secondary auditory cortex: area 22 and part of area 21.

Middle and inferior temporal gyri: areas 21 and 37.

Parietal lobe lesions

These may be associated with:

Contralateral cortical sensory loss, involving joint position sense, two point discrimination, stereognosis or form recognition (appreciation of shape, size, weight and texture) and graphaesthesia.

Dominant hemisphere lesions: communication disorders, or aphasia.

Non-dominant hemisphere lesions: contralateral hemi-spatial neglect and failure to acknowledge the existence of deficits (anosognosia).

Visuospatial abnormalities.

Gerstmann's syndrome (lesion in the left angular gyrus): dyscalculia, dysgraphia, finger agnosia, right–left disorientation.

Agnosia: a disorder of awareness in the presence of normal sensation, vision and motor function.

Apraxia: a disorder of co-ordinated motor activity in the absence of motor or sensory loss.

Temporal lobe lesions

These may be associated with:

Loss of memory for recent events associated with confabulation (medial temporal lobe);

Contralateral superior quadratic hemianopia (optic radiation fibres);

Receptive dysphasia;

Temporal lobe epilepsy.

Occipital lobes

Functions

Processes visual information, allowing visual perception and recognition.

Functional areas

Primary idiotypic visual receptive cortex: area 17: striate cortex; in the walls of the calcarine fissure: has the stria of Gennari – thin myelinated tract in the 4th or granular layer. The region receives the visual pathway from the lateral geniculate body of the thalamus.

Visual association cortex: areas 18 and 19.

Parastriate cortex: area 18.

Peristriate cortex: area 19.

Occipital lobe lesions may be associated with visual seizures and visual agnosia.

Bilateral occipital lobe involvement causes cortical blindness, with lack of awareness of the defect by the patient in the presence of normal pupillary responses. There may also be loss of colour perception, prosopagnosia (inability to identify a familiar face) and simultagnosia (inability to integrate and interpret a composite scene as opposed to its individual elements).

Basal ganglia

The basal ganglia comprise five large interconnected paired subcortical nuclei of grey matter of the forebrain, lying deep to the white matter of the cerebral cortex. They consist of the caudate nucleus, the putamen, the globus pallidus (pallidum), the subthalamic nucleus and the substantia nigra (pars reticulata and pars compacta).

The caudate nucleus and putamen together form the neostriatum.

Functions of the basal ganglia

Receive input from and project to the cortex by way of the thalamus.

Involved in the initiation, sequencing and modulation (smoothness and pre-cision) of motor activity.

Have inhibitory (brake) and switch actions.

Disorders of the basal ganglia

These can be broadly classed as:

Hypokinetic, associated with impaired voluntary movements (bradykinesia and akinesia);

Hyperkinetic, associated with involuntary movements or dyskinesias.

Limbic system

The limbic system comprises a group of interconnected cortical and subcortical regions at the centre of the brain. The component structures form a ring around the brain stem and the diencephalon. The limbic system thereby occupies a bordering zone (limbus) between the diencephalon and telencephalon. It is the only cortical area to receive major projections from the hypothalamus. The limbic cortex functions as a central association area for the control of behaviour. It plays a major role in memory.

The concept of a system that plays a central role in memory and emotion was set out by James Papez in 1937, who described the Papez circuit. This is a reverber-ating circuit involved in short-term memory. The circuit comprises:

Regions of limbic cortex: cingulate gyrus, parahippocampal gyrus, entorrhinal cortex.

Hippocampal formation: dentate gyrus; hippocampus.

Amygdala: basolateral complex; anteromedial complex; parts of stria terminalis and hypothalamus.

Nucleus accumbens.

Mammillary bodies.

Anterior and dorsomedial nuclei of thalamus.

■ Cerebellum

Three anatomical portions of the cerebellum are:

Flocculonodular lobe and fastigial nuclei: archicerebellum.

Anterior lobe: palaeocerebellum: vermis and paravermis; globose and emboliform nuclei.

Posterior lobe: neocerebellum: cerebellar hemispheres, dentate nuclei.

Three functional subdivisions of the cerebellum are:

Flocculonodular lobe (vestibulocerebellum): involved in the maintenance of equilibrium and balance, and in smooth pursuit and saccadic eye movements.

Anterior lobe: involved in the maintenance of posture and muscle tone. Movement is monitored through input from proprioceptors via the posterior spinocerebellar and cuneocerebellar tracts.

Posterior lobe: involved in the learning, co-ordination and execution of skilled movement that is initiated at a cerebral cortical level (trajectory, velocity, acceleration). Co-ordination of movement is achieved by the integration of afferent somatic sensory information with motor output from the cerebrum and brain stem.

This sensory information can be tactile, auditory, vestibular, visual and visceral.

Broadly speaking the cerebellum comprises deep nuclei, which receive excitatory inputs from mossy fibres and climbing fibre collaterals and provide excitatory projections to nuclei in the brain stem and thalamus, and the cerebellar cortex, which receives excitatory inputs from mossy fibres and climbing fibre collaterals and provides inhibitory projections to the deep nuclei via the Purkinje cells.

There are five cell types: the Purkinje, stellate, basket, Golgi and granule cells.

Three types of afferent fibres are identifiable:

Mossy

Climbing

Aminergic:

Dopaminergic

Serotoninergic

The sources of inputs to the cerebellum are from the spinal cord, the vestibular nuclei, the motor cortex and the brain stem (red nucleus, reticular nuclei, inferior olivary nuclear complex).

The cerebellar inputs via the inferior cerebellar peduncle come from the ipsi-lateral spinal cord, inferior olive and the vestibular nuclei. The inputs via the middle cerebellar peduncle arise from contralateral pontine nuclei. The projection fibres in the superior cerebellar peduncle go to the ventro-lateral nucleus of the contralateral thalamus.

■ Hypothalamus

The hypothalamus weighs 4–5 grams, and is bounded rostrally by the midbrain, anteriorly by the optic chiasm and superiorly by a sulcus separating it from the thalamus. It forms the floor and part of the lateral wall of the third ventricle. There are three morphological zones: periventricular; medial (rich in cells); and lateral (rich in axons). The major role of the hypothalamus in the control of autonomic, endocrine, visceral, affective and emotional behaviour is in contrast to its small size.

The hypothalamus possesses three main groups of nuclei:

Anterior: preoptic; supraoptic; paraventricular

Middle: tuberal; arcuate; ventro-medial; dorso-medial

Posterior: mammillary bodies; posterior hypothalamic nuclei

The hypothalamus receives inputs from the nucleus of the tractus solitarius (visceral sensory information), the reticular formation (spinal cord), the circum-ventricular organs, the limbic and olfactory systems and the retina. Optic nerve input from the retina synchronises the body clock in the suprachiasmatic nucleus with the night–day cycle. The two main outputs are neuronal signals to the autonomic nervous system via the lateral medulla and endocrine signals to the pituitary gland.

The functions of the hypothalamus include:

- The head ganglion of the autonomic nervous system, the anterior hypothala-mus being parasympathomimetic and the posterior hypothalamus sym-pathomimetic. The hypothalamus is thereby responsible for the neural control of the internal viscera.

- Circadian and seasonal clock for behavioural and sleep–wake functions, in the suprachiasmatic nuclei. The body clock comprises the paired suprachiasmatic nuclei, which rhythmically influence core temperature, hormonal activity and autonomic function. It is influenced by the light–dark cycle, and by melatonin signals from the pineal gland. It separates body functions associated with daytime from those at night. The basic oscillator in the suprachiasmatic nuclei is an autoregulatory negative feedback system involving cyclical synthesis of period proteins.

- Neural control centre of the endocrine system. Cells in the supraoptic and paraventricular nuclei produce the peptide hormones oxytocin and vasopressin respectively, which are transported to the posterior pituitary. Thirst is mediated by osmoreceptors. A variety of releasing and inhibiting hormones produced by the tuberal and arcuate nuclei affect the anterior pituitary release of hormones.

- Body temperature regulation: The neuronal groups in the anterior hypothalamus co-ordinate heat losing mechanisms, and in the posterior hypothalamus co-ordinate heat conservation. The hypothalamus co-ordinates autonomic (vasoconstriction) and somatic (shivering) responses.

- Hunger is mediated by the satiety centre in the ventro-medial nuclei and the feeding centre in the lateral nuclei.

- Sexual behaviour is controlled by the medial hypothalamus.

■ Pineal gland

The pineal gland is attached to the roof of the third ventricle, and lies outside the blood–brain barrier. It weighs 100–150 mg and has a length of about 9 mm. It is a homologue of the third or parietal eye of the lower vertebrates. The pineal starts to involute just prior to puberty. The gland consists of neurons, neuroglial cells and pinealocytes, which secrete melatonin into the CSF.

The environmental light–dark cycle and autonomic circadial stimulation by the suprachiasmatic nuclei of the hypothalamus (the endogenous circadian oscillator) modulate the secretion of melatonin by the pineal (which takes place in the dark phase of the cycle). This contributes to the maintenance of biological rhythms.

Melatonin is derived from circulating L-tryptophan. It is not stored in the pineal. There is a gradual increase in levels of melatonin at night and a reduction in the morning of serum melatonin levels. Melatonin can induce a phase shift in the circadian oscillation of activity of the suprachiasmatic nuclei. This may help in the amelioration of the symptoms of jet lag.

Thalamus

The thalamus is a paired grey matter mass situated deeply in the forebrain.

The functions of the thalamus include:

Integration modification and relay of motor and sensory (apart from olfactory) inputs to the cerebral cortex;

Awareness of nociceptive stimuli in non-discriminative form;

Control of subjective responses to sensation;

Activation and arousal: processes information that influences electro-cortical activity in the sleep–wake cycle through the ascending reticular activating system;

Modification of the affective component of behaviour upon limbic system communications.

The thalamus comprises several groups of relay nuclei:

Ventral

Medial

Lateral

Intralaminar

Midline

Reticular formation

This is a complex matrix of neurons, which extends from the lower medulla to the upper end of the mesencephalon. The lateral portion is afferent and the medial portion efferent. It includes the sagittally oriented serotonergic raphe nuclei in the midline of the medulla, pons and mesencephalon, and the locus coeruleus, a group of pigmented noradrenergic cells in the floor of the fourth ventricle.

It has afferent connections from:

Spinal cord

Cerebral cortex

Superior colliculus

Basal ganglia

Limbic structures

Hypothalamus

Cerebellum

It has efferent connections to:

Spinal cord

Brain stem nuclei

Cerebellum

Thalamus

Its functions include:

The conscious awareness of, and behavioural responses to, specific sensory stimuli;

Integration of signals from sensory receptors;

Maintenance of the level of wakefulness (fibres that ascend into the intra-laminar nuclei of the thalamus);

Inhibitory and facilitatory effects on skeletal muscle tone and posture, via the reticulospinal tracts;

Inhibitory and facilitatory effects on reflex activity;

Control of ventilation by generation of the respiratory rhythm;

Control of blood pressure;

Control of cardiac output;

Control of the distribution of blood volume to organs.

■ Spinal cord

- The spinal cord extends from the medulla oblongata at the foramen magnum, terminating as the conus medullaris at the level of the L1-L2 interspace. The filum terminale is a prolongation of the pia mater, which attaches to the coccyx.
- The spinal cord is 42–45 cm long in the adult, with a width of 2–3 cm in the cervical enlargement and 3–4.5 cm in the lumbar enlargement. These enlargements allow for innervation of the limbs, the cervical enlargement comprising C4 to T1 segments and the lumbar enlargement L2 to S3 segments.
- The cord is associated with 8 cervical, 12 thoracic, 5 lumbar and 5 sacral motor and sensory rootlets, comprising 30 pairs of spinal nerves.
- The spinal cord receives sensory information from skin, joints and muscles, contains motor neurons responsible for voluntary and reflex movements, conveys sensory information from the viscera and controls visceral function.
- The anterior white column is situated between the anterior fissure and the anterior horn of grey matter. The lateral column is between the anterolateral and posterolateral sulci, and the posterior column between the posterior median septum and the posterior horn of the grey matter.
- The Bell–Magendie law is a statement about the functional distinction between ventral and dorsal nerve roots. Sensory or afferent fibres enter the dorsal root, with their cell bodies in the dorsal root ganglion. Motor or efferent fibres leave via the ventral root, with their cell bodies in the anterior horn of spinal grey matter.

Tracts in the white columns

Ascending
    Anterior column: ventral spinothalamic tract
    Lateral column:
        Ventral and dorsal spinocerebellar tracts
        Lateral spinothalamic tract
        Spino-olivary tract
        Spinotectal tract
    Posterior column:
        Fasciculus cuneatus
        Fasciculus gracilis

Descending
    Anterior column:
        Ventral corticospinal (pyramidal) tract
        Reticulospinal tract
        Vestibulospinal tract
        Tectospinal tract
    Lateral column:
        Lateral corticospinal (pyramidal) tract
        Rubrospinal tract
        Lateral reticulospinal tract
        Olivospinal tract

Spinal cord lesions

Lesions in the spinal cord produce a combination of segmental and long tract (longitudinal) signs.

    Segmental signs are related to:

Lesions of the anterior root or anterior horn cell giving rise to a myotomal distribution of flaccid weakness, atrophy and fasciculations;

Lesions of the dorsal root or dorsal root entry zone giving rise to a dermatomal distribution of sensory loss;

Loss of reflex function, caused by disruption of the mono-synaptic stretch reflex arc;

Dermatomal pain from dorsal root irritation.

Longitudinal signs comprise:

Upper motor neuron lesions characterised by spastic weakness, hyper-reflexia, clonus, extensor plantar responses and loss of superficial cutaneous reflexes (abdominal and cremasteric);

Sensory loss below a sensory level.

■ Electroencephalogram

The electroencephalogram (EEG) is a record of the electrical activity of the brain through the intact scalp. It records the net electrical activity of the cerebral cortex, which is generated by the summated excitatory and inhibitory post-synaptic potentials of the pyramidal cells in the superficial neocortex. The action potentials of these neurons do not contribute directly. The EEG is controlled and paced by subcortical thalamic nuclei and the brain stem reticular formation. It is also partly generated by pacemaker cells within the cortex. The activity is rhythmic, synchronised and oscillatory. Electroencephalography involves amplification, filtering, display, storage and analysis of this activity.

The recordings are obtained by scalp disc electrodes placed bilaterally and symmetrically in standard locations, using the International 10–20 System. The sites for placement are determined by measurement from four standard head positions: nasion, inion, right and left pre-auricular points. The electrodes are coated with conductive paste held in place by adhesives, suction, or pressure from caps and headbands. The scalp-derived EEG is distorted by the presence of CSF, skull and scalp.

Automated EEG processing allows compression of the data obtained and the observation of long-term trends. The computer digitises the time-varying analogue signal. The digitised array of data is divided into epochs which are treated statistically.

The rhythms include:

Beta: > 13 Hz

Alpha: 8–13 Hz

Theta: 4–7 Hz

Delta: < 4 Hz

Electroencephalography is used as a diagnostic neurological tool (classification of seizure type, localisation of epileptogenic focus and recognition of specific epileptic syndromes) and for the intra-operative monitoring of global cerebral hypoxia. Activation procedures in clinical use include:

Hyperventilation for 3–4 minutes;

Natural sleep recording;

24 hour sleep deprivation;

Rhythmic photic stimulation with an electronic stroboscope.

Phases of the EEG

The following EEG phases have been recognised in sleep (a state of increased threshold of response to external stimuli):

Non-rapid eye movement, which involves the following stages:

Stage 1: low amplitude activity, associated with slow rolling eye movements;

Stage 2: sleep spindles (12 Hz); high-voltage discharges or K complexes;

Stage 3: high-voltage and very slow delta waves (1–4 Hz); occasional sleep spindles.

Rapid eye movement sleep, which is characterised by:

Low-voltage mixed-frequency desynchronised EEG pattern, as in the arousal pattern in awake subjects (paradoxical sleep);

3–5 Hz saw tooth waves;

Hippocampal sinusoidal waves at 5–10 Hz;

Phasic bursts of rapid conjugate eye movements;

Reduced or absent skeletal muscle tone;

The occurrence of dreams;

Hyperventilation, tachycardia and fluctuating blood pressure;

Penile erection.

EEG abnormalities

Electroencephalogram abnormalities are, broadly speaking, characterised as:

Focal arrhythmic slow activity;

Intermittent rhythmic slow waves;

General arrhythmic slow activity;

Voltage attenuation;

Epileptiform discharges.

■ Evoked potentials

Evoked potentials are potentials evoked by visual, somatosensory or auditory stimuli. Their production allows real time assessment of sensory information processing in the CNS. They are of two types:

Exogenous sensory, specific for a sensory modality;

Event-related endogenous or cognitive, not specific for a sensory modality.

Description of evoked potentials involves the following information:

The type of eliciting sensory stimulus;

Post-stimulus latency;

Wave amplitude;

The distance between the neural generator and the recording electrodes.

Somatosensory-evoked responses are generated by repetitive electrical stimulation of peripheral nerves.

Brain stem auditory-evoked responses are produced by repetitive auditory click stimulation through headphones or ear inserts.

Visual-evoked responses can be produced by either:

Unpatterned stimuli: stroboscopic flashes;

Patterned stimuli: specific patterns, e.g. checks or gratings.

Evoked potentials generally require enhancement by repetitive stimulation and signal averaging.

■ Autonomic nervous system

This represents the component of the nervous system that is not under voluntary control, innervating the viscera, cardiac and smooth muscle and secretory glands. It helps maintain internal homeostasis, controlling the gastrointestinal and genito-urinary tracts and the cardiovascular and respiratory systems. It regulates visceral, endocrine, immune, behavioural, body temperature and pain functions. The stress response is largely due to autonomic activation. The autonomic nervous system consists of an afferent limb, central integrated elements and an efferent limb.

It subserves the following specific **functions:**

Control of smooth muscle activity in blood vessels and viscera;

Innervation of muscle fibres in the heart and in the uterus;

Control of secretion from salivary, mucus-secreting and eccrine sweat glands;

Activity of the adrenal medulla;

Digestive and metabolic activity of the liver, gastrointestinal tract and the pancreas;

Transmission of visceral pain and organic visceral sensation, e.g. hunger, bladder and bowel fullness, nausea;

Motility of the gastrointestinal tract;

Sexual responses of the genitalia and reproductive organs.

In general, sympathetic and parasympathetic systems produce opposing effects on most viscera. In a few viscera they exert synergistic effects.

Components of the autonomic nervous system

The autonomic nervous system comprises:

Parasympathetic (cholinergic) system

Cranial outflow: 4 cranial nerves (III, VIII, IX, X)

Sacral outflow: S2, S3, S4 segments

Sympathetic (adrenergic) system

Thoracolumbar outflow: T1-L3 segments

Non-adrenergic non-cholinergic (NANC) system

These include the following neurotransmitter systems:

Purinergic: ATP; GABA

Peptidergic: neuropeptides

Nitrergic: nitric oxide

Serotoninergic

Dopaminergic

GABAergic

Enteric nervous system

The enteric nervous system represents collections of nerve plexuses, formed by neurons, axons and dendrites which surround the gastrointestinal tract, pancreas and biliary tract. It can be considered as 'the brain in the gut'. It comprises the myenteric plexus of Auerbach (between the longitudinal and circular smooth muscle layers of the external muscle coat) and the submucosal plexus of Meissner (between the submucosa and the muscularis propria). Fibres project to glands, visceral muscle cells and blood vessels. The system controls gastrointestinal motility, blood flow, water and electrolyte transport, acid secretion, and various local reflexes in the gastrointestinal tract by the generation of stereotyped patterns of electrical activity.

There are three types of component neurons: sensory, associative or interneurons and motor neurons. Motor neurons may be excitatory (parasympathetic postganglionic) or inhibitory (NANC system). The myenteric plexus primarily regulates motility and the submucosal plexus regulates absorption and secretion. Extrinsic nerves supplying the small intestine regulate or modulate the activity of the enteric nervous system.

The central autonomic network

This comprises nuclei within the brain stem and forebrain. The network controls preganglionic sympathetic and parasympathetic neuroendocrine, respiratory and sphincter motor neurons. It is characterised by reciprocal interconnections, parallel organisation, state-dependent activity and neurochemical complexity. The components include:

Insular, anterior cingulate and ventro-medial prefrontal cortices;

Central nucleus of amygdala;

Bed nucleus of the stria terminalis;

Periaqueductal grey matter;

Paraventricular and other hypothalamic nuclei;

Parabrachial nucleus;

Nucleus of the tractus solitarius;

Ventro-lateral and ventro-medial medulla;

Medullary lateral tegmental field: medullary reticular formation.

Components of the sympathetic system

Sympathetic preganglionic neurons:

T1–L2 segments of the intermediolateral cell column of grey matter contain the cell bodies;

The axons emerge through the ventral roots of T1–L2 with the axons of the somatic motor neurons.

Sympathetic chains: 24 pairs of paravertebral ganglia and their connecting trunks

Superior cervical ganglion: C1–C4

Middle cervical ganglion: C5–C6

Inferior cervical ganglion: C7–C8

Stellate: cervicothoracic: ganglion: inferior cervical ganglion fused with T1 or T1 and T2

Sympathetic plexuses

Thorax: cardiac; pulmonary

Abdomen: coeliac; pelvic

Sympathetic postganglionic fibres: small, unmyelinated C fibres

Spinal nerves

Cranial nerves

Arterial walls

Direct visceral nerves

Segmental distribution of sympathetic outflow:

C8–T4: head and neck

T1–T5: heart and lungs

T4–10: upper gastrointestinal tract

T12: lower gastrointestinal tract

T12–L2: pelvic genito-urinary organs

Adrenergic neurons are found in:

Postganglionic sympathetic neurons

Some interneurons
Certain central neurons

Components of the parasympathetic system

Parasympathetic preganglionic neurons:
  Brain stem: cranial outflow: III, VII, IX, X nerves
    Preganglionic fibres:
      Edinger–Westphal nucleus
      Superior and inferior salivatory nuclei
      Dorsal vagal nucleus
      Lacrimal nucleus
      Nucleus ambiguus
    Ganglion cells:
      Ciliary ganglion
      Pterygopalatine ganglion
      Submandibular ganglion
      Otic ganglion
Sacral spinal cord: S2–S4 segments of intermediolateral cell column

Neurotransmitters in the autonomic nervous system

  Acetylcholine: preganglionic sympathetic and parasympathetic neurons; post-ganglionic parasympathetic neurons; postganglionic sympathetic sudomotor fibres.
  Noradrenaline: postganglionic sympathetic neurons.

Neuropeptides and putative neurotransmitters coexist at the various levels of the autonomic nervous system, namely the central autonomic network, the spinal cord and both pre- and postganglionic terminals. They are involved in the regulation of visceral function, and in the modulation of integrated functions such as cognition, locomotion and pain.

Predominant autonomic tone

This varies according to the tissue under consideration:
  Arterioles: sympathetic adrenergic
  Veins: sympathetic adrenergic
  Heart: parasympathetic cholinergic
  Ciliary muscle: parasympathetic cholinergic
  Gastrointestinal tract: parasympathetic cholinergic
  Salivary glands: parasympathetic cholinergic
  Sweat glands: sympathetic cholinergic

Effects of stimulation of adrenergic receptors

Alpha

Arteriolar and venular constriction;

Iris dilatation;

Intestinal relaxation;

Intestinal sphincter contraction;

Pilomotor contraction;

Bladder sphincter contraction;

Contraction of the pregnant uterus;

Ejaculation of seminal fluid.

Beta: The beta receptor is a G-protein-coupled seven transmembrane span polypeptide.

Beta receptor numbers in tissues may decrease with chronic stimulation leading to desensitisation (down-regulation) or increase with chronic blockade (up-regulation).

Beta 1

Cardioacceleration: chronotropic effect

Increased myocardial contractility: positive inotropic effect

Lipolysis

Secretion of renin by the juxtaglomerular apparatus

The cardiac positive inotropic effects result from increased calcium concentration due to phosphorylation of L-type calcium channels and phosphorylation of sarcolemmal calcium pumps.

Beta 2

Vasodilatation

Intestinal relaxation

Uterine relaxation

Bronchodilatation

Calorigenesis

Bladder wall relaxation

Termination of catecholamine action at receptors

This is brought about by:

Reuptake into sympathetic nerve endings: stored and also subject to mono-amine oxidase (MAO) degradation;

Diffusion away from the junctional cleft;

Non-neuronal tissue uptake and enzymatic degradation by extra-neuronal MAO and catechol-O-methyl transferase (COMT) (gut, lung, liver, kidney)

The metabolic transformations undergone by catecholamines include:

Drugs acting on adrenergic receptors

Alpha 1 (postsynaptic)
Catecholamine agonists: dopamine; noradrenaline
Peripheral alpha 1-antagonist: prazosin

Alpha 2 (presynaptic)
Central alpha 2 agonist: clonidine

Beta 1 (predominantly cardiac)
Catecholamine agonists: noradrenaline; isoprenaline; dopamine; dobutamine
Cardioselective blockers: metoprolol; atenolol; acebutolol

Beta 2 (predominantly peripheral)
Catecholamine agonists: adrenaline; isoprenaline; dopexamine; dobutamine
Beta-adrenergic antagonists differ in the following ways:
Selectivity for beta 1 and beta 2 receptors;
Partial agonist activity;
Intrinsic sympathomimetic activity;
Possession of local anaesthetic or membrane-stabilising effects;
Central nervous system penetration.

3-O-methylation (COMT), with transformation into methoxyamines (meta-nephrine and normetanephrine);

Oxidative deamination (MAO) of catecholamines and methoxyamines into vanillylmandelic acid;

Conjugation with glucuronide or sulphate.

Classification of cholinergic receptors

Acetylcholine is an endogenous ligand for two major receptor populations differentiated by their response to the alkaloids nicotine and muscarine.

Nicotinic receptors (nicotine also acts on these receptors):

Autonomic ganglia

Skeletal muscle

Mucarinic receptors (muscarine, a quaternary amine alkaloid also acts on these receptors):

G-protein-linked receptors

M1: parasympathetic ganglia, nasal submucosal glands

M2: heart, postganglionic parasympathetic nerves

M3: airway smooth muscle, submucosal glands

M4: postganglionic cholinergic nerves; possible CNS

M5: possible CNS

Cholinergic nerves, where acetylcholine is the neurotransmitter, are found in:

All motor nerves innervating skeletal muscle;

All postganglionic parasympathetic nerves;

All preganglionic parasympathetic and sympathetic neurons, i.e. all autonomic ganglia;

Postganglionic sympathetic neurons innervating sweat glands and certain blood vessels;

Preganglionic sympathetic neurons innervating adrenal medulla;

Central cholinergic neurons.

Cholinergic-receptor antagonists

These can be classified as:

Anti-muscarinic (parasympatholytic)
Tertiary amines (blocking M1 and M2 receptors): atropine
Quaternary ammonium compounds: propantheline

Antinicotinic
Ganglion blockers
Neuromuscular blocking drugs
Depolarising: succinylcholine
Non-depolarising: d-tubocurarine, atracurium

Autonomic function tests

Sympathetic function
Blood pressure response to:
Head-up tilt or upright posture.
Cold pressor test: the systolic and diastolic blood pressures rise by 10–20 mm Hg with the immersion of one hand in cold water, when blood pressure is measured at 30 seconds and 1 minute.
Mental stress.
Isometric exercise, e.g. handgrip.
Plasma noradrenaline levels in response to head-up tilt or upright posture.

Parasympathetic function:
Beat-to-beat variation in heart rate with deep breathing (respiratory sinus arrhythmia). This can be achieved by R-R interval variability assessment (expiratory: inspiratory ratio). Power spectral analysis of continuous electrocardiographic (ECG) recordings allows determination of heart rate variability.

Sudomotor function
Galvanic skin-resistance test;
Thermoregulatory sweat tests;
Quantitative sudomotor axon reflex test, which involves ionotophoresis of acetylcholine.

Autonomic function testing

Valsalva manoeuvre

This entails forcible expiration against resistance, through a closed glottis. This is mimicked by heavy lifting or straining activities. A normal cardiovascular response involves:

Phase I: increased intrathoracic pressure with pressure on the aorta leading to a small sudden increase in arterial blood pressure.

Phase II: reduced venous return to the heart and reduced cardiac output, leading to a reduction in systolic and diastolic blood pressures and in pulse pressure.

Phase III: return to normal of the intrathoracic pressure, with a sudden transient fall in arterial blood pressure.

Phase IV: rebound and overshoot in systolic and diastolic blood pressures over the baseline level, with a compensatory reflex reduction in heart rate.

A normal response requires preserved baroreceptor reflexes, a functioning central control system, functioning efferent pathways to the heart and peripheral blood vessels and responsive effector organs.

The effects of autonomic neuropathy

These include:

Cardiovascular
Postural hypotension
Cardiac arrhythmia
Resting tachycardia
Loss of diurnal variation in blood pressure

Gastrointestinal
Early satiety
Nocturnal diarrhoea
Abdominal distension
Vomiting of undigested food

Genito-urinary
Feeling of incomplete bladder emptying
Chronic retention of urine with overflow incontinence
Male impotence (erectile dysfunction)
Retrograde ejaculation

Miscellaneous
Recurrent falls
Excessive sweating of the upper body
Sluggish pupillary reaction

■ Motor system

The motor system consists of:

Upper motor neurons, which are the neurons of primary motor, premotor and supplementary motor cortices;

Lower motor neurons, which include:

Alpha and gamma motor neurons of the anterior horn;

Intermediolateral column neurons of lateral horn;

Motor nuclei of III, IV,VI, XII nerves.

Anterior horn cell activity is modulated by the corticospinal (pyramidal) tracts, the extrapyramidal system (basal ganglia and cerebellum) and afferent fibres via the posterior spinal nerve roots.

A motor unit comprises a single anterior horn cell, its motor axon and the muscle fibres innervated by the axon, usually 100–200 in number.

Electromyogram

The **electromyogram** represents spatio-temporal summation of a quasi-random train of motor unit action potentials. Recording involves the use of monopolar or concentric bipolar needle electrodes.

Normal muscle in the resting state is essentially electrically silent but may demonstrate activity related to motor end-plate noise, motor end-plate spikes and insertional activity.

Abnormal electromyographic activity can be classified as:

At rest:

Increased insertional activity, with insertion and movement of the needle electrode

Fibrillation potentials;

Classification of somatic sensation

Epicritic (discriminative)
Fine touch
Joint sensation
Vibration
Two-point discrimination

Protopathic
Pain
Temperature
Crude touch

Fasciculation potentials;

Positive sharp waves;

Myotonic discharges: dive-bomber sound;

Coupled discharges: doublets, triplets and multiplets;

Motor unit action potentials.

With activity:

Motor unit potentials;

Abnormalities of recruitment patterns.

■ Sensory system and pain

Sensory unit

A **sensory unit** comprises a single afferent neuron, all its peripheral nerve endings (the receptive field) and all its ramifications in the CNS. In general, the receptive fields of sensory units overlap with each other.

Sensory receptors transduce environmental stimuli into depolarisation, whose magnitude is related to the intensity of the causative stimulus. Adaptation of receptors is produced by sustained depolarisation, which leads to a reduction in frequency of nerve action potentials generated by stimulation.

Pain

Pain is defined as an 'unpleasant sensory and emotional experience associated with actual or potential tissue damage or described in terms of such damage'(International Association for the Study of Pain, 1994). It is carried in Group A delta fibres (diameter: 2–5 μm), which are responsible for sharp, shooting, intense pain, and Group C fibres (diameter: < 2 μm), which convey steady, slow, constant pain.

Sensory receptors

Pain: free nerve endings
Touch: Meissner's corpuscles; Merkel's discs; hair cells
Cold: Krause's end bulbs
Heat: Ruffini's corpuscles

Sites:
Meissner's corpuscles: glabrous skin
Merkel's discs: all skin and hair follicles
Pacinian corpuscles: subcutaneous tissues, interosseous membranes, viscera

Pain is produced by a variety of mechanisms including:

Ischaemia;

Mechanical damage;

Thermal damage;

Spasm of smooth or striated muscle;

Dilatation of blood vessels at the base of the brain.

Visceral pain is produced by a variety of mechanisms including distension, spasm or contraction, torsion, ischaemia, chemical irritation, and inflammation. The characteristics are:

Poor localisation;

Usually dull and aching, occasional colicky, character;

Associated autonomic symptoms;

Often referred to other parts of the body.

Referred pain is perceived as arising from somatic structures that share an embryologically common spinal segmental origin with the injured viscus.

Pain perception

The perception of and responses to pain comprise the following steps:

Transduction: detection of noxious chemical, mechanical and thermal stimuli by nociceptive receptors, with conversion to a neural response. Nociceptors are specialised nerve endings that respond to high threshold noxious stimuli and generally serve a protective function.

Transmission to the CNS by nociceptive fibres, which terminate primarily in laminae I (marginal zone) and II (substantia gelatinosa) of the superficial dorsal horn of the spinal cord.

Modulation by descending inhibitory responses from the periaqueductal grey matter, nucleus raphe, and reticular formation of the brain stem. These inhibitory pathways descend in the dorso-lateral funiculus to the dorsal horn. The **gate control** represents control of pain perception by the levels of activity in both nociceptive and non-nociceptive afferent fibres. Anti-nociception is mediated by adrenergic, serotoninergic, GABAergic and opioid mechanisms.

Perception as pain.

Pain modulation is a composite of:

Ascending excitatory afferent pain pathways;

Descending inhibitory pain pathways;

Neuromodulation;

Neurotransmitters.

Nociceptor responses may be altered in pathological pain states by the following mechanisms:

Reduced threshold for activation;

Increased receptive field;

Response to normally non-noxious stimuli (allodynia);

Increased intensity of response to noxious stimuli (hyperalgesia);

Prolonged post-stimulus sensation: hyperpathia;

Emergence of spontaneous activity.

Pain pathways

Broadly speaking, the pathways involved in pain perception involve:

The spinal cord–thalamic–somatosensory cortex pathway, which mediates the sensation of pain;

The descending inhibitory pathway, which modulates the pain sensation;

The spinal cord–thalamic–frontal cortex–anterior cingulate gyrus pathway, which is involved with the subjective psychological and physiological response secondary to pain.

Pain pathway to the CNS

Pain fibres enter the spinal cord in the medial portion of the dorsal roots of spinal nerves. They enter in the dorsilateral funiculus, just dorsal to dorsal grey horn. Descending collaterals travel for one to two cord segments in the dorsilateral funiculus as the tract of Lissauer. The main group of fibres ascend in the tract of Lissauer for two cord segments before entering the dorsal horn to synapse in cells in laminae II, III, IV and V on a group of neurons called the nucleus proprius. The Rexed laminae II and III correspond to the substantia gelatinosa. A delta fibres synapse in laminae IV and V, and C fibres in laminae I and II.

The axons of the cells in the nucleus proprius travel across the midline of the cord in the ventral grey and white commissure just below the central canal of the spinal cord. They pass to the ventro-lateral portion of the contralateral lateral funiculus, where they form the ventral and lateral spinothalamic tracts. The lateral spinothalamic tract is topographically laminated.

The neurotransmitters involved predominantly are:

A delta sensory afferents: excitatory amino acids (aspartate and glutamate) and ATP;

C afferents: substance P.

The descending pain inhibitor system comprises the periaqueductal grey matter, the rostral ventro-medial medulla, and the dorsal lateral pontine tegmentum.

Gate control theory

Gating refers to an inhibitory effect on impulse transmission by other sensory modalities, which explains the analgesic effects of counterirritation or transcutaneous electrical nerve stimulation. The substantia gelatinosa in the tip of the dorsal horn of the spinal cord (Rexed's laminae I–III) functions as a gate-controlling mechanism.

The gate can be closed by non-painful sensory input carried by large myelinated A beta fibres from mechanoreceptors responding to low-threshold stimuli. Myelinated non-nociceptive A alpha and A beta fibres (subserving touch and

Components of the spinothalamic pathway

Dorsal horn of the spinal grey matter
Ventral white commissure
Spinothalamic tract
Spinal lemniscus
Reticulothalamic fibres
Ventral posterolateral nucleus of the thalamus
Internal capsule
Primary somatosensory cortex

Components of the medial lemniscal system

Posterior column
Dorsal column nuclei
Gracile and cuneate nuclei
Medial lemniscus
Ventral posteromedial nucleus of thalamus
Internal capsule
Primary somatosensory cortex

Neurotransmitters involved in nociception

Amines: noradrenaline; serotonin
Endogenous opioid peptides: enkephalins; beta-endorphins; dynorphins
Non-opioid peptides: substance P; angiotensin II; vasoactive intestinal peptide (VIP); cholecystokinin (CCK); oxytocin
Excitatory amino acids: glutamate; aspartate
Inhibitory amino acids: GABA; glycine
Nitric oxide

Table 9.3 Endogenous opioid peptides

Precursor peptide	Opioid peptide	Active receptor	Antagonists
Proenkephalin A	leu-enkephalin	delta, mu	naloxone
	met-enkephalin	delta, mu	naloxone
Proenkephalin B	dynorphin	kappa	nalmefene
	dynorphin A(1–8)	mu	naloxone
Pro-opiomelanocortin	beta-endorphin	mu, delta, kappa	naloxone

proprioception) exert inhibitory control on small unmyelinated C afferent fibres. This is brought about by postsynaptic inhibition of the dorsal horn neurons, mediated by inhibitory interneurons. Central descending control of the gating system is achieved primarily through the descending inhibitory or endorphin-mediated analgesia system.

Endogenous opioids

Endogenous opioids are the naturally occurring ligands for the opioid receptors and share a common five amino acid (tetrapeptide) sequence at the amino-terminus of the molecule. They act mainly at nerve synapses, acting as neurotransmitters on interaction with postsynaptic interactors by modulating trans-synaptic membrane potential. At presynaptic receptors they function as neuromodulators, modulating the release of other neurotransmitters.

Endogenous opioids and their inactive precursor proendorphin peptides can be classified as:

Pro-opio-melanocortin (POMC): beta-endorphin. The other members of the POMC family are alpha-melanocyte stimulating hormone (alpha-MSH), adrenocorticotrophin (ACTH) and beta-lipotropin.

Proenkephalin A: methionine-enkephalin; leucine-enkephalin.

Proenkephalin B (prodynorphin): alpha-neo endorphin, beta-neo endorphin, and dynorphin.

The functions of endogenous opioids include:

Spinal cord: pain modulation

Brain stem: vomiting; respiratory depression

Limbic system: euphoria

Hypothalamus: rise in growth hormone (GH) and prolactin (PRL), reduction in thyroid stimulating hormone (TSH), follicle stimulating hormone (FSH) and luteinising hormone (LH)

Gastrointestinal tract: reduction in gut motility

Opioid receptors

These have been characterised on the basis of selectivity of different agonists for different physiological responses. They are G-protein-linked seven transmembrane spanning receptors, which inhibit adenyl cyclase. They include:

Mu (morphine, endorphin, enkephalins): opioid analgesics bind predominantly to these receptors, which are involved in analgesia, respiratory depression, reduced gastrointestinal motility, euphoria, itching. Physical dependence and tolerance characterise these effects.

Delta (enkephalins): analgesia without respiratory depression.

Kappa (dynorphin): analgesia, miosis, dysphoria, agitation, sedation

Sigma

Epsilon

Opioid receptors inhibit signal conduction in the nociceptive pathway. Prevention of calcium influx at presynaptic calcium channels inhibits the release of, and response to, neurotransmitters. Furthermore, activation of potassium channels causes hyperpolarisation of the postsynaptic membrane inhibiting response to neurotransmitters.

■ Skeletal muscle structure

Each skeletal muscle fibre is surrounded by endomysium. Bundles of up to 150 fibres, fasciculi, are surrounded by perimysium. The entire muscle is surrounded by epimysium.

Sarcotubular functional proteins

Slow or L-type calcium channel: dihydropyridine receptor, which has five subunits.

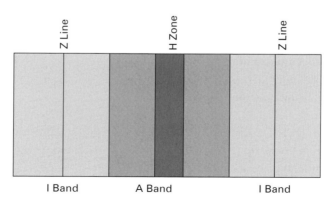

Figure 9.6 Myofibril structure at sarcomere level.

Myofibril structure

Anisotropic (A) bands: overlapping myosin and actin
Isotropic (I) bands: actin
H zone: myosin
Z lines
M lines
The sarcomere extends from Z line to Z line

Structural proteins of the sarcomere

Myofibrils: titin; nebulin
Z lines: desmin; alpha-actin
M lines: myomecin; M protein
Thick filaments: myosin
C stripes: C protein
Thin filaments: alpha-actin; tropomyosin; troponin

Pathophysiology of malignant hyperpyrexia

Impaired calcium binding to sarcoplasmic reticulum;
Increased calcium level in skeletal muscle myoplasm;
Hyperpyrexia, metabolic acidosis and muscle rigidity.

Calcium release channel: ryanodine receptor.
Proteins modulating calcium release channels: calmodulin; FK506-binding protein.
Calcium pump: Ca^{2+}-ATPase.
Proteins modulating calcium pump: phospholamban; sarcolipin.
Integral membrane proteins of the sarcoplasmic reticulum: junctin; triadin; myotonin kinase; calmodulin-dependent protein kinase.
Luminal proteins of the sarcoplasmic reticulum: calsequestrin; calreticulin; histidine-rich calcium-binding protein; sarcolumenin.

Myosin

Myosin is a protein with a molecular weight of 520 kDa. It consists of 6 polypeptide chains, which consist of two identical heavy chains of 220 kDa each, two pairs of light chains of 20 kDa each and a globular cross-bridge head and rod-like tail. The head has a site for binding ATP and also contains an ATPase enzyme.

Limited proteolysis with trypsin results in dissociation into two fragments, light meromyosin and heavy meromyosin. Heavy meromyosin can be further split into two identical globular subfragments and one rod-shaped subfragment by papain. It has ATPase activity.

The biological activities of myosin can be categorised as:

Myosin molecules spontaneously assemble into filaments in solutions of physiological ionic strength and pH.

It acts as an ATPase, hydrolysing ATP to ADP and Pi, being activated when the myosin head binds to actin. This provides the free energy for contraction.

It binds to the polymerised form of actin (F-actin), the major constituent of thin filaments.

Muscle contraction

Excitation–contraction coupling

This refers to the chain of events that intervene between membrane depolarisation and contractile activation. The sequence of events is as follows:

- The detection of transverse tubular membrane depolarisation by a voltage sensor.
- The voltage sensing event is coupled to the intra-cellular release of stored calcium from the terminal cisternae of the transverse tubular system of the sarcoplasmic reticulum. The T-tubules contain voltage-gated Ca^{2+} channels, sometimes called dihydropyridine receptors. The major channel protein is the L-type channel protein.
- The released calcium ions undergo allosteric binding to the regulatory protein troponin and initiate mechanical activity, by removing the inhibitory action of the troponin-tropomyosin complex on the actin-myosin interaction. This causes conformational change in the thin (actin) filament. When calcium binds to troponin, this moves the tropomyosin threads sideways into the groove between the two F-actin chains, thereby uncovering the active binding sites on actin.
- Uncovering of active sites on thin (actin) filaments allows attachment of the myosin heads of the cross-bridges. When the previously activated cross-bridges attach to actin they undergo conformational change. A power stroke causes pulling (sliding) of the thin filaments over the thick filaments.
- Attachment of fresh ATP allows the cross-bridges to detach from actin, with dissociation of the actin-myosin complexes, and to repeat the contraction cycle as long as Ca^{2+} remains attached to troponin.
- Relaxation results from calcium reuptake into the sarcoplasmic reticulum by active transport through a membrane Ca^{2+}-ATPase. The ATPase is activated

by the binding of actin to myosin. The thin filament returns to a configuration in which further cross-bridge cycles are inhibited.

Summary of the sliding filament theory

Muscle shortening is accomplished by the cyclical formation and dissociation of cross-bridges between thick and thin filaments. The thin filament mainly contains actin (and tropomyosin) and the thick filament is mainly myosin.

The thick and thin filaments do not change in length.

The thick and thin filaments slide past each other, shortening the sarcomere.

The sizes of the H^+ zone and the I band are seen to decrease. The Z lines come closer together (shortening of sarcomeres), but the A band remains unaffected.

Adjacent A bands are pulled closer together as the I bands between them shorten.

The cross-bridge detaches from the thin filament.

The cross-bridge returns to its original upright position.

Muscle metabolic systems

Phosphagen system

Glycogen–lactic acid system

Aerobic system

Adenosine s'-triphosphate is needed for both contraction and relaxation of muscle:

Hydrolysis of APT provides energy for movement of cross-bridges between actin and myosin, so that these filaments slide upon each other, bringing the Z lines together and shortening the sarcomere.

Adenosine s'-triphosphate is needed for breakdown of the low-energy actin–myosin complex or rigor complex. Occupation by APT of the vacant site on the myosin head triggers detachment of myosin from actin.

Adenosine s'-triphosphate is used for pumping Ca^{2+} back into the sarcoplasmic reticulum, promoting muscle relaxation.

Skeletal muscle fibres

Classification depends on:

Maximal velocities of shortening: fast and slow. Fast fibres readily fatigue, while slow fibres can maintain smooth tetanic contractions for long periods of time.

Major pathway used to form ATP: oxidative and glycolytic.

Based on the above properties, the following types can be identified:

Slow-oxidative (type I): low myosin ATPase activity; high oxidative capacity

Table 9.4 Skeletal muscle cell types (based on the time between the occurrence of the muscle action fibre potential and the peak of the resulting tension)

	Fast twitch	Slow twitch
Vmax	High	Low
Myosin ATPase activity	High	Low
Glycolytic metabolism	High	Low
Oxidative metabolism	Low	High
Mitochondrial content	Low	High
Myoglobin content	Low	High

Fast-oxidative (type IIa): high myosin ATPase activity; high oxidative capacity

Fast-glycolytic (type IIb): high myosin ATPase activity; high glycolytic capacity

Type I fibres predominate in muscles depending on sustained tone, e.g. postural muscles, and are fatigue-resistant. On the other hand, type II fibres predominate in muscles used for rapid movement and fatigue rapidly from lactic acid accumulation.

Muscle fatigue is related to a reduction in glycogen content of muscle fibres, oxygen lack associated with increased blood and muscle lactic acid levels and fatigue at the neuromuscular junction.

Types of muscle contraction

Isometric

Length of muscle remains constant;

Tension in the muscle increases.

Isotonic

The tension in the muscle remains constant and equals the weight of the load against which the muscle is contracting;

The muscle shortens in length.

The force of muscle contraction is proportional to the physiological cross-sectional area, i.e. the sum of the areas of each fibre in the muscle. The velocity of muscle contraction is proportional to muscle fibre length.

Muscle tension

This depends on:

The tension developed by each individual fibre, which depends on:

Action potential frequency (frequency–tension relationship);

Fibre length (length–tension relationship);

Fibre diameter;

Fatigue.

The number of:

Active fibres;

Fibres per motor unit;

Active motor units.

The smallest motor units have the lowest thresholds for stimulation and the largest motor units have the highest, being recruited only for maximal force of contraction (the size principle of the motor neuron). Individual motor units thus fire asynchronously. Spatial summation refers to an incr-eased number of motor units contracting simultaneously, while temporal summation refers to an increased frequency of contraction of individual motor units.

Exercise training

The **adaptations of skeletal muscle with exercise training** involve:

Increased amounts of enzymes involved in beta oxidation, Krebs cycle meta-bolism and the electron transport chain;

Improved fatty acid transport through the sarcolemma, the plasma membrane of the muscle fibre;

Improved transport of fatty acids within the muscle cell by the action of carnitine and carnitine transferase;

Proliferation of capillaries, represented by an increase in numbers and in their density.

Effects of endurance training

Improved ability to obtain ATP from oxidative phosphorylation;

Increased size and number of mitochondria;

Less lactic acid produced per given amount of exercise;

Increased myoglobin content;

Increased intramuscular triglyceride content;

Increased lipoprotein lipase;

Increased proportion of energy derived from fat, less from carbohydrate;

Lower rate of glycogen depletion during exercise;

Improved efficiency in extracting oxygen from blood;

Decreased number of type IIb fibres; increased number of type IIa fibres.

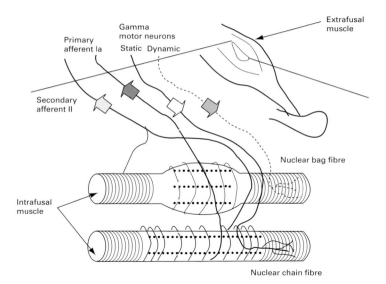

Figure 9.7 Muscle spindle.

■ Muscle spindle

The muscle spindle is a complex, spindle shaped, encapsulated receptor. It monitors muscle length (nuclear chain fibres) and the rate of change of length, i.e. velocity of shortening (nuclear bag fibres). It is a stretch receptor for myotactic reflexes.

The muscle spindle maintains muscles at their most efficient length under variable loads through the gamma loop, which determines muscle tone. Gamma motor neurons control contraction of intrafusal muscle fibres, which are responsible for muscle spindle sensitivity. Spindles are abundant in the anti-gravity muscles, muscles of the neck and in the intrinsic hand muscles.

The **components of a muscle spindle** are:

Fibres:
    Intrafusal: nuclear bag fibres (2–5)
      nuclear chain fibres (6–10)
    Extrafusal
Sensory endings:
    Primary, or annulospiral: responds to both phasic and static stretching; wrap
      around the central regions of the nuclear bag and chain fibres.

Secondary, or flower-spray: responds to static stretch; relatively insensitive to phasic stretch; located over the contracting poles of the nuclear chain fibres.

Spindle afferents inhibit the alpha motor neurons to antagonist muscles via inhibitory internuncial neurons.

Motor nerve supply:

Gamma efferents of Leksell (small motor nerve system).

The gamma motor neuron regulates the sensitivity of the sensory endings to applied stretch.

Two histological types of gamma efferent fibre endings:

Motor end-plate (plate endings on nuclear bag fibres);

Trail endings on nuclear chain fibres.

Two kinds of sensory nerve patterns:

Dynamic;

Static.

The **Renshaw internuncial neuron** or Renshaw cell is a short interneuron in the cord, which is activated by a recurrent collateral from an alpha motor neuron. It synapses with and inhibits other motor neurons. Its system constitutes a feedback loop. The process by which a physiological mechanism controls itself by feeding back information that reflexly governs the action is called a servomechanism.

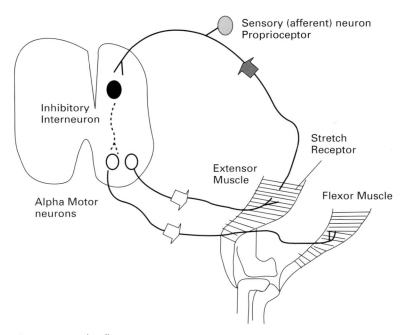

Figure 9.8 Stretch reflex

The **Golgi tendon organ** at the musculotendinous junction comprises collagenous fibres parallel to the extrafusal muscle fibres. Axons from these organs contact inhibitory interneurons in the spinal cord that synapse with alpha motor neurons innervating the same muscle. The circuit is thus a negative feedback system regulating muscle tension.

■ Vision

Structural features of the eye

The eye has three coats:

An outer fibrous layer: the cornea, sclera and the lamina cribrosa.

A middle vascular layer (uveal tract): the iris, ciliary body and choroid. The ciliary body secretes aqueous humour, which is iso-osmotic with plasma, and constitutes the blood–aqueous barrier. The ciliary muscle allows accommodation of vision by producing changes in lens shape.

An inner nervous layer: the retinal pigmented epithelium and the neuroretina (photoreceptors – rods and cones; and retinal neurons). The retinal pigmented epithelium is involved in photoreceptor renewal and in the scavenging of free radicals.

Optical characteristics of the eye

The eye can be considered optically as a positive double-lens arrangement that casts a real image on a light-sensitive surface, the retina. The lens system comprises:

The anterior corneal surface (cornea–air interface), with $+43$ dioptres (D). It has a fixed focal length.

The anterior and posterior surfaces of the lens, with $+15$ D in the accommodated eye.

The iris controls light entry to the retina and reduces intra-ocular light scatter.

The lens has the following properties:

Transparency.

Lamellar structure.

Pliability.

Variation in refractive index from the inner core (lower) to the less dense cortex (higher), constituting a gradient-index system (gradient in the index of refraction).

An adjustable focal length to allow for focussing on objects at different distances. This accommodation is achieved by alteration in shape of the lens,

Refractive defects

Myopia (near-sightedness)
Lengthening of the antero-posterior axis of the eye;
Corrected by placement of a diverging or negative lens in front of the eye.

Hypermetropia (long-sightedness)
Shortening of the antero-posterior axis of the eye;
Corrected by placing a converging or positive lens in front of the eye.

Astigmatism
Due to uneven curvature of the cornea;
Different focal lengths for light rays striking the eye at different planes;
Corrected by cylindrical or sphero-cylindrical (toric) lenses.

produced by the ciliary muscles attaching to the peripheral suspensory ligament. Ciliary muscle relaxation causes flattening of the lens, increasing its focal length. Focussing on a closer object is achieved by ciliary muscle contraction. The closest point on which the eye can focus is the near point. The amplitude of accommodation decreases with age (presbyopia).

Overall, the **refractive power of the eye** depends on:

The refractive power of the cornea, which in turn depends upon its shape;

The depth of the anterior chamber;

The refractive power of the crystalline lens;

The axial length of the eye.

The eye consists of **three compartments:**

The anterior chamber. This contains aqueous humour, which is secreted by the ciliary body into the posterior chamber (between the iris and the lens) and flows through the pupil into the anterior chamber. The fluid is absorbed into the trabecular meshwork, the uveoscleral system and into the episcleral blood vessels. The normal intra-ocular pressure is 10–21 mm Hg.

The posterior chamber.

The vestibular chamber.

There is a protective tear film in front of the eye, comprising an oily surface layer, an aqueous layer and a deep mucoid layer. The pre-corneal tear film has the following properties:

Lubrication of the eyelids;

Smoothening of the optical surface;

Nutrient transfer to the corneal epithelium;

Dilution and removal of irritants;

Antibacterial activity: secretory IgA.

Blood–eye barrier

The **blood–eye barrier** consists of the blood–aqueous and the blood–retinal barriers.

The blood–aqueous barrier is comprised of:

The non-pigmented layer of the ciliary body epithelium;

The endothelium of the blood vessels of the iris.

The blood–retinal barrier is comprised of:

Tight junctions between endothelial cells of the retinal vessels;

Tight junctions in the retinal pigment epithelium.

Eye movements

Four **eye movement systems** determine movements of the eyes at different speeds and in different systems:

The smooth pursuit system, which allows the slow tracking of a moving object.

The saccadic system, which allows fast conjugate eye movements that change the optical axis of the eye from one point of fixation to another with maximal speed.

The vestibular system, which allows eye movements that compensate for head movements.

The vergence system, which allows co-ordinated movement of the two eyes on an approaching or retreating object. This is achieved by changing the visual axes of the eyes relative to each other.

Nystagmus can be described as a rhythmic alteration between saccadic movements and slow pursuit movements.

Visual cycle

The **visual cycle** involves the following mechanisms:

- Retinal rods and cones are photoreceptor cells specialised for the transduction of light stimuli into nerve impulses.

The extra-ocular muscles

These subserve the following primary eye movements:

Lateral rectus:	abduction
Medial rectus:	adduction
Superior rectus:	elevation
Inferior rectus:	depression
Superior oblique:	intorsion
Inferior oblique:	extorsion

- The peripheral retina has more rods and fewer cones. The fovea has no rods, only cones which are densely packed, and is specialised for high-resolution vision.
- The functional regions of the rods and cones include:
  An outer segment specialised for photo-transduction;
  An inner segment with nucleus and most of its biosynthetic machinery: ion pumps, transporters, ribosomes, mitochondria, endoplasmic reticulum;
  A synaptic terminal that makes contact with the photoreceptor's target cells;
  A stalk or cilium connects outer and inner segments;
  Photo-transduction results from a cascade of biochemical events in the outer segment of the photoreceptors.
- Cones detect bright light and colour and provide high resolution. Each cone cell has one of three different colour-sensitive pigments: blue: 430 nm; green: 540 nm; red: 575 nm.
- Rods perceive dim light but do not detect colour, being responsible for black and white vision. They also help in the recognition of movement.
- The disc membrane is rich in rhodopsin, an integral seven transmembrane span protein. Rhodopsin contains 11-cis-retinal, a chromophore, as a prosthetic group, which forms a Schiff base with a free amino group. Retinal, the aldehyde of vitamin A, is the light-sensitive pigment. The discs are loaded with guanosine 3'-5'-monophosphate (cyclic GMP). The inner segment contains the Na^+ pump that is essential in generation of the resting potential.
- The chromophore 11-cis-retinal absorbs light in the visible range (400–700 nm). When one photon of the appropriate energy is captured by 11-cis-retinal, the configuration is changed to 11-trans-retinal by an isomerisation process.
- 11-trans-retinal cannot form a stable complex with rhodopsin. As a result, free 11-trans-retinal and **opsin** (rhodopsin minus retinal) are formed.
- An intermediate, meta-rhodopsin II binds to and activates **transducin**, a G-protein, facilitating a GDP-GTP exchange. The alpha subunit of transducin exchanges its bound GDP for GTP and dissociates from the beta and gamma subunits.
- The free $T\alpha$ -GTP activates a specific cyclic nucleotide **phosphodiesterase**, which catalyses the hydrolysis of cyclic GMP to 5'-GMP.
- In the dark or resting state, cyclic GMP is known to bind to cyclic nucleotide-gated Na^+-channels in the plasma membrane of the rod and stimulates their opening. This causes release of an inhibitory neurotransmitter from their synaptic terminals.
- The decrease in concentration of intracellular cyclic GMP effected by phosphodiesterase activity ensures that it dissociates from the channels, allowing

them to close and causing a hyperpolarisation of rod plasma membrane. Hence the light stimulus has been converted into a nervous electric signal.

- The system is desensitised to allow further photons to be detected because closure of the Na^+-channel prevents entry of Ca^{2+}, to which the Na^+ channel is also permeable.
- The consequent decrease in cytosolic Ca^{2+} concentration ensures its release from the Ca^{2+}-binding protein recoverin.
- The Ca^{2+}-free recoverin stimulates guanyl cyclase, promoting cyclic GMP formation and opening of cyclic GMP-gated channels.
- Changes in intracellular Ca^{2+} underlie light adaptation in the photoreceptors.

Central visual pathways

- The retinal image is an inversion of the visual field. The visual field is what each eye sees.
- Partial decussation of optic nerve fibres in the optic chiasm leads to each optic tract consisting of fibres arising in the temporal retina of the ipsilateral eye and fibres arising in the nasal retina of the contralateral eye.
- The pretectal area of the midbrain controls the pupillary reflexes.
- The superior colliculus controls saccadic eye movements.
- The lateral geniculate nucleus in the thalamus possesses visual information. Neurons in the lateral geniculate nucleus have concentric receptive fields.
- There is point-to-point representation of the retina in the visual cortex, which can be described as being retinotopically mapped.
- The primary visual cortex transforms concentric receptive fields into linear segments and boundaries.
- The primary visual cortex is functionally organised into narrow vertical columns of cells that run from the pial surface to the white matter. These columns subserve a variety of functions: ocular dominance, specific line orientation, direction of movement, spatial frequency and image disparity.

    The most effective stimulus shapes are slits, dark bars, and edges. The cortical columns represent cells with the same receptive-field axis of orientation).
- The columnar units are linked by horizontal connections.

Pupillary light reflex

Pupil size is determined by the balance between sympathetic and parasympathetic innervation of the iris musculature. Pupillary constriction occurs in response to light. The pathway for the reflex involved includes:

An **afferent limb**:

Fibres originate in retinal receptor cells and pass through bipolar cells. They synapse with retinal ganglion cells. Axons of these cells run in the optic nerve and tract. Light reflex fibres leave the optic nerve just rostral to the lateral geniculate body and enter the high midbrain, where they synapse in the pretectal nucleus.

Intercalated neurons give rise to pupilloconstrictor (parasympathetic) fibres, which pass ventrally to the ipsilateral Edinger-Westphal nucleus, some fibres crossing the posterior commissure to the contralateral Edinger–Westphal nucleus.

An **efferent limb**:

There is an efferent two neuron pathway from the Edinger–Westphal nucleus to the pupillary sphincter. Fibres travel in the third nerve and synapse in the ciliary ganglia. Short ciliary nerves supply the ciliary muscles and sphincter pupillae.

Afferent limb lesions do not cause anisocoria. The swinging light test is needed to detect a relative afferent pupillary defect.

Efferent limb lesions cause anisocoria, with a larger pupil on the affected side. A pupil size greater than 4 mm is regarded as being dilated. Physiological anisocoria is usually associated with a difference in pupil size not greater than 1 mm.

■ Hearing

Functions of the ear

Outer ear

The concha forms a resonant cavity which increases sound pressure;
Assists in the localisation of the source of sound, monoaural (vertical plane) and binaural (horizontal plane);
Boosts or amplifies high-frequency sounds;
Protects the middle and inner ears.

Middle ear

The middle ear acts as an acoustic impedance transformer, reducing the reflection of sound energy. It couples the large, low-impedance tympanic membrane to the smaller, higher-impedance oval window. Acoustic impedance refers to the ratio of sound pressure to volume velocity in a transmitting medium.

This transformer function is achieved by:

The smaller area of the stapes footplate and oval window, when compared with the tympanic membrane. The area ratio between the tympanic membrane and the oval window is about 30 to 1.

The lever action of the ossicles, the stiffness of which is controlled by the stapedius and tensor tympani muscles. Contraction of the stapedius muscle pulls the stapes in a direction perpendicular to its normal motion, reducing the amplitude of motion of the stapes. This protects the inner ear from acoustic damage.

The buckling motion of the tympanic membrane. Contraction of the tensor tympani muscle pulls the tympanic membrane inwards.

Inner ear

The inner ear performs frequency analysis of the incoming sounds. The spectral components of a complex sound are separated along the basilar membrane according to their frequency. Each frequency attains its maximal amplitude at a different location on the basilar membrane, the highest frequencies at the base of the cochlea and the lowest at its apex.

Mechanical vibration is converted into electrical energy by the sensory-specific transducing cells of the organ of Corti, the hair cells.

Amplification mechanisms for sound may produce an effective amplification of around 180:

  × 2: pinna and external auditory canal
  × 30: tympanic membrane
  × 3: ossicles

Hearing process

Sound is produced by vibrations resulting in alternating compression and rarefaction of the surrounding air. It is transmitted through the air by a longitudinal pressure wave, in which particles in the medium execute an oscillatory motion parallel to the direction of travel of the wave. The amplitude of the waves is correlated with the loudness of the sound. The frequency (measured in cycles per second or hertz) is the number of times a cycle of compression and rarefaction occurs in one second. The higher the frequency, the higher the pitch of the sound.

Auditory stimuli are transmitted through the tympanic membrane. Amplification is achieved by a chain of small bones, the ossicles, which form a system of pistons and levers. This system matches the impedance of air to that of the cochlea. The malleus and incus act as a lever pivoting on an axis of rotation as a combined unit, concentrating on the footplate of the stapes, which transmits sound to the oval window. Two muscles are attached to the ossicles, the tensor tympani and the stapedius. The wave is transmitted to the round window.

Transmission to the endolymph of the internal ear follows, with conversion into vibrations of this fluid (generation of fluid pressure waves). The organ of Corti rests on basilar membrane in the scala media. Multiple rows of outer hair cells are separated by the columns of Corti from a single row of inner hair cells. The hair cells are the basic physiological unit of the cochlea. Inner hair cells are responsible for the signalling of sound, and the outer hair cells regulate the sensitivity of the cochlea.

Transduction of auditory stimuli into nerve impulses is achieved by the hair cells of the ciliated cells covering the internal ear cavities. The differential pressure between the scala vestibuli and scala tympani is converted into oscillatory movements of the basilar membrane. The basilar membrane of the cochlea vibrates and the crest of the ciliated or hair cells in the organ of Corti is displaced. The progressive travelling wave passes up the cochlea from base to apex. This displacement is accompanied by opening of specific K^+ channels. Potassium ion is the most abundant cation in endolymph, and its entry produces depolarisation of the ciliated cell, as opposed to Na^+ entry as is usually the case. There is a steep potassium gradient and electrical potential gradient across the upper surface of the inner hair cell and its stereocilia.

Depolarisation causes opening of Ca^{2+} channels in the basal part of the cell. Entry of Ca^{2+} triggers fusion of synaptic vesicles with a domain of the plasma membrane of the cell, close to the neuron.

Different regions of the cochlea respond selectively to different frequencies of sound (tonotopic response). The non-linearity of the cochlear response leads to the phenomena of two-tone suppression (reduction in response to one stimulus produced by a second stimulus) and to the generation of combination tones in response to two-tone stimuli. The hair cell vibrations are transformed into electrical signals in the auditory nerve. Auditory nerve fibres near the base of the cochlea respond to high-frequency sounds and those near the apex respond to lower-frequency sounds. The action potential in the neuron is transmitted to the brain where it is interpreted as sound. The human cochlea has 3500 hair cells and 30 000 nerve fibres.

Central auditory neurons are specialised to preserve time and frequency information. Frequency discrimination is the result of temporal coding of sounds in the discharges of auditory nerve fibres. Extraction of vowels, consonants and words from the auditory input occurs in higher language areas.

Testing of hearing

Subjective tests

Tuning fork tests

Rinne's test:

Air conduction > bone conduction in the normal ear and in the ear with sensorineural hearing loss.

Bone conduction> air conduction in the ear with conductive hearing loss.

Weber's test: localisation of the sound to the affected ear occurs with conductive hearing loss; and localisation of the sound to the unaffected ear occurs with sensorineural hearing loss.

Pure tone audiogram.

Objective tests

Electrical response audiometry.

Impedance audiometry (tympanometry).

Otoacoustic emissions: sounds generated by normal outer hair cells that can be recorded in the external auditory canal. They are either spontaneous or evoked by external auditory stimuli.

Acoustic reflex threshold.

Speech recognition threshold.

Speech recognition.

Brain stem auditory evoked potentials.

Electrocochleography.

Audiometry

This tests the threshold for the detection of sounds. The following are normally measured:

Air conduction threshold;

Bone conduction threshold;

Speech reception threshold;

Discrimination scores.

Special tests include:

Tone decay

Speech increment sensitivity

Binaural loudness balance

The loudness of sound is measured on the **decibel scale**, which:

Is logarithmic and non-linear;

Involves a ratio of two sounds;

Uses different reference levels including sound pressure, intensity, hearing and sensation levels;

Has the just noticeable difference in intensity between two sounds as around one decibel;

Has a frequency scale is that based on the musical scale, or octave, a logarithmic scale with a base of two.

■ Vestibular function

Inner ear

The labyrinth lies in the otic capsule in the petrous temporal bone.

The otic capsule consists of three chambers:

The cochlea anteriorly. This is constituted by a spiral of two and a half turns.

The posterior vestibular apparatus, consisting of saccule, utricle and semicircular canals or ducts. These vestibular end organs respond to hair cell movement.

The posterior vestibular chamber. The semicircular canals communicate with this chamber through five round openings.

These chambers of the membranous labyrinth are surrounded by perilymph and are suspended by fine connective tissue strands from the bony labyrinth. Perilymph is continuous with cerebrospinal fluid in the subarachnoid space. The membranous labyrinth contains endolymph. This is formed by the secretory cells of the stria vascularis of the cochlea. It has a high potassium content (145 mmol/l) and a low sodium content (5 mmol/l).

The perilymph has a composition similar to the extracellular fluid and the cerebrospinal fluid. The endolymph resembles intracellular fluid. The two labyrinthine fluids do not mix.

Vestibular apparatus

The spatial orientation of the components of the vestibular apparatus allows analysis of movement. The apparatus comprises:

The **semicircular canals** (pair of lateral or horizontal, anterior), which comprise three pairs orthogonally oriented (i.e. at right angles to each other in the three planes of space) with respect to one another. This orientation allows for maximal detection of movement in three dimensions. Angular velocity of the head, i.e. acceleration of the head along a circular path, is sensed by the cristae

Otolith organs (utricle, saccule). Linear acceleration, and hence angular position relative to gravity, is sensed by the maculae.

Vestibular nuclei.

Central vestibular pathways.

Connections with cerebellum and spinal cord.

Connections within brain stem.

Functions of the vestibular system

Detection of body movement to allow subjective awareness: i.e. linear and angular acceleration, as monitored by movement of the head. Acceleration is detected, and not velocity.

Detection of head tilt in space (spatial orientation).

Maintenance of balance and equilibrium, leading to upright postural stability. This is mediated through vestibulo-spinal reflexes.

Eye position, with gaze fixation during changes of head and body position allowing maintenance of the fovea on the object of visual gaze. Co-ordination of eye movements with head motion is achieved by the vestibulo-ocular reflex.

Balance mechanisms

The **mechanisms of achieving balance** are:

Vestibular hair cells respond to changes in movement or position of the head;

The semicircular ducts respond to angular acceleration in specific directions;

The utricle responds to linear acceleration in all directions;

The lateral vestibular nucleus participates in control of posture;

The medial and superior vestibular nuclei mediate vestibulo-ocular reflexes;

Factors involved in equilibrium

Visual system
Eyes and eye muscles

Proprioceptive system:
Posterior column
Tendons
Joints
Muscles

Statokinetic system
Ear labyrinth
VIII nerve
Brain stem
Cerebellum
Cerebral cortex

These visual, vestibular and statokinetic inputs are integrated in the CNS and modified by input from the extrapyramidal system, reticular formation, cerebellum and cerebral cortex.

Vestibular function testing

Responses to rotational acceleration in the plane of a semicircular canal: Barany chair. With abrupt cessation of rotation, the endolymph continues to circulate for a period of time.

Responses to linear acceleration.

Caloric stimulation: convection currents in the endolymph, with consequent motion of the cupula.

Electronystagmography: based on the corneo-retinal potential difference to allow measurement of eye movement.

Galvanic stimulation.

Vestibular-evoked responses.

The inferior vestibular nucleus integrates inputs from the vestibular labyrinth and the cerebellum;

The vestibulo-collic and vestibulo-spinal reflexes maintain the head vertical with respect to gravity.

Effects of labyrinthine stimulation

Labyrinthine stimulation causes:

Nystagmus

Past pointing

Falling

Cold caloric stimulation causes nystagmus with the fast phase away from the stimulated ear. Warm caloric stimulation causes nystagmus with the fast phase towards the stimulated ear.

Warm caloric test

A head back tilt of 60 degrees brings the lateral semicircular canal into the vertical plane, as it is angled at 30 degrees to the horizontal plane.

Instillation of water at 44 $^{\circ}$C causes heat transfer to the lateral semicircular canal. This produces convection currents in the endolymph.

A slow drift of the eyes away from the stimulated side is followed by a rapid recovery to the resting position.

Functions of the Eustachian tube

Pressure regulation of the middle ear to allow equilibration with atmospheric pressure, i.e. ventilatory function;

Protection from nasopharyngeal sound pressure and secretions;

Clearance of middle ear secretions into the nasopharynx.

■ Special senses

Olfaction

Smell is perceived by bipolar receptor cells in the olfactory neuroepithelium of the superior nasal cavity. The pseudostratified columnar ciliated epithelial cells are located in the region of the superior septum and both superior and middle nasal turbinates. The cilia are organised in 9+2 microtubule arrangement, but lack dynein arms. The receptors for olfactory ligands are of the seven transmembrane domain type.

The second order neurons are in the olfactory bulb.

They continue in the olfactory tract.

The pathways terminate in the primary olfactory cortex and the secondary olfactory cortex of the orbito-frontal region (the rhinencephalon).

The other cells of the olfactory neuroepithelium are the sustentacular or supporting cells and the basal cells.

Taste

There are four basic tastes, sweet, sour, salt and bitter, which are sensed by the taste buds of the tongue.

Taste is subserved by:

The chorda tympani branch of the VIIth nerve, which supplies the fungiform papillae in the anterior two thirds of the tongue;

The IXth nerve, which supplies the circumvallate papillae at the junction of the posterior third and the anterior two thirds of the tongue, as well as the foliate papillae at the base;

The greater superficial petrosal branch of the VIIth nerve, which supplies the palate.

The second order gustatory neurons are located in the rostral half of the nucleus of the tractus solitarius in the medulla oblongata. Their axons enter the ipsilateral central tegmental tract and terminate in the pericellular division of the ventral postero-medial nucleus of the thalamus.

BIBLIOGRAPHY

Ahlquist, R. P. A study of adrenotropic receptors. *Am. J. Physiol.*, **153** (1948), 586–600.

Bernstein, J. Untersuchungen zur Thermodynamik der bioelektrischen Strome (Investigations on the thermodynamics of bioelectric currents). *Pflugers Arch.Ges.Physiol.*, **92** (1902), 521–62.

Carpenter, R. H. S. *Neurophysiology*, 4th edn. London: Arnold, 2003.

Cole, K. S. & Curtis, R. J. Electrical impedance of the squid giant axon during activity. *J. Gen. Physiol.*, **22** (1939), 649–70.

Daube, J. R. (ed.) *Clinical Neurophysiology*, 2nd edn. New York: *Oxford University Press*, 2002.

Eccles, J. C. *The Physiology of Synapses*. New York: Academic Press, 1964.

Fatt, P. & Katz, B. An analysis of the end-plate potential recorded with an intracellular electrode. *J. Physiol.*, **115** (1951), 320–70.

Forrester, J., Dick, A., McMenamin, P. & Lee, W. *The Eye. Basic Sciences in Practice*, 2nd edn. London: W. B. Saunders, 2002.

Gasser H. S. & Grundfest, H. Axon diameter in relation to the spike dimensions and the conduction velocity in mammalian A fibres. *Am. J. Physiol.*, **127** (1939), 393.

Goldman, D. E. Potential, impedance, and rectification in ion channels. *J. Gen. Physiol.*, **27** (1943), 37–60.

Hodgkin, A. L. Chance and design in electrophysiology: An informal account of certain experiments in nerve carried out between 1934 and 1952. *J. Physiol.*, **263** (1976), 1–21.

Huxley, H. E. & Hanson, J. Changes in the cross-striations of muscle during contraction and stretch and their structural interpretation. *Nature*, **173** (1954), 973–6.

Huxley, A. F. & Niedergerke, R. Interference microscopy of living muscle fibres. *Nature*, **173** (1954), 971–3.

Lands, A. M., Arnold, A., Mcauliff, J. P. *et al.* Differentiation of receptors responsive to isoproterenol. *Life Sci.*, **6** (1967), 2241–9.

Mathias, C. J. & Bannister, R. *Autonomic Failure. A Textbook of Clinical Disorders of the Autonomic Nervous System*, 4th edn. Oxford: Oxford University Press, 1999.

Melzack, R. & Wall, P. D. Pain mechanisms: a new theory. *Science*, **150** (1965), 971–9.

Neher, E. & Sakmann, B. Single channel currents recorded from membranes of denervated frog muscle fibres. *Nature*, **260** (1976), 799–802.

   The patch clamp technique. *Sci. Am.*, **266** (1992), 44–51.

Papez, J. W. A proposed mechanism of emotion. *Arch. Neurol. Psychiatry*, **38** (1937), 725–43.

Rexed, B. A cytoarchitectonic atlas of the spinal cord in the cat. *J. Comp. Neurol.*, **100** (1954), 297–380.

Skou, J. C. The influence of some cations on an adenosine-triphosphatase from peripheral nerves. *Biochem. Biophys. Acta*, **23** (1957), 394–401.

10 Endocrine physiology

■ Introduction

Endocrinology deals with the study of chemical messengers that travel via the blood and/or extracellular fluid and regulate tissue function, metabolism, growth, sexual development and reproduction.

■ General concepts

Regulatory systems

The components of **endocrine regulatory systems** are:
- A detector of homeostatic imbalance, usually manifested in altered circulating hormone levels or in alterations in the levels of blood constituents.
- A coupling mechanism to activate the secretory apparatus, usually involving feedback loops.
- The secretory apparatus.
- The hormone.
- An end organ capable of responding to the hormone. The target cells contain specific functional receptors with high specificity and affinity for the hormone. Hormone binding to the receptor causes the formation of an intracellular messenger molecule, which either stimulates or inhibits some characteristic biochemical activity of the target tissue. The coordinated tissue response to hormones involves the regulation, amplification and integration of signalling mechanisms at several levels.
- A detector to recognise that the hormonal effect has occurred.
- A mechanism for removing hormone from target cells and blood.
- A synthetic apparatus to replenish hormone in the secretory cells.

Hormone characteristics

The **characteristics of a hormone** are:

- It is produced by an endocrine or ductless gland, as opposed to an exocrine gland, which releases its products down a tube or duct.
- It acts as a chemical messenger, being secreted by cells into the blood or extracellular fluid, to act on target cells, which possess functional hormone receptors. The receptor consists of a specific binding site, a transduction element and an effector system. Hormones may inhibit, stimulate or regulate the functional activity of target organs or tissues.
- It may act locally, diffusing to adjacent cells (paracrine action).
- It may be carried by the bloodstream to act on distant target cells (endocrine action).
- It may act on the cell that produced it (autocrine action).
- Hormones produce their target cell actions either by enzyme activation or by modulation of gene expression.

Response to hormone

The **magnitude of the response to a hormone** is determined by:

The concentration of the hormone at the surface of the target cell, which in turn depends on the rate of production (under the control of positive and negative feedback loops); the rate of delivery (dependent on blood flow); and the rate of metabolism, degradation and elimination.

The sensitivity of the target cell.

The number of functional target cells.

The availability of cell membrane receptors on target cells

Up-regulation: stimulation of receptor synthesis;

Down-regulation: internalisation of receptors by endocytosis; suppression of receptor synthesis.

Effects of a hormone on a target cell may include:

An alteration in the rate of intracellular protein synthesis;

An alteration in the rate of enzyme activity;

Modification of plasma membrane transport;

Induction of secretory activity.

Regulation of hormone levels involves a balance between:

Spontaneous, or basal, hormone release;

Feedback inhibition by hormones of their synthesis and/or release;

Stimulation or inhibition of hormone release by substances that may/may not be regulated by the same hormones;

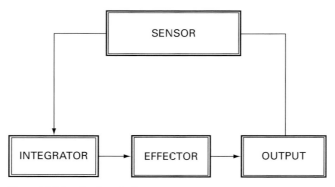

Figure 10.1 Feedback control.

Positive feedback mechanisms

Oestrogens mediate a positive feedback increase in the pulsatile release of gonado-trophin releasing hormone (GnRH), luteinising hormone (LH) and follicle stimu-lating hormone (FSH) prior to ovulation. Ovulation terminates the positive feedback loop abruptly.

Oxytocin release is increased in a positive feedback loop by myometrial contraction during childbirth, with termination of the loop on delivery.

Oxytocin release is also increased via the milk ejection reflex by contraction of mammary duct myo-epithelial cells during suckling at the breast. This loop termi-nates on removal of the stimulus to the nipples.

Establishment of circadian rhythms for hormone release by systems such as brain;

Brain-mediated stimulation or inhibition of hormone release in response to anxiety, anticipation of a specific activity or other sensory inputs.

Mechanisms of endocrine disease

Endocrine disease may be due to:

Hormone deficiency, due to destruction of the gland (infarction, infection, neoplasm, auto-immune processes), genetic defects of hormone production, or inactivating mutations of hormone receptors.

Hormone excess, due to exogenous intake, overproduction by either endo-crine gland or through ectopic hormone production, or activating mutations of cell surface receptors.

Gland enlargement leading to space-occupying lesions producing pressure effects.

■ Classification of hormones

Hormones may be classified chemically as amine hormones (thyroid hormones; catecholamines), peptides and proteins, and steroids.

Based on their affinity for water and lipids, hormones may be further classified as:

- Lipophilic or lipid-soluble with intracellular receptors in the cytoplasm or nucleus: steroid hormones; thyroxine; vitamin D3. Lipophilic hormones mediate allosteric modulation of transcription factors.
- Lipophilic, with target cell-surface receptors in the plasma membrane: prostaglandins.
- Hydrophilic or water-soluble with target cell-surface receptors in the plasma membrane: peptides; glycoproteins; biogenic amines (catecholamines). These receptors are coupled to second messenger systems to allow mediation of hormone action in the target cell, the hormone in question being the first messenger. The hydrophilic properties are related to the presence of numerous polar groups.

Hormone receptors

Plasma membrane receptors are integral membrane proteins with three basic domains:

An extracellular ligand-binding domain;

A transmembrane domain, usually with seven spans of the membrane, with an exposed N-terminal and a C-terminal projecting into the cytosol;

An intracellular or cytoplasmic domain.

Intracellular receptors generally consist of a single polypeptide chain with:

A variable $-NH_2$ terminus domain;

A conserved deoxynucleic acid (DNA)-binding domain (response element), which is a zinc finger motif;

Receptors for molecules used in signalling

Receptors for lipid-soluble signalling molecules
Steroid hormone family of receptors;
Catalytic, cytosolic receptors.

Receptors for water-soluble signalling molecules
Ligand-gated ion channel receptors;
Catalytic, membrane receptors;
Receptors coupled directly to a cytosolic enzyme;
G-protein-coupled membrane receptors.

A variable hinge region;

A conserved ligand-binding domain;

A variable carboxy-terminal region.

These receptors belong to the steroid/thyroid hormone receptor superfamily. The hormone–receptor complex translocates to the nucleus. Here it binds to specific DNA sequences, termed hormone response elements. Alterations in the rate of transcription of the associated gene result. Steroid hormone receptors include numerous isoforms and structurally similar proteins (orphan receptors) of unknown function.

Signal transduction

Signal transduction refers to the mechanism of initiation of a cellular response after an agonist binds to a receptor. The extracellular signal initiates an intracellular signalling **cascade** that transfers, transforms, amplifies and then distributes it.

The mechanisms of signal transduction include:

Membrane depolarisation induced by the opening of a ligand-gated ion channel: neurotransmitters, amino acids;

Activation of a G-protein (guanidine nucleotide-binding protein): peptides, neurotransmitters, prostaglandins;

Synthesis of a second messenger

Cyclic nucleotide: adenosine 3′–5′-monophosphate (cyclic AMP), guanosine 3′–5′-monophosphate (cyclic GMP)

Intermediates of polyphosphoinositide metabolism: diacylglycerol (DAG), inositol-1,4,5-triphosphate (IP3)

Calcium ions

A protein phosphorylation cascade that activates or inhibits intracellular enzymes leading to changes in target cell activity.

G-proteins (GTP-binding transducer proteins)

G-proteins are a family of regulatory proteins involved in both intra- and inter-cellular transduction processes. They are **heterotrimeric**, consisting of three sub units (alpha, beta, gamma), and share structural homology. G-protein-coupled receptors comprise an extracellular ligand binding site and an effector site that extends into the cytosol.

In the resting state, GDP is bound to the alpha subunit, which has GTPase activity at the guanine nucleotide-binding site and separate binding sites for the receptor and effector proteins. The beta and gamma units are shared among G-proteins.

Membrane receptor protein super-families

G-protein-coupled seven-transmembrane (GPCR) proteins
Beta-adrenergic
LH, FSH, thyroid stimulating hormone (TSH)
Glucagon
Parathyroid hormone (PTH), parathyroid hormone releasing peptide (PTHrP)
Adrenocorticotrophic hormone (ACTH), melanocyte stimulating hormone (MSH)
Growth hormone releasing hormone (GHRH), corticotrophin releasing hormone (CRH)
Alpha-adrenergic
Somatostatin
Thyrotrophin releasing hormone (TRH), gonadotrophin releasing hormone (GnRH)

Receptor tyrosine kinase (phosphorylate tyrosines of target molecules)
Insulin, insulin-like growth factor-1 (IGF-1)
Epidermal growth factor, nerve growth factor

Cytokine receptor-linked kinase
Growth hormone (GH), prolactin (PRL)

Serine kinase (phosphorylate serines and threonines of signalling molecules)
Activin, tumour growth factor (TGF)-beta, MIS

Guanylate cyclase (form cyclic GMP in the cytosol)
Atrial natriuretic peptides

Ligand-gated ion channel
Nicotinic: acetylcholine

The **alpha subunit** confers functional and binding specificity to the various types of G-proteins. It is unique for each G-protein. On hormone binding to the receptor, GDP rapidly exchanges for guanosine $5'$-triphosphate (GTP) on the alpha subunit, activating the G-protein. The G-protein dissociates from the receptor. The alpha subunit and beta-gamma complex dissociate to interact with other effector proteins. The alpha subunit modulates the activity of a second messenger system. Guanidine triphosphate is then rapidly hydrolysed to GDP by the GTPase activity of the alpha subunit, with the release of inorganic phosphate. The G-protein heterotrimeric complex is thereupon re-formed. The two **control points** in the G-protein cycle are GDP release from the alpha subunit and hydrolysis of GTP catalysed by the alpha subunit.

G-proteins may be either coupled to adenyl cyclase via either Gs (increased cyclic AMP) or Gi (reduced cyclic AMP); or coupled to Gq or G11 and convert phosphatidylinositol 4,5-biphosphate into two second messengers, inositol 1,4,5-triphosphate (which increases intracellular Ca^{2+} concentration by causing release from endoplasmic reticulum) and diacylglycerol (which activates protein kinase C).

They are monomeric proteins of the rhodopsin family, which sense external environmental signals such as light, taste and odour, and signals transmitted by hormones. They possess seven membrane spanning domains with four intracellular loops responsible for direct interaction with the G-protein. There is an N-terminal extracellular domain and a C-terminal intracellular domain.

Properties of second messengers

Increases in concentration following binding of hormone to receptor;

An increase in messenger concentration precedes biological effects of hormone;

When the hormone is removed the concentration of the second messenger and the biological response proportionately decline.

Second messenger (intracellular mediator) pathways

Cyclic AMP

Diacylglycerol-IP3 (inositol-1,4,5-triphosphate)

Arachidonic acid

Cyclic GMP

Tyrosine kinases

Second messengers

Components of the **second messenger system**, which constitutes a molecular cascade amplification system, include:

A first messenger

A receptor for the first messenger;

A second receptor: a G-protein, which acts as a connecting protein, interacting with the receptor for the first messenger;

Enzyme activation by a binary complex of the two receptors;

A second messenger, which is produced by enzyme activity.

Cyclic AMP pathway

Activated beta1 and alpha2 adrenergic receptors, for example, act via Gs or Gi proteins to stimulate or inhibit adenyl cyclase respectively. Adenyl cyclase induces cAMP synthesis.

Cyclic AMP stimulates target gene expression (tyrosine hydroxylase, somatostatin) via protein kinase induction and phosphorylation of transcription factors (cAMP-responsive element (CRE)-binding protein, CREB). It is a tetramer of two

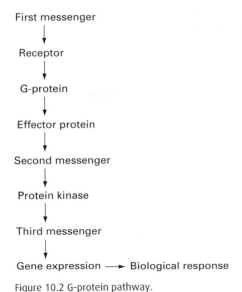

First messenger

↓

Receptor

↓

G-protein

↓

Effector protein

↓

Second messenger

↓

Protein kinase

↓

Third messenger

↓

Gene expression ⟶ Biological response

Figure 10.2 G-protein pathway.

identical catalytic subunits and two identical regulatory subunits. It binds directly to certain plasma membrane proteins that function as cation channels: cyclic AMP-gated cation channels, the function of which is not understood. Protein kinase A is activated. This catalyses the transfer of the terminal phosphate group of ATP to the hydroxyl groups of serine or threonine residues of other enzymes, increasing or decreasing their catalytic activity.

Cyclic AMP is the second messenger for a number of hormones, including ACTH, adrenaline, calcitonin, chorionic gonadotrophin (CG), FSH, glucagon, lipotrophin, LH, MSH, noradrenaline, PTH, TSH and vasopressin.

Adenyl cyclase is composed of three protein units, which comprise three functional parts:

The **receptor**, GM1 ganglioside receptor.

A guanyl nucleotide regulatory unit: a **coupling protein**, regulated by GTP, called GTP-binding protein or G-protein: attached by farnesyl bonds to the plasma membrane. It both binds GTP and can act as a GTPase, constituting a molecular 'on-off' switch for signal transduction.

A **catalytic unit**, the enzyme adenyl cyclase itself, which converts ATP to cyclic AMP.

Sequence of events involving cyclic AMP as a second messenger

Hormone binds to its receptor on the outer surface of the target cell membrane. Hormone–receptor interaction stimulates the activity of adenyl cyclase on the

Effects of cyclic AMP in cholera

- At villus: inhibits entry of water, sodium and chloride.
- In the crypt: promotes pumping out into the gut lumen of water, sodium, chloride and bicarbonate.

Inositol 1,4,5-triphosphate pathway

Activated alpha1 adrenergic receptors act via G-proteins to stimulate phospholipase C. Phospholipase C cleaves phosphoinositide to give inositol 1,4,5-triphosphate and 1,2-diacylglycerol.

Inositol 1,4,5-triphosphate mobilises Ca^{2+} from intracellular stores.

Ca^{2+} and 1,2-diacylglycerol activate calmodulin kinases and protein kinase C.

These in turn phosphorylate a number of important proteins (epidermal growth factor receptor, glycogen synthase)

cytoplasmic side of the membrane. Activated adenyl cyclase catalyses the conversion of ATP to cyclic AMP within the cytoplasm. Cyclic AMP activates protein kinase enzymes that are already present in the cytoplasm in an inactive state.

Activated cyclic AMP-dependent protein kinase transfers phosphate groups (phosphorylates) to other enzymes in the cytoplasm. The activity of specific enzymes is either increased or inhibited by phosphorylation. Altered enzyme activity mediates the target cell's response to the hormone.

Phosphoinositide cascade
The effects mediated by the phosphoinositide cascade include:

Glycogenolysis in liver cells;

Histamine secretion by mast cells;

Serotonin release by blood platelets;

Aggregation of blood platelets;

Insulin secretion by pancreatic islet cells;

Adrenaline secretion by adrenal chromaffin cells;

Smooth muscle contraction.

Sequence of events involving the Ca^{2+} second-messenger system
The hormone binds to its receptor on the outer surface of the plasma membrane of the target cell. Hormone–receptor interaction stimulates the activity of a membrane enzyme, phospholipase C. Activated phospholipase C catalyses the conversion of certain membrane phospholipids to IP3 and another derivative, diacylglycerol.

Inositol triphosphate enters the cytoplasm and diffuses to the endoplasmic reticulum, where it binds to its receptor proteins and causes the opening of Ca^{2+} channels. Since the endoplasmic reticulum accumulates Ca^{2+} by active transport, there exists a steep Ca^{2+} concentration gradient favouring the diffusion of Ca^{2+} into the cytoplasm. Calcium ion that enters the cytoplasm binds to and activates a protein called calmodulin.

Activated calmodulin activates protein kinase, which phosphorylates other enzyme proteins. Altered enzyme activity mediates the target cell's response to the hormone.

Steroid-hormone receptor mechanism

The specific glucocorticoid receptor in the cytoplasm exists as a heterocomplex that contains the receptor in association with two subunits of the heat shock protein hsp 90, one subunit of the heat shock protein hsp 56, one subunit of the heat shock protein hsp 70 and an acidic 23 kDa protein.

The hormone binds to the hormone-binding domain that has been kept in an inactive state by the various heat shock proteins. Activation of the hormone–receptor complex by conformational change follows dissociation of heat shock proteins. Dimerisation of the hormone–receptor complexes relieves them from protection by the heat shock protein. The hormone-activated receptor translocates to the nucleus. Binding of dimer occurs to special DNA sequences known as hormone-responsive elements by the zinc finger area of the DNA-binding domain.

Classification of protein kinases

Cyclic nucleotide-dependent kinases
cAMP-dependent protein kinases, types I and II
cGMP-dependent protein kinases

Calcium-dependent kinases
Calcium/calmodulin-dependent protein kinases, types I, II, III
Calcium/phospholipid-dependent protein kinases (protein kinase C): 9 isozymes

Cyclic nucleotide- and calcium-independent kinases
Casein kinases
Pyruvate dehydrogenase kinase
Glycogen synthase kinase 3
Rhodopsin kinase: beta-adrenergic receptor kinase

Tyrosine-specific kinases
Growth factor receptors
Non-receptor tyrosine kinases

Stimulation of transcription is mediated by transcription activation functions and influenced by the protein content of the cell, and by phosphorylation (messenger ribonucleic acid (mRNA) synthesis and transport to ribosomes). The transcription rate of a specific protein's mRNA can be induced (up-regulated) or suppressed (down-regulated). Stated otherwise, the expression of genes can be either inhibited or enhanced by the hormone–receptor complex. Cytoplasmic protein synthesis results in a specific cellular activity.

■ Thyroid

Introduction

The thyroid gland is located in the anterior neck and consists of two lateral lobes joined by a midline isthmus. The weight of the adult gland is around 10–25 grams. The gland is involved with the synthesis, storage and secretion of thyroid hormones.

The functional unit is the **follicle** or acinus, which is lined with cuboidal epithelium. Cell height varies with the degree of TSH stimulation. The lumen of the follicle is filled with colloid, which consists almost entirely of thyroglobulin. The follicles are held together by loose reticular fibres.

Parafollicular or C cells lie between the basement membrane of the follicles and the follicular cells. They are of neural crest origin, being derived from the ultimobranchial bodies of the 4th and 5th branchial pouches. The thyroid gland also possesses a lymphatic network and a network of short, fenestrated capillaries surrounding the follicles.

Ninety per cent of the total body iodine is stored in the thyroid gland, in the form of iodinated amino acids and thyroid hormone. Ten per cent is located in the extracellular pool. Dietary iodine is derived primarily from fish, seafood and seaweed. In goitre endemic regions, iodinated salt or iodinated vegetable oil are employed in prophylaxis.

Thyroid hormone synthesis

This involves the following steps:
- Dietary iodine is largely converted to iodide in the gut and absorbed into the circulation. The main sources of dietary iodine are iodised salt, iodated bread and dairy products. Iodine is also present in medications, disinfectants and radiographic contrast media.
- **Iodide trapping** by the thyroid gland (iodide pump in the basolateral membranes of the follicular epithelial cells: sodium-iodide co-transport-symport)

is an active transport mechanism, stimulated by TSH. The TSH receptor on the basolateral membrane surface is a G-protein-coupled receptor. The iodide carrier is a 643 amino acid transport protein with 13 transmembrane domains, known as the sodium iodide symporter. The concentration of free iodide achieved is around 30 to 40 times that in plasma.

- **Iodide oxidation** to free iodine (peroxidase-H_2O_2 system). Thyroid peroxidase is a membrane-bound glycoprotein with a molecular weight of 102 000 and a hame compound as the prosthetic group. It is synthesised in the rough endoplasmic reticulum.

- **Thyroglobulin synthesis** by the endoplasmic reticulum of the thyroid cells. Thyroglobulin is a homo-dimeric glycoprotein with 5496 amino acids and a molecular weight of 660 000. The glycosylation of thyroglobulin is completed in the Golgi apparatus prior to secretion into the colloid of the follicular lumen.

- **Iodination of tyrosine residues** in thyroglobulin to give monoiodotyrosine (MIT) and diiodotyrosine (DIT).

- **Coupling of the iodotyrosines** to give iodothyronines: MIT + DIT = triiodothyrosine (T3); DIT + DIT = thyroxine (T4). The iodination and subsequent coupling reactions are catalysed by thyroid peroxidase.

- The synthesis of thyroid hormone occurs at the apical membranes of the follicular epithelial cells.

- Storage takes place extracellularly in the colloid of the thyroid follicles.

- Secretion of thyroid hormones follows **proteolysis of thyroglobulin** within endocytotic vesicles by endosomal and lysosomal enzymes. Proteolysis is initiated by cathepsins D, B and L. Exopeptidases release free T3 and T4. The thyroid predominantly produces T4, which is converted in peripheral tissues to the metabolically active form T3.

- The iodotyrosines MIT and DIT are deiodinated by an iodotyrosine deiodinase and their iodide re-enters the intra-thyroidal pool where it is recycled.

   The control of thyroid hormone secretion and action occurs at three levels:

   The hypothalamic–pituitary–thyroid axis;

   Autoregulation within the thyroid depending on organic iodine content;

   Peripheral hormone conversion.

   Increasing iodide intake may occasionally either reduce total organic iodine (Wolf–Chaikoff effect) or increase organic iodine, especially in iodine deficiency areas (Jod–Basedow phenomenon).

   Iodothyronines in the circulation are bound to thyroxine-binding globulin (70% of T4 and 80% of T3), albumin (20% of T4 and 10% of T3) and transthyretin (10% of T4 and 10% of T3). Only about 0.03% of T4 and 0.3% of T3 is free in the circulation.

Characteristics of the iodide pump

Located in the basal plasma membrane of follicular cells;
Concentrates iodide against chemical and electrical gradient;
Saturable and obeys Michaelis–Menten kinetics;
Depends on ATP availability (derived from oxidative phosphorylation or glycolysis);
Concentrates other monovalent anions;
Inhibited by anions (bromide, perchlorate, pertechnetate, thiocyanate) and Na^+-K^+ activated; ATPase inhibitors (ouabain).

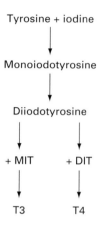

Figure 10.3 Pathway for thyroid hormone synthesis

The half-life of T4 is from 5 to 7 days, and that of T3 is from 1 to 3 days.

Thyroid hormone actions

These can be broadly classified as nuclear (on nuclear receptors) and non-nuclear or non-genomic (on plasma membrane, cytoskeleton, sarcoplasmic reticulum, cytoplasm and mitochondria). The actions of thyroid hormone are primarily produced by the interaction of T3 with the nuclear thyroid hormone receptor. The effects include:

Metabolic effects
Protein metabolism
   Increased amino acid uptake and synthesis of protein
   Increased protein degradation and turnover

Serum thyroxine

Comprises the following components:
  Free thyroxine: 0.03%;
  Bound to thyroxine-binding globulin (TBG) (an alpha 1-alpha 2-glycoprotein) (70%);
  Bound to thyroxine-binding pre-albumin (TBPA) or thyretin (comprised of four identical polypeptide units) (20%);
  Bound to albumin (10%).

Carbohydrate metabolism
  Increased glucose uptake by adipose, liver and muscle cells
  Increased glycolysis
  Increased gluconeogenesis and glycogenolysis in the liver
  Increased insulin secretion
Fat metabolism
  Increased fat mobilisation and lipolysis
  Increased fat oxidation
Increased oxygen consumption in all cells except brain, anterior pituitary, spleen and testes: **calorigenic action**, increasing the basal metabolic rate. This is achieved by stimulation of synthesis of the cell membrane Na^+/K^+-ATPase system.
CNS maturation in utero and in early infancy.

Skeletal growth and maturation
Promotion of the activities of other hormones, e.g. catecholamines and steroids. Thyroxine increases the responsiveness of tissues to catecholamines.

Hypothalamic–pituitary–thyroid axis

The **hypothalamic–pituitary–thyroid axis** is an integrated organ complex providing for the regulated production of thyroid hormones. It is affected by the following factors:
Hypothalamic TRH production:
  Increased: dopamine, noradrenaline
  Decreased: T3, T4, glucocorticoids
Pituitary TSH production:
  Increased: TRH
  Decreased: dopamine, oestrogens, T3, T4, glucocorticoids
Thyroid gland hormone production:
  Increased: TSH, iodine, human chorionic gonadotrophin (HCG), catecholamines

Thyroid function tests

Serum thyroid hormones: T4, free T4, T3, free T3, thyroglobulin.

Tests of the thyroid–pituitary axis:

Basal serum TSH: a normal level virtually rules out thyrotoxicosis or hypothyroidism;

Serum TSH response to exogenous TRH.

Dynamic tests of thyroid activity:

In vivo radionuclide uptake studies: ^{99}Tc m, ^{123}I, ^{131}I;

T3 suppression tests;

TSH stimulation test.

Table 10.1 Hypothalamic–pituitary–thyroid axis dysfunction

	T4, T3	TSH	TSH response to TRH
Primary hypothyroidism	Low	High	Exaggerated response
Secondary hypothyroidism (pituitary failure)	Low	Low	No increase in TSH
Tertiary hypothyroidism (hypothalamic failure)	Low	Low	Normal/exaggerated TSH secretion
Primary hyperthyroidism	High	Low	Blunted or no response
Secondary hyperthyroidism	High/normal	High	Normal

Decreased: iodine, medications (lithium; anti-thyroid medication); dietary goitrogens

Thyroid stimulating hormone is a glycoprotein, with an alpha chain of 89 amino acids and a beta chain of 112 amino acids.

Causes of alterations in TSH levels in the serum

Low TSH levels

Hyperthyroidism (negative feedback);

Pituitary gland failure (secondary hypothyroidism);

Reduced pituitary function (sick euthyroid syndrome): low total and free T4, low normal TSH, and raised reverse T3.

High TSH level

Low T4 and T3 levels (primary hypothyroidism; with reduced negative feedback).

Mechanisms of hyperthyroidism

Stimulation of TSH receptor: thyroid-stimulating immunoglobulin; HCG; TSH.

Autonomous overproduction of thyroid hormone: adenoma, multi-nodular goitre.

Increased thyroid hormone release: subacute granulomatous and lymphocytic thyroiditis.

Extra-thyroidal sources of thyroid hormone: exogenous administration; ectopic production.

Mechanisms of hypothyroidism

Primary reduction in thyroid gland tissue: autoimmune, iatrogenic, infiltrative;
Thyroid hormone biosynthetic defects;
Secondary to pituitary or hypothalamic failure;
Generalised resistance to thyroid hormones.

■ Pituitary gland

The pituitary gland lies in the sella turcica of the sphenoid bone and is connected to the median eminence of the hypothalamus by a stalk, the infundibulum. It measures 0.6 cm in height and 1 cm in width, and weighs about 500–800 mg. The sella turcica has an antero-posterior diameter of 15 mm and a supero-inferior diameter of 12 mm. The diaphragma sella, a dural extension, separates the pituitary from the chiasmatic cisterns and the floor of the anterior portion of the third ventricle.

Structural components of the pituitary gland

Adenohypophysis (anterior pituitary)

This comprises about 80% of the gland.
Pars tuberalis
Pars intermedia
Pars anterior (distalis; glandularis)

Neurohypophysis (posterior pituitary)

Median eminence in the floor of the third ventricle, and parts of the wall of the third ventricle. The supraoptic and paraventricular nuclei of the hypothalamus include the cell bodies of magnocellular neurosecretory neurons that synthesise and secrete vasopressin and oxytocin.

Infundibular stem or pituitary stalk.

Infundibular process or pars posterior (nervosa), which consists of 100 000 unmyelinated axons of secretory neurons from the supraventricular and para-optic nuclei.

Hypothalamic–pituitary axis

The **hypothalamic–pituitary axis** regulates the function of the thyroid, adrenal, and reproductive glands, by allowing fine tuning of the pituitary–thyroid, –adrenal and –reproductive axes. It also controls somatic growth, lactation and water balance. Evaluation of hypothalamic function entails the documentation of circadian rhythm of hormone secretion, stress testing induced release of hormones and feedback blocking procedures.

Intermittent stimulation of the pituitary gland is caused by pulses of hypothalamic releasing hormones, which are the result of episodic neuronal discharge. The ultra-pulsed secretion of the hypophysiotrophic hormones is smoothed terminally to the circadian rhythm of pituitary hormone secretion. The hypothalamic–pituitary–end organ axis is a sequential amplification cascade mechanism. Feedback inhibition by target hormones on proximal centres constitutes the primary regulatory mechanism of the axis.

A circadian rhythm of pituitary hormone release is superimposed on the pulsatile release mechanisms. This rhythm is generated by the paired suprachiasmatic nuclei in the anterior hypothalamus, which receive afferent information from the retina and convey efferent information to the pineal gland, thereby affecting melatonin release. Sleep–wake cycles thereby influence pituitary hormone release. The pulsatile release of pituitary hormones is altered at puberty, during ovulatory menstrual cycles and with advancing age.

Characteristics of hypothalamic releasing hormones

Pulsatile secretion;

Action on specific plasma membrane receptors;

Transduction of signals through calcium, membrane phospholipid products and cAMP as second messengers;

Hypothalamic releasing and inhibitory hormones

Vasopressin (antidiuretic hormone; ADH)

CRH

GnRH

TRH

GHRH

Somatostatin (growth hormone inhibitory hormone; GHIH)

Dopamine (PRL-inhibiting factor): PRL is the only pituitary hormone to be suppressed by a hypothalamic factor

Stimulation of release of stored target anterior pituitary hormones via exocytosis;

Stimulation of synthesis of target anterior pituitary hormones at the transcriptional level;

Modification of biological activity of target anterior pituitary hormones by posterior translational effects such as glycosylation;

Stimulation of hyperplasia and hypertrophy of target cells;

Modulation of effects by up- and down-regulation of their own receptors.

Levels of feedback to the hypothalamus

Long loop feedback: circulating target gland hormones;

Short loop feedback: negative feedback by pituitary hormones;

Ultra-short loop feedback: hypothalamic releasing hormones effecting feedback on their own secretion.

Features of the hypophyseal portal tract

Portal veins are veins interposed between two capillary networks. In this case they are interposed between the capillaries of the median eminence of the ventral hypothalamus and the sinusoids of the anterior pituitary.

The hypophyseal portal venous system carries releasing hormones from peptidergic neurons in the hypothalamus directly to target cells in the anterior pituitary cells, without dilution in the systemic circulation. It is formed by superior and inferior hypophyseal branches of the internal carotid artery, which form a complex capillary plexus in the median eminence of the hypothalamus. Hormones reach the median eminence via axoplasmic transport through axons of the tubero-infundibular tract.

Six to ten long portal vessels descend along the anterior surface of the pituitary stalk, opening into sinusoids between secretory cells in the anterior pituitary. Eighty-five per cent of the blood supply for the anterior pituitary is carried by the hypophyseal portal tract, the remaining 15% from the superior hypophyseal artery.

The **median eminence** is a specialised region of the floor of the third ventricle, which gives rise to the pituitary stalk. It is characterised by:

High vascularity;

Fenestrated endothelium;

Lack of neuronal perikarya;

Specialised astrocytes interposed between ependymal cells, called tanycytes, which can transfer hormones between the cerebrospinal fluid and the pituitary portal system.

Anterior pituitary gland

The anterior pituitary gland comprises five types of **secretory cells**, arranged in nests and cords. These cells are distinguished by histochemical and immuno-cytochemical staining, and by electron microscopic appearances, into:

Somatotrophs: GH

Lactotrophs: PRL

Thyrotrophs: TSH

Gonadotrophs: LH and FSH

Corticotrophs: ACTH

Somatotrophs and lactotrophs are acidophilic, while thyrotrophs, gonado-trophs and corticotrophs are basophilic.

Furthermore, there are inactive secretory cells called chromophobe cells.

Life cycle

The **life cycle of anterior pituitary peptide hormones** involves the stages of:

Pre-prohormone;

Prohormone, which is the storage form in the anterior pituitary;

The biologically active hormone;

Degradation fragments of the hormone.

Growth hormone

Growth hormone is a single chain polypeptide comprising 191 amino acids and containing two intramolecular disulphide bonds. It has a molecular weight of 21 500. The plasma half-life is 20–50 minutes.

Anterior pituitary hormones

The number of amino acid residues are as follows:

Somatotrophic hormones
GH 191
PRL 198

Corticotrophin-related peptides
ACTH 39
Beta-lipotrophin (LPH) 91
Beta-LPH 61–91 31 (beta-endorphin)
Alpha-MSH 13

Glycoprotein hormones
TSH alpha chain 89; beta chain 112
FSH alpha chain 89; beta chain 115
LH alpha chain 89; beta chain 115
The beta subunit is the hormone-specific subunit.

Growth hormone is secreted in an irregular and intermittent pulsatile fashion by somatotrophs. Secretion shows diurnal variation, peak secretion occurring during sleep. Secretion is stimulated by GHRH and inhibited by somatostatin. This represents dual control by opposing hypothalamic peptides. Stimuli for GH secretion include increased plasma amino acid concentrations and decreased plasma concentrations of fatty acids and carbohydrates.

Growth hormone stimulates the synthesis and release of somatomedin C (insulin-like growth factor 1), a 70 amino acid peptide, from the liver and kidneys. Somatomedin C mediates most of the effects of GH on target tissues. Somatomedin antagonises GH release by antagonising the effect of GHRH on pituitary somatotrophs and by the stimulation of somatostatin release in the hypothalamus.

Growth hormone actions

Promotes linear growth:
Induces precursor cells to differentiate and secrete IGF-1, which stimulates cell division.

Stimulates protein synthesis: increases amino acid transport into muscle, liver and adipose cells and accelerates transcription and translation of mRNA.

Anti-insulin effects:
Adipocytes more responsive to lipolytic stimuli;
Stimulation of gluconeogenesis;
Reduced ability of insulin to stimulate glucose uptake.

Muscle:
Reduced glucose uptake;
Increased amino acid uptake;
Increased protein synthesis;
Increased lean body mass.

Metabolism:
Increased plasma glucose;
Increased plasma free fatty acids;
Reduced plasma amino acids;
Reduced plasma urea.

Chondrocytes:
Increased amino acid uptake;
Increased protein synthesis;
Increased DNA, RNA synthesis;
Increased chondroitin sulphate synthesis;

Collagen synthesis;

Increased cell size and number;

Increased linear growth.

Adipose tissue:

Reduced glucose uptake;

Increased lipolysis;

Reduced adiposity.

Prolactin

This is a 198 amino acid single chain polypeptide, encoded by a gene on chromosome 6. It has a molecular weight of 23 000. Prolactin is synthesised in ribosomes and rough endoplasmic reticulum of lactotrophs of the adenohypophysis. It is concentrated in the Golgi apparatus and stored in cytoplasmic granules. Secretion occurs in a sleep-related circadian rhythm in both males and females. Hypothalamic control of secretion is primarily inhibitory, mediated by PRL-release-inhibiting factor (dopamine). Thyrotrophin releasing hormone stimulates PRL secretion. The plasma half-life is 15–20 minutes. The actions are mediated by a dimeric tyrosine kinase-linked receptor.

Actions

Increased sensitivity of the testis to LH stimulation, sustaining testosterone levels. Normal corpus luteum function.

Initiation and maintenance of lactation in the post-partum period: it induces lobulo-alveolar growth of the breasts and stimulates lactogenesis after parturition.

Osmoregulation.

Immune regulation.

Effects of hyperprolactinaemia

Women

Galactorrhoea

Amenorrhoea or oligomenorrhoea

Infertility

Men

Galactorrhoea and gynaecomastia

Hypogonadism with reduced sex drive

Impotence

Both sexes

Pituitary mass effects

Secretion is stimulated by breast-feeding, mediated by stimulation of the nipple during suckling, stress, sexual intercourse, hormones (oestrogens), sleep, dopamine antagonists and TRH.

Secretion is inhibited by somatostatin and by dopamine agonists.

Oxytocin

Oxytocin is released as a consequence of depolarisation of oxytocinergic cells of the supraoptic and paraventricular nuclei of the hypothalamus. Propagation of action potentials along the hypothalamiconeural–hypophyseal tract to posterior pituitary gland nerve terminals leads to calcium influx, which stimulates release of oxytocin by exocytosis. Release is stimulated by suckling at the breast leading to nipple stimulation, activation of stretch receptors in the walls of the uterus and vagina, pregnancy and at parturition.

Actions

Causes the release of milk by contraction of myo-epithelial cells of the breasts (milk let-down);

Responsible for the contraction of uterine smooth muscle at parturition.

These actions are mediated by binding to specific G-protein-coupled cell surface receptors, linked to calcium channels, on target cells.

■ Adrenal glands

Structural features

- Paired retroperitoneal organs, in close proximity to the superior poles of the kidneys, anterior to the diaphragmatic crura at D11 level. The right gland is pyramidal in shape, and the left gland semilunar.

Anterior pituitary function testing

Indirect, i.e. tests of end-organ function: plasma T4 (TSH); plasma cortisol (ACTH); ovulation (LH, FSH); spermatogenesis (LH, FSH).

Direct, static: plasma levels of ACTH, TSH, LH, FSH, GH, PRL.

Direct, dynamic: TSH (iv TRH); LH, FSH (iv GnRH); ACTH (insulin hypoglycaemia); GH (stimulation: sleep; iv arginine; insulin hypoglycaemia); PRL (iv TRH).

Combined sequential stimuli testing with a triple intravenous bolus of hormones: soluble insulin (0.15 unit/kg); TRH (200 μg) and GnRH (100 μg). This involves venous blood sampling for glucose, cortisol, GH, LH, FSH, PRL and TSH prior to administration, and at 20, 30, 45, 60, 90 and 120 minutes thereafter.

- Each gland weighs 5–10 g in the adult and measures 4–5 cm in length, 2–3 cm in width and 1 cm in thickness.
- The cortex is of mesodermal origin, and the medulla of neuro-ectodermal origin.
- The cortex comprises 80%–90% of the total weight of the gland.

Adrenal medulla (15%)

The adrenal medulla is the most prominent part of the chromaffin system, which consists of aggregates of chromaffin cells, which stain brown with chrome salts. It is derived from ectodermal chromaffin tissue, and can be considered to be a modified sympathetic ganglion with post-ganglionic cells but no axons.

Ovoid and columnar chromaffin cells are arranged in clumps and cords, around blood vessels. The **chromaffin cells** contain dense-cored chromaffin vesicles storing catecholamines, which are synthesised by the hydroxylation and decarboxylation of phenylalanine and tyrosine. The process of amine precursor uptake and decarboxylation is a feature common to a variety of embryologically related neuroendocrine tissues derived from the neural crest. Tyrosine hydroxylase activity is the rate limiting step in catecholamine synthesis. It catalyses the para-hydroxylation of tyrosine to form hydroxyphenylalanine (DOPA).

The adrenal medulla is unique in containing phenylethanolamine N-methyl transferase (PNMT), which catalyses N-methylation of noradrenaline to adrenaline. The adrenal medulla secretes mostly adrenaline, containing 80% adrenaline-secreting cells and 20% noradrenaline-secreting cells.

Catecholamine release results from **stimulus-secretion coupling**. Acetylcholine is released by preganglionic nerve impulses. This increases membrane permeability, producing depolarisation and leading to calcium influx. Exocytosis of the secretory granules ensues.

Glucocorticoids

Cortisol is the primary glucocorticoid in man. It is synthesised from cholesterol in the zona fasciculata of the adrenal cortex. Synthesis of cortisol involves the

Zones of the adrenal cortex (85%)

Zona glomerulosa (15%): 21 carbon mineralocorticoids (aldosterone)
Zona fasciculata (70%): 21 carbon glucocorticoids (cortisol, dehydroepiandrosterone (DHEA)); and 17 and 18 carbon androgens
Zona reticularis (15%): DHEA, an androgen precursor

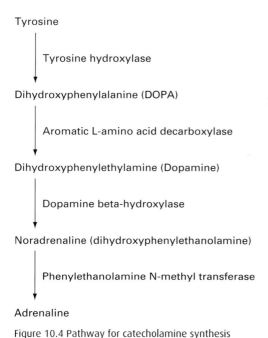

Tyrosine

     Tyrosine hydroxylase

Dihydroxyphenylalanine (DOPA)

     Aromatic L-amino acid decarboxylase

Dihydroxyphenylethylamine (Dopamine)

     Dopamine beta-hydroxylase

Noradrenaline (dihydroxyphenylethanolamine)

     Phenylethanolamine N-methyl transferase

Adrenaline

Figure 10.4 Pathway for catecholamine synthesis

cytochrome P450 system. Secretion is episodic and variable, demonstrating a diurnal circadian rhythm. In the circulation, cortisol is largely bound to a specific glucocorticoid binding $\alpha 2$-globulin called corticosteroid-binding globulin, with the remainder being either bound to albumin (15%–20%), or unbound (5%). **Stimuli to cortisol secretion include stress**, hypoglycaemia, ACTH, haemorrhage.

The high-affinity **glucocorticoid receptor** in target cells is a 94 kDa single-chain polypeptide in the cytosol. After glucocorticoid binding, the hormone–receptor complex translocates to the nucleus and binds to DNA. Gene transcription is affected, stimulating the synthesis of specific proteins.

Adrenocorticotrophic hormone (ACTH)

Adrenocorticotrophic hormone is a 39 amino acid peptide which is secreted by corticotroph cells of the anterior pituitary, being cleaved from a precursor molecule, pro-opiomelanocortin (POMC). It is secreted in a pulsatile fashion, with a diurnal rhythmicity. Peak secretion is in early morning, with a trough in late evening. Secretion of ACTH is controlled by closed loop feedback responsive to changes in serum cortisol, and by an open-loop component related to neurally mediated stimuli such as stress.

Corticotrophin releasing hormone, a 41 amino acid hypothalamic peptide, stimulates secretion and release of pro-opiomelanocortin and its derivatives from the anterior pituitary. Pro-opiomelanocortin is the precursor for ACTH, α-, β-, and γ-MSH, β-lipoprotein and endorphins. ACTH binds to cell membrane receptors in the adrenal cortex, activating adenyl cyclase. Steroidogenesis is initiated in the mitochondria by the binding of cholesterol to a C27 side chain cleavage enzyme, thereby starting its step-wise conversion to pregnenolone.

Secretagogues for ACTH include CRH, vasopressin, catecholamines, angiotensin II, atrial natriuretic peptide and serotonin.

Actions of glucocorticoids

- Permissive homeostasis, permitting the full expression of metabolic and circulatory processes without initiating them:

   Sensitises vascular smooth muscle to alpha and beta catecholamines, increasing vascular reactivity and facilitating adrenergic vasoconstriction of small vessels.

   Permits muscle resistance to fatigue, especially cardiac muscle, leading to a positive inotropic effect on myocardium.

   Facilitates mineralocorticoid action on renal tubules, with retention of sodium and excretion of potassium.

   Permits ADH activity on renal collecting duct, allowing excretion of a water load.

   Increased gluconeogenesis in the liver, along with inhibition of peripheral glucose utilisation, produces hyperglycaemia.

   Permits GH action on cells to facilitate growth.

   Plays a role in parturition.

- Bone marrow effects

   Allows bone marrow response to increase in neutrophil, red cell and platelet production.

   Reduces T cell number and function.

   Reduces B cell clonal expansion.

   Increases neutrophil count.

   Reduces eosinophil and basophil counts.

   Reduces lymphocyte and monocyte counts.

- Stress response

   Agonism of catecholamine effects.

   Promotes protein catabolism: with increased protein breakdown in plasma, muscle, skin and bone to amino acids. This increases urea concentration.

   Promotes peripheral lipolysis.

   Increases neuronal excitability.

- Metabolic effects: Both anabolic and catabolic effects are produced, with the catabolic effects predominating:

  Enhances lipid mobilisation, by enhancing peripheral lipolysis and by reducing re-esterification, especially in the liver. The deposition of additional fat in the central or truncal area is stimulated.

  Increases glucose synthesis in the liver.

  Increases hepatic glycogen synthesis and storage, and peripheral glycogenolysis.

  Reduces peripheral utilisation of glucose, inhibiting glucose transport into fat cells, fibroblasts and lymphoid cells.

  Increases peripheral protein catabolism.

  Increases protein synthesis in the liver and reduces peripheral protein synthesis.

- Alters mood and behaviour, producing euphoria.

- Inhibits formation of, and stimulates resorption of, bone. Bone formation is inhibited by the inhibition of osteoblast replication and of bone marrow synthesis, and by the induction of osteoblastic apoptosis. Bone resorption is increased by the stimulation of osteoclast synthesis.

- An anti-inflammatory response, which may be produced by the inhibition of transcription of several cytokines relevant to the response, namely interleukins 1,3,4,5,6, and 8, tumour necrosis factor-alpha, and granulocyte-mediated colony stimulating factor. Most anti-inflammatory effects require supra-physiological doses of glucocorticoids. The components of this response include:

  Inhibition of white cell mobilisation to areas of inflammation;

  Inhibition of capillary dilatation and reduced exudation of serum;

  Reduced histamine release from tissue mast cells and circulating basophils;

  Inhibition of synthesis and release of prostaglandins;

  Stabilisation of intracellular lysosomes.

Hypothalamic–pituitary–adrenal axis

Regulation of the hypothalamic–pituitary–adrenal axis is achieved by:

Long and short negative feedback loops: feedback inhibition by CRH, ACTH and glucocorticoids.

An ACTH-dependent diurnal rhythm of cortisol release with increased plasma levels in the early morning and low levels in late evening and early sleep. Peak levels are achieved between 3 am and 8 am. The circadian diurnal rhythm is abolished in Cushing's syndrome.

Stress activation of the axis by severe illness, trauma or surgery.

Actions of aldosterone

Increased sodium reabsorption in the distal tubule and cortical collecting duct with increased hydrogen and potassium secretion;

Increased sodium reabsorption by epithelial cells of the intestine, salivary and sweat glands;

Net sodium and water retention;

Increased intravascular volume.

Adrenocortical disorders

Mechanisms of glucocorticoid deficiency

Adrenocorticotrophic hormone-independent: destruction of the gland (infection; infiltration; autoimmune reaction; haemorrhage); congenital adrenal hyperplasia.

Adrenocorticotrophic hormone-dependent: hypothalamus–pituitary–adrenal axis suppression by exogenous glucocorticoids or ACTH, or by endogenous glucocorticoid; hypothalamus–pituitary lesions.

Mechanisms of glucocorticoid excess

Adrenocorticotrophic hormone-independent: adrenal adenoma, carcinoma, micronodular dysplasia, macronodular hyperplasia; iatrogenic causes.

Adrenocorticotrophic hormone-dependent: pituitary adenoma; ectopic ACTH syndrome.

Cushing's syndrome

The diagnosis of Cushing's syndrome requires the demonstration of:

An increased cortisol secretion rate, with raised 24 hour urinary free cortisol levels.

Features of primary hyperaldosteronism

Hypertension;

Polyuria and polydipsia;

Muscle weakness and spasm;

Hypokalaemia;

Metabolic alkalosis;

Increased urine potassium excretion, which is greater than 30 mmol/24 hours in the absence of diuretic therapy;

Reduced plasma renin activity;

A high aldosterone:renin ratio.

Adrenocortical function testing

Blood levels
Plasma steroids: cortisol (9 am and 11 pm levels); aldosterone.
Plasma peptides: ACTH; angiotensin II.

Urine levels
Urine 24 hour steroid metabolite excretion: free cortisol; 17-hydroxycorticosteroids; 17-ketosteroids.

Suppression tests
Hypothalamic–pituitary suppression: dexamethasone suppression test: low dose; high dose.
Mineralocorticoid suppressibility: extracellular fluid volume expansion leading to reduced plasma renin activity.

Stimulation tests
Glucocorticoid reserve: ACTH infusion.
Mineralocorticoid reserve and renin–angiotensin–aldosterone system stimulation: programmed volume depletion (e.g., upright posture; sodium restriction; diuretic administration).

Tests of pituitary adrenal responsiveness
Insulin-induced hypoglycaemia;
Metyrapone test;
CRH test.

Loss of circadian rhythm of cortisol secretion, with raised midnight serum cortisol levels.

Loss of negative feedback of increased glucocorticoid levels on the pituitary, with failure of inhibition of pituitary ACTH secretion and thence of serum cortisol by the administration of low-dose dexamethasone. High-dose dexamethasone will significantly lower serum cortisol in pituitary-dependent Cushing's disease but not in ACTH-independent Cushing's syndrome. High-dose suppression has no effect on ectopic ACTH syndromes.

■ Endocrine pancreas

The functional unit is the **islet of Langerhans**. There are about one million islets, comprising about 1%–1.5% of the total pancreatic mass and weighing about 1–2 grams in the adult.

The islets of Langerhans comprise:
Alpha cells: glucagon.

Beta cells: insulin. These cells comprise 70%–80% of the cell population of the islets.

Delta cells: somatostatin; gastrin.

Pancreatic polypeptide cells: pancreatic polypeptide.

Insulin

Insulin is the principal anabolic hormone of the body. It is a polypeptide with a molecular weight of 5808, consisting of a 21 amino acid alpha chain, linked by two disulphide bridges to a 30 amino acid beta chain.

Synthesis

Insulin is synthesised as a single polypeptide pre-prohormone on rough endoplasmic reticulum of pancreatic B cells. Cleavage of signal sequence yields 86 amino acid peptide proinsulin, which is the storage form of insulin.

Proinsulin is converted to insulin, immediately before secretion, in clathrin-coated prosecretory vesicles, with the excision of C peptide. Mature secretory vesicles in beta cells of the pancreatic islets contain equimolar amounts of insulin and C peptide. Circulating C peptide levels reflect beta cell activity.

Insulin is released by exocytosis of the secretory vesicles, stimulated by raised plasma glucose levels. The circulating half-life of endogenous insulin is 5–20 minutes.

Effects on cellular metabolism

Liver

Increased uptake of amino acids and glycerol;

Increased production of nicotinamide adenine dinucleotide phosphate dehydrogenase (NADPH);

Increased synthesis of glycogen, proteins, triglycerides and very low density lipoproteins (VLDLs);

Inhibition of glycogenolysis, promoting glycogen storage;

Inhibition of gluconeogenesis;

Inhibition of ketogenesis, i.e. conversion of fatty acids and amino acids to keto acids.

Skeletal muscle

Increased uptake of glucose and amino acids;

Increased synthesis of glycogen;

Inhibition of ketone body formation;

Inhibition of triglyceride utilisation;

Inhibition of proteolysis: reduced protein catabolism;

Increased protein synthesis.

Adipose tissue

Increased uptake of chylomicrons and VLDLs and of glucose;

Increased uptake and utilisation of glucose;

Inhibition of lipolysis;

Increased triglyceride synthesis.

Metabolic effects of insulin

Insulin is an anabolic hormone with widespread effects.

Carbohydrate metabolism

Increased glucose entry in adipose tissue and muscle cells. Glucose entry into cells is brought about by a family of sodium-independent facilitative glucose transporters, known as GLUT-1 to GLUT-5. Insulin stimulates translocation of glucose transporters from intracellular pools to the cell membrane.

Increased glycolysis in muscle and adipose tissue.

Increased glycogen synthesis in adipose tissue, muscle and liver cells.

Reduced gluconeogenesis and glycogenolysis in the liver.

Fat metabolism

Increased synthesis of free fatty acids in adipose tissue cells;

Increased synthesis of glycerol phosphate;

Increased synthesis and deposition of triacylglycerols in liver and adipose tissue;

Activation of lipoprotein lipase in adipose tissue;

Reduced ketogenesis (ketone body formation) by fatty acid oxidation in liver;

Increased rate of cholesterol and VLDL synthesis in the liver.

Protein metabolism

Increased amino acid uptake by cells, especially in muscle, liver and adipose tissue;

Increased rate of protein synthesis in muscle, adipose tissue and liver;

Inhibits protein degradation in muscle;

Reduced glucogenic amino acid release from hepatocytes;

Reduced rate of urea production;

Positive nitrogen balance.

Electrolytes

Uptake of K^+ into muscles and adipose tissue.

The metabolic actions of insulin on target tissues are mediated by the specific **insulin receptor**, located in the plasma membrane. It is an integral transmembrane glycoprotein with a molecular weight of 450 000 daltons. The receptor functions as an enzyme of the tyrosine protein kinase receptor class. It comprises two alpha sub-units of molecular weight 130 000 each, and two beta sub-units with molecular weights of 95 000 each.

Blood glucose homeostasis

Fasting blood glucose ranges between 3.5 and 5.5 mmol/l. The renal threshold for glucose is around 10.5 mmol/l.

Blood glucose homeostasis depends on:

Insulin, whose secretion is stimulated by glucose, glucagon, amino acids, ketoacids and other gastrointestinal tract hormones. Secretion is inhibited by adrenaline and somatostatin.

Counter-regulatory hormones – glucagon, catecholamines, cortisol and growth hormone – which antagonise the metabolic actions of insulin.

Blood glucose levels depend on a balance between intake, utilisation and production of glucose:

Glucose is utilised in cellular transport and phosphorylation, as well as in glycolysis and glycogen synthesis.

Glucose is produced by glycogenolysis and gluconeogenesis.

Dietary glucose intake can be from glucose itself, glucose-containing polysaccharides (starch and glycogen), glucose-containing disaccharides (sucrose, maltose, lactose), sugars readily converted to glucose (fructose), gluconeogenic amino acids and the glycerol moiety of triglycerides.

Hypoglycaemia

This is defined as a plasma glucose under 2.5 mmol/l. Broadly speaking, it can be either:

Fasting, related to:

Increased glucose utilisation: insulin; oral hypoglycaemics; insulinoma.

Reduced glucose production: severe liver disease; adrenocortical deficiency; pituitary failure; glycogen storage disease.

Non-fasting or reactive:

Postprandial: glucose; galactose; fructose

Alcohol
Leucine

Ketoacidosis

The pathogenesis of **diabetic ketoacidosis** involves the following sequence:
A relative or absolute deficiency of insulin.
Hyperglycaemia, which leads to glycosuria when the renal threshold for glucose is exceeded.
Glucose in the urine leads to osmotic diuresis, causing dehydration and electrolyte depletion.
Increased lipolysis, leading to increased plasma free fatty acids. These are used in ketogenesis in the liver, with consequent ketonaemia and ketonuria.
The use of base in buffering ketoacids (acetoacetate and beta-hydroxybutyrate) leads to metabolic acidosis. The presence of ketoacids creates a large anion gap.
Insulin deficiency produces hyperglycaemia by the following mechanisms:

Increased glycogenolysis and gluconeogenesis;
Increased proteolysis, with increased circulating amino acids;
Reduced peripheral utilisation of glucose.

Glucagon

Glucagon is a single chain 29 amino acid polypeptide with a molecular weight of 3485. It is encoded for on chromosome 2. Synthesis occurs in A cells of the islets of Langerhans and L cells of the ileum and colon. It is derived from 169 amino acid proglucagon, which is stored within granules in alpha cells.

Glucagon is secreted in response to hypoglycaemia and low free fatty acid levels. Secretion is inhibited by glucose.

It has the following actions:

Liver
Increased glycogenolysis in the liver;
Reduced glycogenesis;
Increased gluconeogenesis;
Reduced glycolysis;
Increased ketogenesis by fatty acid oxidation.

Adipose tissue
Increased lipolysis;
Stimulation of insulin secretion.

Gastro-intestinal tract

Inhibition of gastric acid secretion;

Inhibition of pancreatic exocrine secretion;

Inhibition of intestinal peristalsis.

■ Reproductive system

The reproductive system is concerned with the propagation of the human species and is controlled by the hypothalamic–pituitary–gonadal axis.

Gonadotrophin releasing hormone

Gonadotrophin releasing hormone is a 10 amino acid peptide, with N- and C-terminals blocked to enzymatic degradation. It is synthesised as a 92 amino acid pre-prohormone comprising a 23 amino acid signal peptide, the 10 amino acid GnRH sequence, and a 56 amino acid GnRH-associated peptide.

It is secreted by hypothalamic neurons in the arcuate nucleus and the organum vasculosum lamina terminalis. The neurons responsible arise as precursor peripheral sensory neurons of the nasal epithelium, from the medial olfactory placode, and migrate into the hypothalamus. Failure of migration of the neurons is associated with Kallman's syndrome of hypogonadotrophic hypogonadism and anosmia. The neurons do not have any axonal connections with other neuronal networks. Their axons are directed into the median eminence, where they are apposed to the hypophyseal portal vessels.

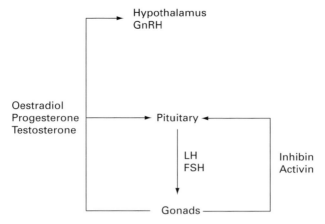

Figure 10.5 Hypothalamic–pituitary–ovarian pathway. GnRH, gonadotrophin releasing hormone; LH, luteinising hormone; FSH, follicle stimulating hormone.

The neurons have rhythmic intrinsic depolarisation and secretory activity with self-generated pulsatile secretion, involving short periods of abrupt secretion separated by large periods of low or undetectable secretion.

Gonadotrophin releasing hormone travels by axonomic flow to the axon terminals of the median eminence. It binds to anterior pituitary gonadotrophs that secrete FSH and LH. The activation mechanism is calcium-dependent activation of a specific membrane receptor adenyl cyclase-cyclic AMP process. The GnRH receptor is a member of the seven transmembrane domain G-protein-coupled family of receptors.

The reproductive cycles commence at puberty as a hypothalamic pulse generator is activated and stimulates the GnRH neurons. Gonadotrophin releasing hormone simultaneously regulates FSH and LH secretion. It has a short plasma half-life, of 2–4 minutes due to rapid proteolytic cleavage. Follicle stimulating hormone and LH are glycopeptides consisting of two subunits, alpha and beta. They share the alpha subunit. Specificity resides in the beta subunit.

Target tissues for gonadotrophins

Luteinising hormone

Leydig cells
Thecal cells: antral follicles
Granulosa cells: pre-ovulatory follicles
Luteal cells: corpus luteum
Interstitial glands of ovary

Follicle stimulating hormone

Sertoli cells
Granulosa cells: follicles

Chorionic gonadotrophin

Luteal cells

Oestrogens

17 beta-oestradiol: E2
Oestriol: E3
Oestrone: E1

Oestrogen actions

Stimulate secondary sexual characteristics of females;

Growth, development and maintenance of fallopian tubes, uterus, vagina and external genitalia;

Stimulation of follicular growth;

Prepare uterus for spermatozoal transport;

Increased vascular permeability and tissue oedema;

Stimulate growth and activity of mammary glands and of endometrium in the proliferative phase of the menstrual cycle;

Prepare endometrium for progestogen actions;

Increase the amount of contractile proteins in the myometrium;

Secrete thin, plentiful, cervical mucus;

Mildly anabolic;

Stimulates calcification, bone growth and epiphyseal closure;

Regulation of gonadotrophin secretion;

Stimulate synthesis of transport globulins in the liver;

Reduce serum cholesterol and increase serum high density lipoprotein (HDL) levels;

Reduce glucose tolerance;

Increase clotting factor production.

Androgens

5 alpha-dihydrotestosterone

Testosterone

Androstenedione

Dehydroepiandrosterone

Sources of androgen in the female are:

Peripheral conversion of androstenedione in the liver, adipose tissue and skin: 50%.

Ovarian stimulation by serum LH: 25%.

Adrenal cortical stimulation by serum ACTH: 25%.

Hormonal effects of oestrogen levels

Low levels
Increased synthesis and storage of oestrogens;
Little effect on LH secretion;
Inhibit FSH secretion.

High levels
Induce mid-cycle LH surge;
High steady levels lead to sustained increase in LH secretion.

Androgen actions

Induce and maintain differentiation of male somatic tissues. Regulate the differentiation of male internal and external genitalia in the fetus.

Induce and maintain secondary sex characteristics of males and body hair of females.

Induce and maintain the function of the accessory sex organs in males: seminiferous tubules; ductuli efferentes; epididymis; vas deferens; ejaculatory duct; seminal vesicles; prostate gland; bulbo-urethral glands.

Initiate and maintain spermatogenesis.

Induce sexual and aggressive behaviour in males and females.

Promote protein anabolism, linear growth, muscle development and ossification, and epiphyseal closure.

Regulate gonadotrophin secretion: testosterone.

Anti-corticosteroid effects: dehydroepiandrosterone.

Responsible for male pattern hair growth.

Cause laryngeal enlargement.

Stimulate synthesis of androgen-binding protein.

Modes of androgen action

Intracellular conversion of testosterone to dihydrotestosterone;

Testosterone itself;

Intracellular conversion of testosterone to oestradiol (aromatisation).

Progestagens

Progesterone
  17 alpha-hydroxyprogesterone
  20 alpha-hydroxyprogesterone

Progestagen actions

Responsible for the secretory phase of the endometrium in the menstrual cycle;

Prepare the uterus to receive the conceptus;

Maintain the uterus during pregnancy;

Reduce the frequency and amplitude of myometrial contractions;

Stimulate the secretion of scanty, viscous cervical mucus;

Stimulate the growth of the lobules and alveoli of the mammary glands;

Suppress milk secretion;

Promote sodium loss in the distal convoluted tubules;

Generalised mild catabolic effect;

Regulate gonadotrophin secretion;

Cause elevation of basal body temperature after ovulation.

Hormonal effects of changes in progestagen levels

Low levels:

Enhance LH secretory response to GnRH.

High levels:

Inhibit pituitary secretion of gonadotrophins, in the presence of oestrogens.

Other peptide hormones involved in the hypothalamic–pituitary–ovarian feedback cycle are activin and inhibin, members of the transforming growth factor-beta superfamily of glycoproteins.

Inhibin is a heterodimer of alpha and beta sub-units linked by disulphide bonds. There are two forms, A and B. The molecular weight is 32 kDa. It is synthesised and secreted by the granulosa and luteal cells.

Activin is a homodimer of inhibin beta subunit linked by disulphide bridges. There are three types, A, B and AB. The molecular weight ranges from 26 to 28 kDa. It is synthesised by the granulosa cells.

Male reproductive system

This consists of the hypothalamus, other CNS sites, the pituitary gland, the testes, sex steroid-responsive end organs and sites of androgen transport and metabolism.

Normal sexual function in men comprises normal desire or libido, along with erectile, ejaculatory and orgasmic capacity.

Testis

The testes are 35–45 grams in weight and around 4.5 cm in length. They are involved in spermatogenesis and steroidogenesis and consist of two functional units, the interstitial or Leydig cells and the seminiferous tubules. The three major cell types are the germ cells, the Sertoli cells and the interstitial cells. Testicular activity is under endocrine control via the gonadotrophins and under autocrine/paracrine control mediated by tissue growth factors.

The products of the testes include:

Spermatozoa-seminiferous tubules, which house the Sertoli cells;

Hormones;

Leydig cells: androgens; oxytocin; relaxin-like factor;

Sertoli cells: inhibin; activin; Mullerian inhibiting substance.

Spermatogenesis refers to the process by which the spermatogonial germ cell is converted to a mature spermatozoon.

The accessory sexual glands consist of:

Seminal vesicles;

Prostate;

Bulbo-urethral glands of Cowper.

The epididymis is involved with post-testicular maturation of spermatozoa and with the storage of spermatozoa.

Components of semen

Seminal plasma

Prostate gland: acid phosphatase; citric acid; zinc; fibrinolytic enzymes.

Seminal vesicles: prostaglandins; fructose; ascorbic acid; phosphorylcholine.

Spermatozoa

Functions of Sertoli cells

The tight junctions between the Sertoli cells form the **blood–testis barrier**, maintaining the gradient of ions, small molecules and proteins between the blood and the tubular fluid;

Production of Mullerian inhibitory substance;

Aromatisation of androgen to oestrogen;

Secretion of androgen-binding protein, growth factors, transferrin, caerulo-plasmin, hormones (inhibin, activin, steroids) and seminiferous tubule fluid.

Functions of Leydig cells

Secrete testosterone as a result of LH stimulation and thus contain a large amount of smooth endoplasmic reticulum. This is responsible for the development of secondary sexual characteristics. The LH receptor is a G-protein-coupled receptor.

Seminal fluid fructose production.

Semen analysis

Volume of ejaculate: 2–6 ml

Sperm concentration: 20–250×10^{6}/ml

Motility (0.5–2 h post-ejaculation): >50% motile

Vitality: 75% or more live

pH: 7.2–8.0

Total acid phosphatase: >200 U/ejaculate

Penile erection

Basic features

Erection is initiated by local genital sensory stimulation, or by cerebral stimulation produced by visual, auditory, psychogenic, tactile or gustatory stimuli. Penile vascular vasodilatation is mediated by neurotransmitters of the non-adrenergic, non-cholinergic system.

Erection commences with blood accumulation in the lacunar spaces of the paired corpora cavernosa, caused by dilatation of the cavernosal and helicine arteries. Continued accumulation of blood is facilitated by relaxation of the trabecular smooth muscle. A corporeal veno-occlusive mechanism traps blood inside the corpora cavernosa, by compression of the sub-tunical arterial plexus with reduction in venous outflow from the lacunar spaces.

Vascular phases of erection

Flaccid: a tonic low blood flow state resulting from cavernosal smooth muscle contraction.

Latent (filling): relaxation of arteries and of smooth muscle of cavernosa

Tumescence: increasing inflow of blood, with commencing increase in intra-cavernosal pressure.

Full erection: impedance of outflow of blood, with intracavernosal pressure equalling mean systolic arterial blood pressure.

Rigid erection: intracavernosal pressure exceeds systolic blood pressure

Detumescence: contraction of cavernosal smooth muscle and relaxation of ischio-cavernosus muscles.

Mediators of smooth muscle activity in the penis

Smooth muscle relaxation: nitric oxide; acetylcholine; vasoactive intestinal peptide (VIP); prostaglandin E; ATP; adenosine.

Smooth muscle contraction: noradrenaline; endothelins; prostanoids; angio-tensin; vasopressin.

Ovary

Functional constituents of the adult ovary

Follicles
  Primordial
  Secondary follicles
    Pre-antral (growing)
    Antral (liquor-filled antral cavity)

Pre-ovulatory

Single dominant ovulatory, which tends to alternate in each ovary in successive cycles

Corpus luteum

Atretic follicles

Stromal component

Hilar medulla

The primary monthly ovarian cycle of follicular development, steroid biosynthesis and ovulation, is mediated by GnRH, pituitary gonadotrophins and ovarian steroid feedback on the adenohypophysis. This finely tuned process maintains cyclicity and synchronicity. A secondary neuroendocrine control system modulates the primary system in relation to environmental changes such as light, smell and temperature. This involves neural inputs from higher CNS centres.

At **puberty**, a sequence of events ensues, including:

Primarily an increase in pulsatile secretion of GnRH and gonadotrophins;

Changes in ovarian and adrenal steroid production;

Maturation of the hypothalamic–pituitary–ovarian axis;

Development of secondary sexual characteristics;

Acceleration of linear growth;

Bone maturation;

Changes in body composition, including lean body mass skeletal mass and body fat mass.

The **ovarian cycle** comprises:

Pre-ovulatory recruitment from pool of primordial follicles.

Orderly development of a single dominant follicle.

Proliferation and differentiation of granulosa cells.

Follicular synthesis of oestrogens. Follicle stimulating hormone receptors are present on the granulosa cells. Luteinising hormone receptors are present on the theca cells. As the follicle grows, FSH induces the appearance of LH receptors on the granulosa cells.

Ovulation is triggered by the mid-cycle LH surge, itself triggered by the sustained high circulating levels of oestradiol produced by the pre-ovulatory follicle. It can also be triggered by exogenous HCG after FSH priming of the pre-ovulatory follicle.

Follicular rupture.

Luteal development with secretion of progesterone, oestradiol and inhibin by the corpus luteum.

Regression of the corpus luteum (luteolysis).

Luteal rescue by human chorionic gonadotrophin occurs if conception results, with delay in regression.

Menstrual cycle

Phases

Menstrual phase: 0–3 days

Proliferative phase: 3–14 days

Secretory phase: 14–20 days

Preparation for implantation: 21–26 days

Endometrial breakdown: 24–28 days

Follicular or proliferative phase

Endocrine:

Rising LH, with mid-cycle peak;

Falling FSH, with a small mid-cycle rise;

Rising oestrogen, with a pre-ovulatory peak;

Rise in progesterone at mid-cycle.

Endometrium:

Proliferation of glandular, stromal and luminal epithelium;

Proliferation of vascular elements: spiral arterioles.

Breast:

Epithelial proliferation;

Ductal epithelial sprouting.

Luteal or secretory phase

Endocrine:

Declining LH after mid-cycle peak;

Declining FSH after mid-cycle peak, rising at the end;

Oestrogen peak in mid-cycle, decreasing by the end;

Increasing progesterone, declining by the end.

Endometrium:

Early: elongation; filling of lumina with glycogen-rich secretions; coiling of spiral arterioles.

Late: saw tooth glands; stromal oedema caused by fluid accumulation in the extracellular matrix.

Breast:

Secretory changes;

Ductal dilatation.

Functions of the Fallopian tubes

Pickup of the ovum
Transport of gametes
Transport of the early embryo

Menstruation is caused by withdrawal of ovarian steroid support from the decidualised endometrium. Spiral arteriolar vasospasm causes endometrial ischaemia. Lysosomal enzyme release ensues. Shedding of the decidua functionalis of the endometrium occurs. Control of menstrual bleeding is achieved by platelet plug formation, prostaglandins (PGE2, PGF2α) and endometrial repair.

Fertilisation

This is achieved by:

Penetration of the zona pellucida by the spermatozoon;

Binding of sperm head receptors and ligands of the zona pellucida;

Fusion of sperm and oocyte membrane;

Enzyme-induced zona reaction;

Cell division.

At the menopause ovarian follicle maturation begins to decline prior to its eventual cessation. This is associated with increased pituitary secretion of FSH and LH.

Hypogonadism

This is defined as inadequate gonadal function, manifested by defects in gametogenesis and/or secretion of gonadal hormones. The manifestations vary according to the sex of the subject, and whether the onset is pre- or post-pubertal. The features of pre-pubertal hypogonadism are those of pubertal delay, while the features of post-pubertal hypogonadism are often more subtle.

Mechanisms of hypogonadism

These can be categorised as:

Primary or hypergonadotrophic hypogonadism due to ovarian or testicular failure, with lack of sex steroid production by the gonads;

Secondary or hypogonadotrophic hypogonadism, due to either failure of the hypothalamic GnRH pulse generator, or to pituitary failure to secrete gonadotrophins;

End organ resistance to sex steroids.

Physiological changes in pregnancy

These can be described as follows:

- Circulatory system: a gradual and progressive increase in cardiac output, with an increase of 40% by the third trimester. An increase in blood volume by about one-third is related to a disproportionate increase in plasma volume as compared with red cell volume, resulting in the physiological anaemia of pregnancy. A reduction in systemic and pulmonary vascular resistances counterbalances the increased volume load. Systolic arterial blood pressure is unaltered, while diastolic blood pressure falls in the first two trimesters, returning to non-pregnant levels in the third trimester. The cardiovascular stress of pregnancy is maximal at labour, during delivery, and in the immediate post-partum period.

- Respiratory system: an increase in respiratory rate, associated with reduction in $paCO_2$ and in buffering capacity, leads to increased minute ventilation. There is also a reduction in functional residual capacity. Splinting of the diaphragm reduces lung volumes.

- A hypercoagulable state in the blood is the result of increased plasma concentrations of clotting factors, fibrinogen and fibrin degradation products.

Placenta

The human placenta is circular and disc-like, and of the haemomonochorial type, with the fetal–maternal barrier comprising trophoblastic cells, fetal connective tissue and fetal endothelium. This provides direct contact between the fetal chorionic villi and the maternal bloodstream. The villi are composed of a superficial layer of syncytiotrophoblast, which surrounds the villous stroma. Maternal blood circulates in the diffuse inter-villous space. Utero-placental flow is not subject to autoregulation. Flow through the inter-villous space depends on maternal blood pressure and is inversely proportional to uterine vascular resistance.

Functions of the placenta

Feto-maternal transport of:

   Respiratory gases: oxygen and carbon dioxide
   Nutrients: carbohydrates (glucose); amino acids; lipids; minerals; trace elements
   Water
   Immunoglobulin G
   Waste products for excretion

Endocrine: synthesis of hormones that maintain pregnancy and regulate fetal growth, maturation and development.

   Peptide hormones: human chorionic gonadotrophin; human placental lactogen; activin; inhibin; CRH; ACTH; insulin-like growth factors.

Factors affecting placental transfer of drugs

These include:
- Molecular weight
- Lipid solubility
- Degree of ionisation
- Protein binding
- Maternal–fetal concentration gradient
- Placental surface area
- Placental blood flow
- These factors need to be taken into consideration while prescribing medications during pregnancy.

Steroids: progesterone; oestrogens; glucocorticoids.

Immune barrier between the mother and the fetal allograft

The **mechanism of placental transport** depends on the nature of the transported substance:

Lipophilic substances are transported by diffusion.

Hydrophilic substances are transported by:
- Pores
- Transport proteins or carriers
- Ion channels
- Pumps
- Vesicular endocytosis

Trans-placental respiratory gas exchange depends on:
- The trans-placental concentration gradient of the gas;
- Gas carrying capacities of fetal and maternal blood;
- Rates of fetal and maternal placental blood flow;
- The permeability and surface areas of the membranes involved.

■ Calcium metabolism

Calcium is the most abundant cation in the body (1–1.5 kg; around 25–35 moles), 99% being present in bones and teeth. The exchangeable pool of calcium comprises 1%–2% of the total, around 0.1% being in the extracellular fluid and 0.5% in the intracellular fluid in the soft tissues. Calcium regulation involves three tissues (bone, intestine and kidney), three hormones (PTH, calcitonin and activated vitamin D3) and three cell types (osteoblasts, osteocytes and osteoclasts).

The regulatory mechanisms comprise:

Intestinal absorption (vitamin D dependent): duodenum and proximal jejunum;

Renal tubular reabsorption and excretion;

Exchange of calcium between plasma and bone:bone remodelling.

Plasma calcium homeostasis depends on a balance between the hypocalcaemic effects of calcitonin and the hypercalcaemic effects of PTH, vitamin D and calcium intake.

Functions of calcium

- Structural integrity and metabolism of bone (bone growth and remodelling)
- Tooth formation.
- Synaptic transmission.
- Coenzyme function, e.g. in haemostatic (clotting cascade) and complement systems.
- Control of excitability of nerve and muscle cells: stabilisation of membrane potentials by modulation of permeability to sodium and potassium.
- Excitation–contraction coupling in muscles.
- Stimulus–secretion coupling: nerve terminals; endocrine and exocrine glands (exocytosis).
- Regulation of transmembrane ion transport. Bidirectional calcium transport occurs across the plasma membrane and across the membranes of organelles such as the endoplasmic reticulum, sarcoplasmic reticulum and mitochondria.
- Second or third messenger in intracellular signal transduction pathways. The low cytosolic content of calcium plays a part in explaining this mechanism.
- Cell motility.

Components of plasma calcium

The plasma calcium is kept tightly regulated at between 2.30 and 2.60 mmol/l, implying an important regulatory role. It consists of the following fractions:

Body calcium pools

Bony skeleton (mineral component)
Intracellular pool
Extracellular pool
Plasma/serum: ionic; protein bound; citrate bound

Corrected calcium

Albumin < 40 g/l.
Corrected calcium (mmol/l)= (Ca) + 0.02 × (40−albumin)
Albumin > 40 g/l
Corrected calcium (mmol)= (Ca) + 0.02 × (albumin−40)

Protein bound (45%), predominantly to albumin (35%), the remainder (10%) to globulins.

Ultrafilterable calcium:

Complexed with anions – phosphate, sulphate, citrate, lactate (10%);

Free or ionised (45%) (1.16–1.30 mmol/l).

Ionised calcium is the physiologically active fraction, and the focus for metabolic control by the parathyroid gland through its membrane-bound extracellular calcium receptor. Total plasma calcium is unreliable as a measure of ionised calcium. The use of a correction factor for albumin may allow an indirect estimate of ionised calcium. Ionised calcium is reduced by an alkaline pH and by low temperature and increased by acid pH, high temperature and by blood cell metabolism.

Calcium homeostasis

Calcium absorption

Calcium absorption in the small intestine occurs by both active transport and by diffusion. Active transport predominates in the duodenum and jejunum, and diffusion in the ileum. Calcium absorption occurs down an electrochemical gradient across the brush border of the duodenal and jejunal enterocytes, through transmembrane calcium channels at the apical membrane. Intracellular transport involves carrier proteins, intestinal calcium-binding protein and cytosolic calcium-binding protein. Active transport across the basolateral membrane is mediated by a Mg^{2+}-dependent Ca^{2+}-ATPase (primary active transport), and a $Ca^{2+}/3Na^{+}$ exchanger (secondary active transport). Vitamin D (1,25 dihydroxyvitamin D3 – calcitriol) regulates the amount of cytosolic calcium-binding protein and activates the active transport systems. Parathyroid hormone indirectly increases small intestinal absorption by enhancing 25-OH D-1α hydroxylase activity and calcitriol synthesis.

Reabsorption of calcium

The majority of filtered calcium is reabsorbed in the proximal tubule by transcellular (20%) or para-cellular (80%) pathways. Transcellular absorption

Factors affecting intestinal calcium absorption

Increased
Vitamin D3
Some amino acids, e.g. lysine

Decreased
Glucocorticoids
High calcium diet
High phosphate diet
Low intestinal pH
Fat malabsorption
Liver disease

involves entry via calcium channels in the apical membrane, down the electro-chemical gradient produced by calcium extrusion at the basolateral membrane. Calcium extrusion across the basolateral membrane is achieved by Ca^{2+}-ATPase and a $Ca^{2+}/3 Na^{+}$ anti-porter, acting against the electrochemical gradient. Para-cellular absorption takes place across the tight junctions between epithelial cells. Further absorption takes place in the thick ascending limb of the loop of Henle. Absorption in the distal tubule is transcellular, through voltage-sensitive calcium channels activated by PTH. This is the stage subject to hormonal regulation.

Seventy per cent of filtered calcium is reabsorbed in the proximal tubule, 20% in the loop of Henle, and 9% in the distal tubule. The remaining 1% is excreted in the urine. Parathyroid hormone stimulates calcium reabsorption in the loop of Henle and in the distal tubule.

Hypercalcaemia

This can be broadly classified as being:

Parathyroid hormone related: primary hyperparathyroidism; secondary hyperparathyroidism in chronic renal insufficiency; tertiary hyperparathyroidism; ectopic PTH secretion.

Vitamin D related: vitamin D toxicity; granulomatous diseases associated with excess 1,25-dihydroxyvitamin D3 production.

Malignancy: increased osteoclastic activity due to bone destruction by primary or metastatic tumour; PTH-related protein or peptide.

Medications: thiazide diuretics; lithium; vitamin A and analogues.

Endocrine disorders: thyrotoxicosis; adrenocortical insufficiency.

Hypocalcaemia

This can be encountered in the following situations:

Factitious hypocalcaemia
Hypoalbuminaemia
Hypomagnesaemia

True hypocalcaemia
Vitamin D deficiency or target organ resistance;
Dietary deficiency or malabsorption;
Impaired 25-hydroxylation: liver disease;
Impaired 1 alpha-hydroxylation: renal failure;
Accelerated loss: anticonvulsants;
PTH deficiency or target organ resistance;
Hyperphosphataemia;
Loss of calcium from the circulation: excessive deposition in the skeleton (osteoblastic metastases; hungry bone syndrome); chelation.

Phosphorus metabolism

The total body phosphorus content is distributed between bone (90%), other intracellular locations (9%) and in the extracellular fluid (1% or under). Phosphate circulates as the free ion (55%), complexed ion (33%) or the protein-bound form (12%). Phosphate is the principal intracellular anion. Dietary phosphate is absorbed in the duodenum and jejunum. Ninety per cent of filtered phosphate is reabsorbed in the kidneys. Reabsorption in the renal proximal tubule is achieved by passive co-transport with sodium, involving a 2 Na^+/Pi symport mechanism in the apical membrane. This is regulated by the dietary phosphate intake, PTH levels and insulin-like growth factors. Parathyroid hormone inhibits phosphate reabsorption in the proximal tubule by increasing cyclic AMP levels, increasing urinary phosphate excretion.

Functions of phosphate

These include:
Formation of high energy compounds: e.g. ATP, creatinine phosphate;
Formation of second messengers, e.g. cyclic AMP, inositol phosphates;
Component of DNA/RNA, phospholipid membranes, bone;
Phosphorylation (activation/inactivation) of enzymes;
Intracellular anion.

Parathyroid glands

Structural features

The parathyroid glands are usually four in number: two superior and two inferior. They are located on the posterior aspect of the lateral lobes of the thyroid or in its fibrous capsule. Each gland weighs about 35 mg. They originate from the third and fourth branchial pouches. The cells that constitute the gland are the chief cells, oxyphil cells and water clear cells.

Parathyroid hormone (PTH)

Parathyroid hormone is an 84 amino acid polypeptide, with a molecular weight of 9500. The molecule has no disulphide bridges. Biological activity is confined to the NH_2-terminal 34 amino acid sequence. It is encoded for on chromosome 11. The serum level ranges from 10–60 pg/ml and the circulating half-life is 2–4 minutes.

It is secreted by parathyroid chief cells as a prepro-PTH, a 115 amino acid precursor. A 25 amino acid hydrophilic leader peptide is cleaved from the $-NH_2$ terminus to yield a prohormone. Further cleavage of a basic, $-NH_2$-terminal hexapeptide yields the mature 84 amino acid hormone. Parathyroid hormone is cleaved at the 33–34 and 36–37 positions in the liver and kidneys to yield an amino terminal and a carboxyl terminal fragment.

Parathyroid hormone maintains the plasma ionised calcium level, the PTH level being controlled by a negative feedback mechanism. The calcium sensing receptor is a glycoprotein with molecular weight of 500 000 and is located on the parathyroid cell surface. Magnesium is required for PTH release and for its effects on target tissues. Serum PTH levels show a diurnal circadian variation. For the correct interpretation of the significance of serum levels, simultaneous measurement of serum calcium and phosphate concentrations is required.

It has a direct effect on bone and renal tubules and an indirect effect on small intestine. Parathyroid hormone binds to plasma membrane G-protein-coupled receptors on target cells in bone and the kidneys, where they are concentrated at the basolateral surface of the cortical thick ascending limb of the loop of Henle. The calcium-sensing receptor (CSR) is a 1079 amino acid membrane protein, with seven α-helical transmembrane domains, an extracellular domain and an intracellular carboxyl-terminal G-protein-binding domain. The extracellular domain binds Ca^{2+} and Mg^{2+}. The calcium-sensing receptor detects the serum calcium concentration, and determines the set point for the serum PTH concentration.

Parathyroid hormone increases bone resorption (osteolysis) by increasing the numbers and activity of osteoclasts, and by increasing calcium transport from bone to the extracellular fluid. It increases proximal renal tubular reabsorption of calcium and reduces tubular reabsorption of phosphate (cyclic AMP mediated).

Parathyroid hormone stimulates renal hydroxylation of 25-hydroxy vitamin D3 to 1,25-dihydroxyvitamin D3, which increases intestinal calcium absorption by inducing a calcium-binding protein in the duodenal and jejunal mucosae.

There is no direct effect on intestine. Parathyroid hormone acts synergistically with calcitriol to absorb calcium and phosphate.

Calcitonin

Calcitonin is a 32 amino acid polypeptide, with a disulphide bridge between the cysteine residues in positions 1 and 7. It is secreted by the parafollicular or C cells of the thyroid gland, which comprise 0.1% of the thyroid mass.

The **calcitonin receptor** is a seven transmembrane domain G-protein-coupled receptor in the osteoclast and in the kidneys. Receptor down-regulation may explain the self-limiting nature of calcitonin action.

Calcitonin inhibits osteoclastic activity by increasing intracellular cyclic AMP levels. It diminishes osteolytic activity of osteoclasts and osteocytes. Other actions include:

Antagonism to the effect of PTH on bone;

Inhibition of gastric motility and gastrin secretion;

Inhibition of jejunal absorption of calcium and phosphate;

Inhibition of tubular reabsorption and promotion of urinary excretion of phosphate, calcium and sodium;

Inhibition of renal 1 alpha-hydroxylase activity, with decreased synthesis of calcitriol.

Calcitonin is used for the treatment of hypercalcaemia and for osteoporosis. Salmon calcitonin possesses 100 times the potency of human calcitonin.

Vitamin D

Vitamin D3 (cholecalciferol) is produced by ultraviolet irradiation of provitamin D3 (7-dehydrocholesterol) in the skin, and can also be obtained from dietary sources. Vitamin D2 (ergocalciferol) is produced by the ultraviolet irradiation of the plant sterol, ergosterol.

In the liver, vitamin D3 is converted by hydroxylation at the C-25 position to 25-hydroxyvitamin D3 (calcidiol).

In the kidneys, 25-hydroxyvitamin D3 is hydroxylated at the C-1alpha position to the hormonally active metabolite, 1,25-dihydroxyvitamin D3 (calcitriol). This reaction is catalysed by 1alpha-hydroxylase in the proximal tubule cells, and

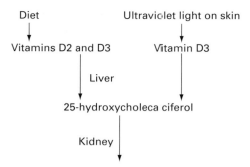

Figure 10.6 Pathway for vitamin D synthesis.

promoted by PTH. Hydroxylation can also lead to 24, 25-dihydroxyvitamin D3. The biological activity of calcitriol is 100 times greater than that of 25-hydroxycholecalciferol.

The hydroxylases in the liver and kidneys are all cytochrome P450 mixed function oxidases. The most important control point is the activity of renal 1-hydroxylase, which modulates the production of 1,25 dihydroxyvitamin D3.

Calcitriol acts by binding to the nuclear vitamin D receptor, a 427 amino acid protein encoded by an 11 excn gene located at chromosome 12. It stimulates absorption or reabsorption of calcium in the small intestine, bone, and kidneys.

Vitamin D actions

These can be categorised as:

Classical:

Increased calcium-binding proteins;

Increased calcium pumps on basolateral surface of intestinal villus and crypt cells;

Stimulated production of paracrine signals on osteoblasts, which recruit and activate osteoclasts;

Increased alkaline phosphatase and osteocalcin for bone mineralisation;

Increased 24-hydroxylase activity.

Non-classical:

Reduced production of interleukin-2, gamma-interferon and other cytokines in monocytes and activated T lymphocytes;

Inhibition of cell cycle of proliferating T and B lymphocytes; proliferating keratinocytes; smooth muscle cells, cardiac myocytes; myometrium and endometrium of uterus.

Vitamin D disorders

These may be produced by:
    Alterations in availability of vitamin D;
    Altered conversion of vitamin D3 to 25-hydroxyvitamin D3;
    Altered conversion of 25-hydroxyvitamin D3 to 1,25-dihydroxyvitamin D3 and/or
        24,25-dihydroxyvitamin D3;
    Altered end organ responsiveness.

The **vitamin D receptor** is a member of the steroid/thyroid receptor super-family. It is a nuclear receptor that is found in all target tissues on which vitamin D acts. The wide distribution of the receptor explains the wide range of activity of the vitamin. The receptor acts as a ligand-induced transcription factor regulating the rate of expression of genes involved in the regulation of calcium homeostasis, the control of bone cell differentiation as in remodelling, the modulation of immune responses, the control of hormone secretion, inhibition of cell growth and the induction of cell differentiation.

Bone function

The human body comprises 208 bones. The axial skeleton includes the skull, vertebral column and the thoracic cage, while the appendicular skeleton consists of the bones in the upper and lower limbs. Cortical bone is found in the shafts of long bones of the appendicular skeleton. Cancellous or trabecular bone is found in the marrow cavity. Seventy per cent to 80% of bone by mass is cortical or compact bone. The remaining 20%–30% is trabecular or spongy or cancellous bone. Bone marrow consists of stroma, myeloid tissue, fat cells, blood vessels, sinusoids and lymphatic tissue.

The structural unit of cortical bone is the **osteon**. This consists of irregular, branching and anastomosing cylinders, which are composed of a central neuro-vascular Haversian canal. The canal is surrounded by concentric lamellae of cell permeated layers of the bone matrix. The cylinders are between 200 and 300 μm in diameter. Six to seven concentric osteocyte rings comprise up to 20 lamellar plates.

The osteons are oriented in the long axis of the bone. They are connected to one another by perpendicularly oriented Volkmann's canals. Cortical bone is a complex structure of adjacent osteons and their interstitial and circumferential lamellae.

Bone is a dynamic tissue with the capacity for continuous remodelling. It has the following functions:

    Provision of mechanical support and the structural framework for the body;

Provision of a site for muscle attachment;

Protection of the viscera;

Contains the bone marrow and is a site for haematopoiesis;

Provides a metabolic reserve of calcium and phosphate ions, thereby contributing to mineral metabolism.

Remodelling provides a constant and rapid source of calcium for the maintenance of homeostasis of serum levels, and allows enhancement of skeletal strength and elasticity. It is an integrated process of coupled bone resorption and bone formation that results in the maintenance of net skeletal mass with the renewal of mineralised matrix. This allows regeneration in response to injury, particularly micro-damage from exposure to physiological loads. The remodelling sequence can be considered to be one of activation, resorption and formation.

The components of bone

The extracellular organic matrix (osteoid), which contains calcium in the form of hexagonal hydroxyapatite crystals;

A cellular component of bone-forming osteoblasts and bone-resorbing osteoclasts. The cells are embedded in the matrix.

The extracellular matrix

This comprises:

Collagen, mainly type I. This has a triple helical structure, with two identical alpha 1 chains and one unique alpha 2 chain cross-linked by hydrogen bonding between hydroxyproline and other charged residues.

Other proteins and proteoglycans:

Proteoglycans I and II

Matrix Gla protein

Osteonectin

Osteocalcin (bone Gla protein)

RGD (arg-gly-asp)-containing glycoproteins:

Thrombospondin

Fibronectin, laminin: adhesive proteins

Vitronectin

Osteopontin

Fibrillin

Bone sialoproteins I and II

Bone cells

The **bone cells** include:

Osteoblasts, arising from multi-potential mesenchymal stem cells. They possess abundant rough endoplasmic reticulum and Golgi apparatus, reflecting their ability to synthesise and secrete type I collagen and the proteoglycan complexes that constitute the organic matrix. Osteoblasts play a role in mineralisation of the matrix.

Osteocytes arise from osteoblasts. They maintain mineral exchange in the bone matrix, and act as transducers of mechanical loading of bone, transmitting information about mechanical stress. This helps detect microdamage to bone.

Osteoclasts arise from haematopoietic cells of the monocyte–macrophage lineage. They are giant multinucleated cells, located in Howship's lacunae, and contain large amounts of tartrate-rich acid phosphatase. Osteoclasts act in promoting bone resorption and remodelling.

The bone remodelling cycle

Remodelling is designed to renew old bone and to replace bone with microfractures. The process leads to loss of bone mass and to disruption of the trabecular network with increasing age. In the shorter term, remodelling allows bone to be reshaped to adapt to mechanical stresses on the skeleton.

During the remodelling process, the osteoclasts and osteoblasts work closely together in time and space (coupling) in units known as bone multi-cellular units. Activation of resting osteoblasts on the surface of bone and stromal cells in the bone marrow is followed by a cascade of signals to stimulate recruitment and differentiation of osteoclasts from haematopoietic stem cells.

Activated osteoclasts resorb a discrete area of mineralised bone matrix, with the release of matrix components into the microenvironment. Capillary endothelial cells provide the microvasculature. Osteoblasts migrate into the resorption site and deposit new bone matrix (osteoid). They become embedded in osteoid and mature into osteocytes.

Mechanism of bone repair

Bone break or fracture leads to haematoma formation from the vessels of the periosteum, endosteum and surrounding soft tissues. An acute inflammatory response ensues that comprises:

Arrival of systemic factors: e.g. platelet-derived growth factor (PDGF);

Arrival of phagocytic cells;

Bone mineral density > 2.5 standard deviations below the mean for young adults: osteoporosis.

Bone mineral density 1–2.5 standard deviations below the mean for young adults: osteopenia.

Formation of clots;

Demineralisation of bone.

Simultaneously, the following processes ensue:

Mesenchymal cell attraction;

Mesenchymal cell multiplication;

Stem cell differentiation into chondrocytes;

Hypertrophy of chondrocytes;

Cartilage mineralisation;

Osteogenesis.

Bone repair may be primary (without callus formation), which is obtained with stable rigid bone fixation with close approximation of the bone ends, or secondary (with abundant callus formation), which is the usual process.

Osteoporosis

This is defined as a disease characterised by low bone mass and microarchitectural deterioration of bone tissue leading to enhanced bone fragility and a consequent increase in fracture risk.

Methods for the measurement of bone mineral density

Biopsy of the iliac crest allows direct quantification of bone and osteoid volumes, trabecular and cortical widths, trabecular number, bone formation, mineralisation, and resorption surfaces, and the rates of bone formation and mineralisation (after labelling with tetracycline or calcein).

Photon absorptiometry: single photon; dual photon.

X-ray absorptiometry: single energy; dual energy (DEXA).

Quantitative computed tomography scan.

Quantitative ultrasound.

Biochemical markers of bone turnover

Bone formation (osteoblast products)

Alkaline phosphatase – serum: total activity/bone-specific enzyme;

Osteocalcin – serum;

Procollagen type I C and N terminal extension peptides – serum.

Bone resorption (osteoclast products)

Propeptides of type I collagen – serum:

C-propeptide

N-propeptide

Tartrate-resistant acid phosphatase – serum;

Hydroxyproline – urine;

Hydroxylysine glycerides – urine;

Collagen cross-links – urine and serum

Total pyridinolines

Free pyridinolines

Cross-linked N- and C-telopeptides of collagen

Articular cartilage

Articular cartilage consists of hyaline cartilage. It is composed of a large extracellular matrix with only one cell type, the chondrocyte. Chondrocytes occupy less than 10% of the total volume of the cartilage. The matrix is composed of water, collagens (proteins with a characteristic triple-helical structure), proteoglycans (complex macromolecules that consist of protein and polysaccharides) and non-collagenous proteins and glycoproteins. The chemical composition and physical properties of the cartilage are primarily determined by the extracellular matrix.

Structural heterogeneity is reflected by changes in structure from the joint surface proceeding to the depth. These changes affect collagen fibre and chondrocyte arrangement. There are four distinct histological zones or layers. There are no blood vessels, lymphatic vessels or nerves. The cartilage obtains nourishment from the synovial cavity by diffusion of fluid.

While it is meant to function over the lifetime of the joint, it only possesses a limited capacity for growth and repair. A limited process of remodelling occurs in articular cartilage in response to injury. This process originates in the chondrocytes, which are responsible for synthesis and degradation of the extracellular matrix. However, this process does not restore the matrix to normal. Injury can result from acute and/or chronic loading. Acute injury is usually the result of excessive impact loading. Chronic injury results from either interfacial wear caused by impaired lubricating mechanisms, or from repetitive loading over a long period of time.

Cartilage is metabolically active. The chondrocytes secrete matrix molecules and metalloproteases capable of matrix degradation. The breakdown and synthesis of matrix by the chondrocytes is regulated by cytokines, including

Functions of intra-articular fibrocartilaginous **menisci** (present in the knee, wrist, temporomandibular, acromioclavicular, sternoclavicular and costovertebral joints)
Load bearing, with weight distribution over a large surface;
Shock absorption;
Facilitation of rotatory movement;
Limitation of translatory movement;
Protection of the articular surfaces;
Joint lubrication.

interleukin-1 (with catabolic effect) and transforming growth factor-beta (with anabolic effect). Chondrocytes respond to changes in mechanical load by alteration of matrix, probably mediated through cytokine expression.

The functions of articular cartilage include:

Load bearing, with weight transmission and distribution over the underlying bone at high loads;

Mechanical shock absorption;

Formation of articular surfaces of diarthrodial joints. It allows relative movements between articular surfaces with minimal friction.

Synovial membrane

This lines the joint cavity and consists of two cell types: type A cells with a prominent Golgi apparatus, numerous vesicles and vacuoles, and many mitochondria; and type B cells, with a large endoplasmic reticulum and a few vacuoles that secrete hyaluronan.

The functions of the synovial membrane include:

Secretion of sticky mucoid substance into synovial fluid, which lubricates the joint and nourishes the avascular articular cartilage;

Allows for changes in the joint cavity shape and size associated with normal joint movement, as a result of flexibility, loose synovial folds, villi and marginal recesses;

Aids in removal of substances from the joint cavity.

BIBLIOGRAPHY

Berridge, M. J. Inositol triphosphate and calcium signalling. *Nature*, **361** (1993), 315–25.
Gilman, A. G. Guanine nucleotide-binding regulatory proteins and dual control of adenyl cyclase. *J. Clin. Invest.*, **73** (1984), 1–4.

Hadley, M. E. *Endocrinology*. Upper Saddle River, NJ: Prentice-Hall, 2000.

Hafez, E. S. E., Hafez, B. & Hafez, S. D. *An Atlas of Reproductive Physiology in Men*. New York: The Parthenon Publishing Group, 2003.

Harris, G. W. *Neural Control of the Pituitary Gland*. London: Edward Arnold, 2000.

Nussey, S. S. & Whitehead S. A. *Endocrinology. An Integrated Approach*. Oxford: Bios Scientific Publishers Ltd, 2002.

Speroff, L., Glass, R. H. & Kase, N. G. *Clinical Gynecologic Endocrinology and Infertility*. Philadelphia: Lippincott, Williams & Wilkins, 1999.

11 Gastrointestinal physiology

■ Introduction

The function of the gastrointestinal tract depends on the coordination and integration of secretory activity, motility and epithelial transport in order to allow the digestion of food with subsequent absorption of nutrients, minerals, vitamins and electrolytes.

■ Saliva

Saliva is produced by three paired major salivary glands, and minor salivary glands in the lip and palate:

Parotid glands: serous, enzyme-rich saliva;
Sublingual and submandibular glands: mixed serous and mucous saliva;
Minor salivary glands: mucin-rich saliva.

The rate of production is around 550 ml per day. Over 99% of saliva is constituted by water. Less than 1% consists of solids. Saliva is characterised by low osmolality and a high potassium concentration.

Functions of saliva

Moistens and lubricates food in preparation for swallowing.
Helps in food bolus formation.
Solubilises dry food, facilitating taste.
Aids speech.
Antimicrobial actions comprise the body's first barrier against infection: lysozyme, lactoferrin, lactoperoxidases, mucin, secretory IgA. Saliva helps to control the bacterial counts of the oral cavity.
Digestive actions: contains alpha-amylase, initiating the digestion of starch.

Salivary protein families

Statherin
Acidic proline-rich proteins
Histatine
Cystatine
Mucins (mucous glycoproteins)
Digestive enzymes: alpha-amylase, lipase
Kallikrein
Immunoglobulins

Deficient salivary production

This can lead to:
Difficulty in chewing and swallowing;
Difficulty with speech;
Alteration in taste sensation;
Halitosis;
Difficulty with the wearing of dentures;
A predisposition to caries and periodontal disease.

Cleanses the mouth mechanically of food debris and cellular and bacterial remnants.

Buffering activity: saliva contains bicarbonate, protein and phosphate buffer systems. This helps neutralise refluxed gastric material in the oesophagus. A non-irritating oral pH is maintained in spite of daily exposure to acidic influences.

Secretion of saliva

Saliva can be considered as an ultrafiltrate of plasma. This fact has allowed the use of saliva as a medium for the diagnostic testing of levels of ethanol, drugs of abuse and other substances.

Afferent input to stimulate secretion may arise from chemoreceptors in taste buds on the tongue, mechanoreceptors in periodontal ligament, and the sight and smell of food.

The efferent pathway involves the auriculotemporal nerve, which conveys parasympathetic fibres via the otic ganglion to the parotid gland, and the chorda tympani nerve, which supplies the submandibular and sublingual glands.

■ Swallowing

The process of swallowing is initiated voluntarily and followed by the swallowing reflex. It comprises the following phases:

Oral phase

The food is chewed, mixed with saliva and formed into a bolus; a rounded, smooth, lubricated portion of food. The tongue facilitates formation, containment and propulsion of the bolus backward and upward into the pharynx.

Pharyngeal phase

Nasopharyngeal closure, preventing the reflux of food, is brought about by retraction and elevation of the soft palate with approximation of the palatopharyngeal folds.

Laryngeal closure is brought about by elevation of the larynx upwards and forwards against the epiglottis, along with approximation of the vocal cords. This prevents food entering the trachea.

The upper oesophageal sphincter opens and relaxes:

Pharyngeal clearance is brought about by peristaltic activity, which begins in the superior constrictor muscles of the pharynx and moves towards the oesophagus. Sequential contraction of the superior, middle and inferior constrictors of the pharynx allows onward propulsion of the bolus.

Respiration is reflexly inhibited.

Oesophageal phase

The food bolus is transported by gravity and by peristaltic propulsion, depending on its consistency and the position of the subject.

Reflex constriction of the upper oesophageal sphincter takes place.

Primary peristaltic waves propel the bolus distally. Secondary peristalsis may be initiated by oesophageal distension due to food remnants within the oesophagus if primary peristalsis is insufficient to allow oesophageal clearance. Tertiary contractions may also occur. The lower oesophageal sphincter relaxes.

■ Oesophagus

The oesophagus extends from the lower border of the upper oesophageal sphincter to the upper border of the lower oesophageal sphincter and is 20–24 cm long. It has virtually no absorptive or secretory function, and is lined by non-keratinising squamous epithelium.

Characteristics of the upper oesophageal sphincter

A high pressure zone, 2–4 cm long;
Opened by the thyrohyoid and geniohyoid muscles;
Closed by cricopharyngeus, thyropharyngeus and cervical oesophagus.

Gastro-oesophageal competence

The anti-reflux mechanism of the gastro-oesophageal junction separates the neutral pH of the oesophagus from the low pH of the stomach. The oesophageal mucosa is protected from the adverse effects of exposure to gastric secretion (acid, pepsin, trypsin), alkaline duodenal secretions and bile acids.

Contributory mechanisms to **competence at the gastro-oesophageal junction** include:

The physiological lower oesophageal sphincter, which demonstrates a mean resting end-expiratory pressure of 10–25 mm Hg and a mean resting mid-expiratory pressure of 15–35 mm Hg.
Oesophageal compression by muscle fibres of the right crus of the diaphragm as it passes through the oesophageal hiatus.
Valve-like effect of the acute angle of entry of the oesophagus into the stomach.
Mucosal folds at the gastro-oesophageal junction act as a valve.
The intra-abdominal portion of the oesophagus is subjected to intra-abdominal pressure that compresses the walls of the intra-abdominal segment of the oesophagus.
The hormone gastrin causes contraction of the muscle at the lower end of the oesophagus.

Characteristics of the lower oesophageal sphincter

A high pressure zone, with an average pressure of 15–25 mm Hg;

Extends from approximately 2 cm above the diaphragm to 2 cm below, thus being partly intrathoracic and partly intra-abdominal;

Cannot be identified anatomically (physiological sphincter);

Competence prevents gastric juice reflux from stomach into the oesophagus;

It relaxes in response to primary or secondary peristalsis, as well as to intra-luminal distension;

It contracts in response to active contraction of abdominal muscles, abdominal compression and to the presence of acid placed just proximal to the sphincter.

Assessment of gastro-oesophageal reflux

Tests to prove gastro-oesophageal reflux

Ambulatory pH monitoring, using glass or antimony electrodes with either combined or external reference electrodes. For a 24-hour monitoring period, the exposure of oesophageal mucosa to a pH less than 4 for more than 5% of the duration of the test indicates pathological acid reflux.

Barium swallow (air-contrast or double-contrast).

Scintigraphy, which usually involves the use of $^{99}T_c$ m and gamma camera scanning.

Oesophageal manometry. This is achieved with a multi-lumen, low-compliance, water-perfused catheter with radially oriented orifices at multiple positions along the catheter. This allows the recording of pressure at each position and the tracking of peristaltic waves from the pharynx to the lower oesophageal sphincter. The information obtained includes oesophageal motility, along with length, resting pressure, ability to relax, and location in relation to the diaphragm of the lower oesophageal sphincter. Gastro-oesophageal reflux is evidenced by low basal lower oesophageal sphincter tone, with complete relaxation following a successful wet swallow.

Tests to prove oesophagitis

Barium swallow

Oesophagoscopy with biopsy

Acid perfusion tests

Vomiting

This is a reflex consisting of a sequence of events:

Reverse peristalsis from the mid-small intestine to the duodenum;

The relaxation of the pyloric sphincter;

Forced inspiration against a closed glottis, thereby reducing intrathoracic pressure and increasing intra-abdominal pressure;

Forceful contraction of the abdominal musculature, allowing the passage of gastric contents into the oesophagus;

Contraction of the pyloric sphincter and relaxation of the oesophageal sphincter, associated with anti-peristalsis within the oesophagus forcibly expelling the gastric contents through the mouth.

This is associated with vagal and sympathetic activity leading to salivation, sweating, pallor, lacrimation and bradycardia

The vomiting centre lies in the region of the nucleus of the tractus solitarius in the medulla, close to the fourth ventricle. The vomiting reflex is produced by afferent stimulation from the chemoreceptor trigger zone (in the area postrema of the medulla), from the glossopharyngeal, hypoglossal and vagal nerves and from the cerebral cortex. Efferent signals are directed to the glossopharyngeal, hypoglossal, trigeminal, accessory and spinal segmental nerves.

▪ Stomach

The stomach consists of the following portions:

Proximal: cardia; fundus; proximal body.

Distal: distal body; antrum.

Pylorus: sphincter. Has a narrow lumen, limited distensibility and a redundant folded mucosal lining.

Functions of the stomach

- Reservoir function: storage of food in the body and antrum. Receptive relaxation allows large volumes to be accommodated with small increases in intragastric pressure.
- Mixing of gastric secretions with food. This is aided by reduction of the size of solid particles in the meal (fragmentation), which is brought about by antral contractions.
- Secretion of hydrogen ions (protons) to activate pepsinogen and to kill or suppress the growth of micro-organisms (sterilisation of contents).
- Digestion of protein: pepsinogen (secreted by chief cells) is cleaved in the presence of hydrogen ions to pepsin I, II or III, initiating peptic hydrolysis of dietary proteins.
- Initiation of hydrolysis of dietary triglycerides, mediated by gastric lipase.
- Gastrin production by antral G cells.

Factors affecting gastric emptying	
Gastric distension	increases
Duodenal content osmolarity	
High	reduces
Low	reduces
Acidity of duodenal contents	
High	reduces
Low	0
Fat content of duodenal fluid	
High	reduces
Low	0

- Intrinsic factor production by parietal cells. This binds to vitamin B12 to allow terminal ileal absorption and is the only essential function of the stomach.
- Secretion of mucin and bicarbonate to form the gastric mucosal barrier, which protects against noxious agents such as acid, alcohol, bile salts and pepsin. Mucin is a high molecular weight glycoprotein secreted by the surface mucous cells, the mucous neck cells and glandular mucous cells.
- Conversion of ferric iron to ferrous iron to enable ileal receptor-mediated uptake.
- Regulation of emptying of contents at a controlled rate into the duodenum. Antral contractions cause gastric emptying.

Mechanism of gastric acid secretion

Gastric parietal cells secrete HCl into the gastric lumen. A magnesium-dependent H^+/K^+ exchanging-ATPase (**gastric proton pump**) is involved in the mechanism of active pulsatile secretion of HCl. The enzyme is unique to the parietal cell and is found only in the luminal (apical) region of the plasma membrane. It is a heterodimer consisting of a larger catalytic alpha subunit and a smaller glycosylated beta subunit. It couples adenosine 5-triphosphate (ATP) hydrolysis to an electrically neutral obligatory exchange of K^+ for H^+, secreting H^+ and moving K^+ into the cell. (One mole of transported H^+ and K^+ for each mole of ATP.) Under steady state conditions, HCl secretion into the gastric lumen is coupled to movement of HCO_3^- into the plasma. The proton pump is capable of secreting protons against a large electrochemical gradient. While parietal cell cytosolic pH is 7.2, acid is secreted at a pH of 0.8, representing a 2.5 million-fold hydrogen ion concentration. Equivalent amounts of base are delivered by the parietal cell to maintain normal intracellular pH, through a Cl^-/HCO_3^- exchange mechanism in the basolateral membrane of the parietal

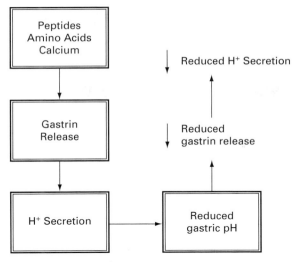

Figure 11.1 Gastric acid secretion.

Gastric mucosal homeostasis

This is maintained by the following mechanisms:
Defence mechanisms:
    Mucus-bicarbonate barrier
        Mucus (mucopolysaccharide and glycoprotein)
        Bicarbonate
        pH gradient
Prostaglandins:
    Inhibit gastric secretion
    Prevent deep tissue injury
    Increased bicarbonate secretion
    Preserve vascular flow
    Restore epithelial surface
Adaptive cytoprotection:
    Epithelial resistance to mild injury
Adequate circulatory flow, with reactive hyperaemia

cell. Back-diffusion of acid is prevented by the apical membrane and the tight intercellular junctions.

The four physiologically relevant stimuli for acid secretion are histamine, acetylcholine, gastrin and extracellular calcium. The H2 receptor is a 70 kDa glycoprotein belonging to the G-protein-coupled receptor superfamily. Acetylcholine is the physiological agonist for the muscarinic cholinergic receptor on the basolateral membrane of the parietal cell. Gastric acid secretion is inhibited by cholecystokinin, somatostatin, prostaglandins and secretin.

Stomach cells

Parietal cells

The structural and functional features are:

An intracellular secretory canalicular network, lined by microvilli;

The canaliculi communicate with the luminal surface;

An abundance of large mitochondria;

A high oxidative capacity;

A limited amount of rough endoplasmic reticulum, which secretes intrinsic factor.

Chief cells

The structural and functional features are:

Abundant rough endoplasmic reticulum;

Zymogen granules containing pepsinogen, which is released by exocytotic fusion of the granules with the luminal or apical plasma membrane into the gastric lumen.

Gastrin cells

These are in the antral glands.

The structural and functional features are:

Pyramidal shape;

Gastrin storage granules, with release of gastrin by exocytotic fusion of the granules with the basal plasma membrane into the submucosal capillaries.

Phases of gastric acid secretion

Resting or interprandial phase;

Stimulated or postprandial phase, which consists of:

Cephalic phase

Initiated by the thought, sight, smell and taste of food, by conditioned reflexes, and by insulin-induced hypoglycaemia. This phase is mediated by cholinergic vagal fibres. The areas of the brain stem that relay information to the stomach are the area postrema, nucleus tractus solitarius and the dorsal motor nucleus. Acetylcholine directly stimulates parietal cells to produce acid. It also indirectly stimulates acid secretion by releasing gastrin from G cells and histamine from enterochromaffin-like cells in the gastric mucosa.

Gastric phase

The presence of food or fluid in the stomach releases gastrin by:

Mechanical stimulation: distension of the body or antrum (short intramural cholinergic reflexes and long vasovagal reflexes).

Chemical stimulation: products of protein digestion–peptides and L-amino acids in the antrum stimulate receptors on G cells.

Pyloric distension enhances gastrin release through a local intramural cholinergic reflex. Once the buffering capacity of the gastric contents is saturated, gastric pH falls rapidly and inhibits further acid release.

During the gastric phase, distal gastrointestinal tract responses include stimulation of pancreatic secretion, contraction of the gall bladder along with relaxation of the sphincter of Oddi and increased colonic motor activity.

Intestinal phase

Gastric secretion is brought about by duodenal distension and the presence of protein digestion products, i.e. peptides and amino acids. The presence of acid, fat digestion products and hypertonicity in the duodenum and proximal jejunum inhibit gastric acid secretion and gastric emptying. Acid in the duodenum causes secretin release, which inhibits gastrin release by G cells and inhibits the response of parietal cells to gastrin. Fatty acids in the duodenum release two hormones, cholecystokinin (CCK) and gastric inhibitory peptide (GIP). Cholecystokinin inhibits acid secretion by parietal cells. Gastric inhibitory peptide suppresses gastrin release and also directly inhibits acid secretion by parietal cells.

Gastric acid secretion control mechanisms

These may be:

Long reflex or cephalo-vagal arcs;

Local intra-gastric reflex arcs;

Mediated by humoral substances, by endocrine and paracrine pathways.

Tests of gastric acid secretion

Pentagastrin test
Augmented histamine test
Insulin (Hollander) test

Gastrin

Gastrin represents a family of peptides, secreted by antral G cells. Secretion is regulated by luminal, paracrine, endocrine and neural stimuli. The biologically active forms are 17 and 34 amino acid peptides. Gastrin 17 or 'little gastrin' (a heptadecapeptide) accounts for 90% of gastrin produced by the antral G cells. Gastrin 34 is also known as 'big gastrin'. The critical information for biological activity is contained in the carboxy-terminal tetrapeptide-amide.

Effects of gastrin

Stimulates acid secretion by the parietal cells. This is achieved by direct stimulation of the parietal cells, and by inducing the release of (from gastric enterochromaffin-like cells) and potentiating the action of histamine.

Stimulates pepsin and intrinsic factor secretion.

Stimulates mitotic activity in the mucosa of the stomach, small intestine and colon (trophic effect).

Contraction of the musculature of the lower oesophageal sphincter.

Stimulation of insulin, glucagon and calcitonin secretion.

Stimulation of pancreatic enzymes and bile flow.

Stimulation of small intestinal secretion.

Stimulation of gastric, small and large intestinal and gall bladder motility.

The gastrocolic reflex.

Inhibition of contraction of the pylorus and sphincter of Oddi.

Stimuli for gastrin secretion

Luminal: peptides and amino acids
distension of the antrum
Neural: increased vagal discharge, probably non-cholinergic
Blood borne: calcium
adrenaline

Causes of hypergastrinaemia

Gastrinoma
Antral G cell hyperplasia
Gastric outlet obstruction
Following massive small bowel resection
Pernicious anaemia

Gastrointestinal regulatory peptides

These are hormones that regulate intestinal and pancreatic function. The gastrointestinal tract can consequently be regarded as the largest endocrine organ in the body. The physiological roles of many of these hormones await elucidation. The modulation of gastrointestinal hormone release is achieved by either a direct effect on the endocrine cells or by the activation of intrinsic neural reflexes.

Endocrine

Gastrin: 17 amino acids; 34 amino acids
Cholecystokinin
Secretin: 27 amino acids
Gastric inhibitory peptide: 43 amino acids
Glucagon
Enteroglucagon
Pancreatic polypeptide: 36 amino acids
Peptide tyrosine
Motilin: 22 amino acids
Neurotensin: 13 amino acids

Neurocrine

Vasoactive intestinal peptide: 28 amino acids
Gastrin-releasing peptide: 27 amino acids
Neuromedin K
Substance P: 11 amino acids
Neurokinins alpha and beta
Endorphins
Neuropeptide Y
Calcitonin gene-related peptide

Paracrine

Somatostatin

Structural classification of gastrointestinal peptides

Gastrin/cholecystokinin family: gastrin; cholecystokinin.

Secretin family: secretin; vasoactive intestinal peptide; gastric inhibitory peptide; glucagon-like peptide.

Pancreatic polypeptide family: pancreatic polypeptide; peptide YY; neuropeptide Y.

Miscellaneous: neurotensin; motilin; galanin; somatostatin.

Classes of gastrointestinal hormone receptors

Receptors are dynamic molecules, which are characterised on the basis of biological activities and on receptor-binding characteristics.

Single transmembrane receptors, e.g. ligand-triggered protein kinases

Receptors with subunits that traverse the membrane multiple times and form pores or ligand-gated channels

G-protein-coupled receptors that traverse the membrane seven times

Cholecystokinin

This is a peptide produced by I cells of the small intestine. Its actions are mediated by binding to CCK-A receptors in the gall bladder, pancreas, smooth muscle and peripheral nerves.

Effects of cholecystokinin

Stimulation of pancreatic acinar cell secretion of zymogens, in response to amino acids and fatty acids in the duodenum;

Potentiation of the primary effects of secretin;

Stimulation of contraction of smooth muscle of gall bladder, for which it is the major hormonal regulator;

Relaxation of the sphincter of Oddi, which allows bile to enter the duodenum;

Stimulation of contraction of pylorus to slow gastric emptying;

Satiation of the appetite via activation of CCK-A gut receptors and vagal pathways projecting to the nucleus of the tractus solitarius, the lateral para-branchial nucleus, amygdala, and higher sites. This leads to suppression of food intake.

Secretin

This is a 27 amino acid peptide. It is produced in specialised entero-endocrine S cells in the small intestine.

Effects of secretin

Stimulation of pancreatic ductal cell release of water and bicarbonate;

Stimulation of bile flow; stimulation of biliary ductular secretion of fluid and bicarbonate;

Inhibition of release of gastrin;

Inhibition of gastric acid secretion;

Inhibition of gastrointestinal motility;

Reduction of lower oesophageal motility.

Somatostatin

Somatostatin is a 14 amino acid peptide. Isolated from the ovine hypothalamus in 1973 as a growth hormone release inhibiting factor.

It acts in paracrine function to inhibit gastric, intestinal and pancreato-biliary secretion and cell growth.

Inhibits secretion of hormones by pancreatic islets: insulin; glucagon.

Inhibits gastrin secretion.

Somatostatin acts as a neurotransmitter in the CNS.

It inhibits splanchnic blood flow by inhibiting the release of vasodilatory peptides, including glucagon, vasoactive intestinal peptide (VIP) and substance P.

Long-acting somatostatin analogues include octreotide acetate (half-life: 90–120 minutes) and lanreotide.

Vasoactive intestinal peptide

Vasoactive intestinal peptide is a 28 amino acid peptide, released from nerve terminals.

It acts on cells bearing VIP receptors, which are G-protein-coupled receptors. Vasoactive intestinal peptide acts as a neurotransmitter throughout the central and peripheral nervous systems. It is a major component of the non-adrenergic non-cholinergic nervous system in the gut. Stimulation of blood flow in the gastrointestinal tract is associated with epithelial secretion and absorption and smooth muscle relaxation.

Gastro-intestinal neuroendocrine tumours
Carcinoid
Gastrinoma
VIPoma
Glucagonoma
Somatostatinoma

It also promotes the secretion of fluid and bicarbonate from cholangiocytes in the bile ducts.

■ Small intestine

The small intestine consists of the duodenum, jejunum and ileum, which possess structural and functional differences. It extends from the pylorus to the ileocaecal valve and is between 12 and 20 feet long. The epithelial cells of the small intestine form an interface between the body and an external or luminal environment comprising digestive enzymes, bacteria and toxins and potentially toxic chemicals.

Digestion and absorption

Small intestinal epithelium is characterised by:

A large absorptive and secretory surface area created by villous processes and by microvilli on the luminal brush border;

Intercellular tight junctions, joining the lateral borders of adjacent enterocytes;

A basolateral membrane in close contact with the vasculature of the villi;

Functional polarity, with asymmetrical distribution of proteins involved in solute transport between the apical (luminal) and basolateral (serosal) surfaces of the cell;

Digestive enzymes are located on the apical surface and the ATPase sodium pump on the basolateral surface;

A characteristic electrochemical potential profile.

Electrolyte transport proteins

These include:

ATPase pumps
Na^+K^+-ATPase
K^+/H^+-ATPase

Exchangers and co-transporters
Na^+ solute co-transporters
H^+ solute co-transporters
Na^+/H^+ exchangers
Cl^-/HCO_3^- exchangers
$Na^+/K^+/2Cl^-$ co-transporter

Ion channels
Na^+
K^+
Cl^-

The **epithelial cell types are**:

Enterocytes, with absorptive and secretory functions;

Goblet cells, which secrete mucus;

Paneth cells, which produce antibacterial substances;

Enteroendocrine cells;

Owing to the nature of distribution of cells, there is functional heterogeneity in electrolyte, fluid and nutrient transport along the crypt–villus axis.

Carbohydrate digestion

- Luminal hydrolysis of starch and glycogen by salivary and pancreatic alpha-amylases, yielding maltose, maltotriose and alpha-limit dextrins.
- Brush border membrane disaccharidases:

Lactase-phlorizin hydrolase: beta-galactosidase

Alpha-glucosidases:

Sucrase-isomaltase

Maltase-glucoamylase

Trehalase

- Absorption into the enterocyte as monosaccharides, utilising the following transport mechanisms:

Passive diffusion across the epithelium, both transcellular and paracellular

Na^+-coupled glucose and galactose active transport: sodium-linked glucose transporter 1 (SGLT1) is the transport protein responsible. It is a 664 amino acid protein with a molecular weight of 73 kDa and has 12 membrane-spanning domains. The Na^+ gradient is maintained by Na^+K^+-ATPase.

Facilitated diffusion (Na^+ independent):

GLUT 2: basolateral membrane associated glucose transport into the portal circulation.

GLUT 5: apical membrane fructose transport.

Lipid digestion

- Dietary fat is primarily composed of the triglycerides of long chain (16–18 carbon) fatty acids.
- Luminal digestion processes involve:

Emulsification;

Lipolysis (hydrolysis of triglycerides) by pancreatic lipase;

Formation of micelles, which possess a hydrophobic core and a hydrophilic outer surface;

Micellar uptake;

Delivery of products of lipolysis to the brush border of the enterocyte.

- Intracellular events within the enterocyte:

  Uptake across the brush border membrane of long-chain fatty acids and monoglycerides.

  Intracellular transport by association with low molecular weight cytosolic fatty acid-binding proteins (apoproteins).

  Re-esterification in the smooth endoplasmic reticulum of fatty acids and beta-monoglycerides to triglycerides through the monoglyceride acylation pathway and the phosphatidic acid pathway.

  Lipoprotein synthesis and chylomicron formation in the Golgi apparatus. The core of chylomicrons contains triglycerides and cholesterol, and the surface is made up of phospholipids and apoproteins.

- Chylomicron transport to the basolateral cell membrane and uptake into the lymphatic system by reverse pinocytosis. Chylomicrons are transported to the blood via the thoracic duct.

  Micelles are spherical or disc-shaped molecular complexes. Amphipathic bile salts and phospholipids are arranged with their hydrophilic poles facing outwards and their hydrophobic poles inwards. Fatty acids and other lipids are incorporated between the bile salts and in the interior, forming mixed micelles.

Protein digestion

Gastric phase: pepsins form oligopeptides and free amino acids, which stimulate secretin and cholecystokinin secretion.

Intestinal phase:

Luminal phase: pancreatic proteases and peptidases (three endopeptidases and two exopeptidases).

Brush border phase: amino acid absorption. Aminopeptidases in the brush border membrane hydrolyse oligopeptides further. Amino acid transport systems transport free amino acids. A peptide transport system transports dipeptides and tripeptides.

Fat-soluble vitamin absorption

Vitamin A: passive diffusion
Vitamin D: passive diffusion
Vitamin E: passive diffusion
Vitamin K:
    K1 or phytomenadione: carrier mediated uptake
    K2 or multiprenyl menaquinones: passive diffusion

Tests for intestinal absorption

Fat absorption
 72 hour stool fat: >6 grams per day on a 60–100 gram fat diet is abnormal
 C14-triolein breath test
 Prothrombin time and international normalised ratio
 Serum vitamin D

Carbohydrate absorption
 Stool pH < 5.5
 Lactose/hydrogen breath test
 Flat oral glucose tolerance curve

Vitamin B12
 Schilling test

Bile acid
 SeHCAT test

There are five major sodium-dependent amino acid transport systems in the brush border of the enterocyte:

 Neutral amino acids
 Anionic amino acids
 Imino acids
 Neutral amino acids
 Cationic amino acids and cystine

Basolateral membrane amino acid transport systems export amino acids into the portal circulation.

Barrier function

The gastrointestinal tract performs a **barrier function**, which helps prevent microbial translocation (bacteria and endotoxins) from the tract into the systemic circulation. The barrier function consists of anatomical and functional components. These include:

 Intestinal motility from peristalsis. Bacterial stasis from ileus leads to overgrowth and translocation. The basal electrical rhythm of rhythmic oscillations of the membrane potentials of smooth muscle cells acts as a pacesetter for small intestinal motility.

 Epithelial cells and intercellular matrix and the mucus layer

 Inhibition of microbial adherence to epithelial cells by goblet cells, secretory IgA and the normal gastrointestinal microflora.

Patterns of gastrointestinal motility

Peristalsis:
    Propulsive: transport
    Non-propulsive: mixing
Rhythmic segmentation
Pendular activity
Tonic contraction: sphincters

Cell-mediated immunity from the gut-associated lymphoid tissue, repre-sented by Peyer's patches in the muscularis mucosa of the small intestine.

Furthermore, microbial translocations into the portal circulation may be dealt with by the phagocytic function of Kupffer cells in the liver.

Splanchnic ischaemia results in failure of the gut barrier, leading to intracel-lular acidosis secondary to inadequate oxygen delivery. The gastric pH may hence be a marker of barrier function.

Motility of small intestine

Gut smooth muscle demonstrates variable tone on which are superimposed spontaneous rhythmic contractions, driven by cycles of depolarisation and repolarisation that originate in the pacemaker cells, or interstitial cells of Cajal.

The basic electrical rhythm is responsible for the cylindrical and propa-gated pattern of evacuation controlling the smooth muscle in the stomach and small intestine. The frequency of the rhythm depends on the location, and is related to the density, of interstitial cells of Cajal locally. These cells are located at the interfaces of circular and longitudinal muscle and act as an interface between the smooth muscle and motor neurons. Propagation of intestinal slow wave activity requires continuity of the circular and longitu-dinal muscle layers.

■ Liver

The liver plays a central role in metabolic homeostasis, and is involved in the synthesis as well as detoxification of a wide range of compounds. It is anatomi-cally coupled to the gastrointestinal tract through the biliary tree and the portal circulation.

Structural features

- It is the largest solid organ in the body. Weight in the adult ranges from 1200–1700 grams, comprising 2%–5% of the total body weight. It consists of 8 segments.
- The liver is supplied by two vascular beds; 75% of the blood supply being from the portal vein and the remaining 25% from the hepatic artery. The portal vein is interposed between the intestinal and hepatic capillary beds. Venous and arterial blood mix in the sinusoids and flow towards the central vein.
- It contains 25–30 ml blood per 100 grams of tissue, i.e. 10%–15% of the total blood volume. The total resting blood flow is around 1200–1400 ml/min, i.e. around 25% of the cardiac output.
- The liver has considerable regenerative capacity, achieved by both cell pro-liferation (hyperplasia) and by increase in cell size (hypertrophy) in response to cell destruction by chemical or infective stimuli.

Segmental anatomy of the liver

The liver is divided into right and left lobes by the middle hepatic vein. Cantlie's line demarcates the lobes on the surface of the liver, connecting the fundus of the gall bladder to the insertion of the middle hepatic vein into the inferior vena cava.

The right hepatic vein divides the right lobe into anterior and posterior segments.

The left hepatic vein divides the left lobe into medial and lateral segments.

Each of the four segments is divided by an imaginary transverse line through the right and left portal veins into anterior and posterior sub-segments.

The segments are numbered in anti-clockwise fashion from the inferior vena cava.

The caudate lobe is segment one. It is located between the portal vein and inferior vena cava and is supplied by vessels from both left and right branches of the portal vein and hepatic artery. Its draining veins flow directly into the inferior vena cava.

Cells of the liver

These can be categorised as:

Parenchymal: hepatocytes. Hepatocytes radiate from the central vein, forming anastomosing plates or trabeculae, and rows of cells. The sinusoids are interposed between the rows.

Non-parenchymal:

Sinusoidal endothelial cells, which are involved in macromolecular clearance, storage of vitamin A and the metabolism of lipoprotein. The endothelial cells are fenestrated and do not contain a basement membrane.

Kupffer cells (derived from macrophages).

Peri-sinusoidal lipocytes (fat storage, stellate, or Ito cells), which store fat and vitamin A and synthesise collagen.

Bile duct epithelial cells.

Characteristics of hepatocytes

- Polarised epithelial cells bounded by three distinct membrane domains:

  Sinusoidal, or basolateral, membrane, oriented along the sinusoids and lined with microvilli. This allows active and bidirectional transport of proteins, water, organic solutes.

  Apical, or bile canalicular, membrane, which are joined by tight junctions to form canaliculi, long and narrow channels less than 1 μm in diameter. This maintains canalicular shape and is involved in bile formation.

  Lateral hepatic membrane, between adjacent hepatocytes. This contains structural proteins that allow attachment and communication between cells. Tight junction complexes separate the sinusoidal space from the bile canaliculi.

- Arranged in cords on a basement membrane in the liver lobule.
- Possess highly developed endoplasmic reticulum, mitochondria, peroxisomes, lysosomes, Golgi complex and cytoskeleton.
- The liver microsomal fraction comprises the smooth and rough endoplasmic reticulum and the Golgi complex.

Kupffer cells

The Kupffer cells represent the largest population of fixed macrophages in the body.

The functions of the Kupffer cells include:

Phagocytosis and clearance of:

Micro-organisms, including bacteria and viruses

Endotoxins

Immune complexes

Tumour cells

Lipid assemblies

Fibrin degradation products

Other particulate matter

Modulation of the synthesis of acute phase proteins and lipoproteins;

Cytokine secretion;

Antigen processing;

Catabolism of glycoproteins and lipids.

Units of the liver

Lobule: a histological and functional unit.

Hexagonal in cross-section with interlobular portal triads (portal vein, hepatic artery and bile duct branches) at the angles of the hexagon.

In the centre of the lobule is the central vein or terminal hepatic venule.

Hepatocytes form single cell plates radiating from the central veins to the portal triads.

The plates are located between the endothelial-lined sinusoids that carry blood from the portal triad vessels to the central vein. The endothelial cells are fenestrated and highly permeable to macromolecules.

Acinus: a structural model.

The portal triad is at the centre of the acinus.

The terminal hepatic venules are at the periphery.

Cells are grouped into three zones, depending on their distance from the central portal triads.

The acinus is a portion of the liver parenchyma that receives blood from a single portal venule and hepatic arteriole and delivers bile into a single small duct in the same portal tract. It lies between two hepatic venules, into which its blood drains.

The acinus can be divided into three zones based on heterogeneity of function. These are:

The peri-portal hepatocytes, which are involved in gluconeogenesis, amino acid utilisation, oxidative energy metabolism and bilirubin excretion.

The intermediate hepatocytes.

The peri-venular hepatocytes (surrounding the central vein), which are involved in glucose uptake and glycogen synthesis, lipogenesis, ketogenesis, glutamine formation, ammonia detoxification, urea synthesis and biotransformation.

Liver function

The functions of the liver consist of:

Bile synthesis and secretion; bilirubin conjugation and excretion.

Storage: glycogen, vitamins (A, D, E, K, B12), metals (iron, copper).

Metabolism of protein (plasma protein synthesis; urea formation; amino acid interconversions - deamination). The albumin synthesis rate is around 12 g per day.

Metabolism of carbohydrate (glycogen synthesis and breakdown; gluconeogenesis).

Metabolism of fat (synthesis of cholesterol, bile acids, lipoproteins, fatty acids and enzymes, e.g. lecithin acyl transferase (LCAT); catabolism of chylomicrons and very low density lipoprotein (VLDL) remnants, low density lipoprotein (LDL) and high density lipoprotein (HDL) (excretion in the bile of cholesterol and phospholipids).

Detoxification and inactivation of hormones (steroid hormone detoxification and conjugation; polypeptide hormone inactivation; 25-hydroxylation of vitamin D), drugs and toxins.

Kupffer cells – part of the reticuloendothelial system.

Hydrogen ion homeostasis: decrease in ureagenesis and increased glutamine synthesis in acidosis.

The **serum protein changes** that may be associated with liver disease include:

The presence of acute phase reactants: in acute hepatitis;

Reduction in serum albumin;

Release of integral cell membrane enzymes:

Transaminases: aspartate aminotransferase (AST), alanine aminotransferase (ALT)

Bile ductular enzymes: alkaline phosphatase, gamma-glutamyl transferase and 5-nucleotidase

Increased serum immunoglobulins: IgG, IgA, IgM;

Appearance of abnormal protein antigens (marker export proteins): alpha-fetoprotein, ferritin, alpha 1-antitrypsin.

Liver function tests

Indicators of uptake, conjugation and excretion of anionic compounds

Serum total (direct; indirect) bilirubin: normally less than 17 μmol/l in females and less than 23 μmol/l in males.

Plasma proteins synthesised by the liver

These include:
Albumin
Vitamin K-dependent blood coagulation factors: II, VII, IX, X; proteins C and S
Fibrinolysis proteins
Protease inhibitors: Alpha 1-antitrypsin, alpha 2-antiplasmin, antithrombin III
Caeruloplasmin
Alpha-fetoprotein
Iron storage and binding proteins
Acute phase proteins

Urine bilirubin/urobilinogen.

Serum bile acids: levels rise with impaired hepatocyte extraction from portal venous blood.

Tests reflecting hepatocellular damage

Aspartate and/or alanine aminotransferase: aminotransferases catalyse amino group transfer from aspartic acid or alanine to ketoglutaric acid to produce oxaloacetic acid and pyruvic acid, respectively. Alanine aminotransferase is a cytosolic enzyme that is relatively liver specific. Aspartate aminotransferase has both cytosolic and mitochondrial isoenzymes and is also found in skeletal and cardiac muscles, the kidneys, brain, pancreas and in blood cells. An AST/ALT ratio greater than 2 is typical of alcoholic liver injury, while ALT>AST is found with viral hepatitis.

Glutathione-S-transferase.

Serum ferritin.

Vitamin B12.

Clearance tests.

Tests indicating bile flow obstruction

Alkaline phosphatase: this can originate from liver, bone, intestine and placenta. It is present in both the apical or canalicular domain of the hepatocyte plasma membrane and in the luminal domain of bile duct epithelium.

Gamma glutamyl transferase (GGT) is derived from both hepatocytes and biliary epithelium.

5′ nucleotidase.

Leucine aminopeptidase.

Lipoprotein X.

Tests of synthetic function

Serum albumin: normally 35–50 g/l. Albumin has a half-life of 20 days and about 10 g is synthesised and secreted by the hepatocytes each day. The level correlates with prognosis in chronic liver disease.

Serum prealbumin.

Serum cholinesterase.

Lecithin-cholesterol acyltransferase.

Serum protein electrophoresis.

Prothrombin and partial thromboplastin time.

Serum ammonia: normally less than 1 mg/l.

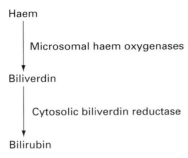

Haem

Microsomal haem oxygenases

Biliverdin

Cytosolic biliverdin reductase

Bilirubin

Figure 11.2 Production of bilirubin

Techniques to measure liver blood flow

Parenchymal clearance techniques;

Reticuloendothelial clearance of radiolabelled colloidal particles;

Indicator dilution techniques.

The uses of liver function tests include the detection of liver disease, the placement of liver disease in specific diagnostic categories and following the progress of liver disease.

Bilirubin

Bilirubin is a linear tetrapyrrole. It is a product of the breakdown of circulating mature red blood cells in Kupffer cells of the liver and in the reticuloendothelial system. Immature and defective red cells are destroyed in the bone marrow. The average rate of production in the adult is 4 mg/kg per 24 hours, about 250–400 mg being produced daily. Eighty per cent of the total production of bilirubin is derived from the haem moiety of haemoglobin. The remainder of the bilirubin (shunt bilirubin) is produced from the catabolism in the liver of other haem-containing proteins such as myoglobin, cytochromes and catalases.

Increases in circulating bilirubin may arise from increased production, impaired hepatocyte uptake, defective conjugation in the hepatocyte and interference with the binding of bilirubin by albumin.

Pathway for bilirubin metabolism

Free or unconjugated bilirubin is lipid soluble, and does not undergo glomerular filtration and does not appear in the urine as a result.

Bilirubin is processed in the liver according to the following sequence:

Tight and reversible binding to albumin of unconjugated bilirubin allows transport in the plasma.

Bilirubin is taken up by hepatocytes by a process of facilitated (carrier-mediated) diffusion that requires inorganic anions.

Intracellular storage of bilirubin is achieved by binding to cytosolic proteins: ligandins and Z protein.

Conjugation with glucuronic acid of one or both propionic acid carboxyl groups. This is mediated by uridine diphosphate-glucuronyl transferase to form a diglucuronide and a monoglucuronide. Conjugation makes bilirubin water soluble.

Active transport across the bile canalicular membrane, which is formed by the apical membranes of the hepatocytes.

Bilirubin undergoes degradation by intestinal bacteria into urobilinogen and related compounds.

Detoxification of drugs in the liver

Phase 1

Oxidation: oxidation is largely a function of the cytochrome P450 system, which is part of the non-specific mixed function oxidase system in the endoplasmic reticulum. The P450 system is further classified into families, subfamilies and isoforms.

Reduction.

Hydrolysis.

Phase 2

Conjugation with:

Glucuronic acid

Glycine

Sulphates

Acetic acid

The extraction ratio is the fraction of the drug removed from the blood by the liver, and depends on hepatic blood flow, uptake of drug into hepatocytes and enzyme metabolic activity within the hepatocyte.

Bile

Bile is an isotonic aqueous solution of bile acids, cholesterol, phospholipids, bile pigments and inorganic electrolytes. It is secreted by hepatocytes into the bile canaliculi and undergoes further modification in bile ductules or ducts. The rate of bile production is around 1.5 l/24 h. Eight per cent is secreted by hepatocytes: canalicular bile. Twenty per cent is secreted by bile duct epithelial cells: ductular bile

Components of bile

Bile salts: a family of amphipathic steroids that contain a cyclopentanoperhydrophenanthrene nucleus and a variable length side chain at the C17 position.

Lecithin (phosphatidylcholine).

Cholesterol.

Inorganic electrolytes: bicarbonate ions.

Bile pigments.

Trace metals.

Bile acids

Over 70% of circulating bile acids are primary bile acids. The secondary bile acids are produced in the ileum and colon by anaerobic bacterial degradation of primary bile acids.

Primary:

Cholic acid

Chemodeoxycholic acid

Secondary:

Deoxycholic acid

Lithocholic acid

Bile salt production

Bile salt synthesis occurs in the canalicular membrane of the hepatocyte, and in bile ductules or ducts. Conjugated bile salts are transported across the canalicular membrane by a carrier. The rate-limiting step in the hepatocellular transport of bile salts from the portal blood to the bile is at the canalicular membrane.

Functions of bile salts

Negative feedback role on their own rate of synthesis by inhibition of cholesterol 7 alpha-hydroxylase in the liver.

Resecretion into bile.

Stimulate bile acid-dependent mechanisms: choleresis.

Increase secretion of phospholipids.

Cholesterol solubilisation by incorporation into micelles. The stability of a solution of bile salts, lecithin and cholesterol can be shown in a triangular graph with an ordinate for each component of the micelle.

Emulsification of dietary lipid into micelles, increasing the surface area accessible to lipid hydrolysing enzymes.

Aid absorption of fat-soluble vitamins.

Stimulate pancreatic secretion by releasing cholecystokinin-pancreozymin (CCK-PZ).

Inhibit pancreatic lipase.

Inhibit electrolyte and water absorption into the colon.

Increase colonic motility.

Enterohepatic circulation

The components of the enterohepatic cycle are the liver, biliary tract, intestine and the portal venous system. Ninety per cent to 95 % of the bile acids entering the gut are actively absorbed in the terminal ileum by a Na-anion co-transporter. The energy for uptake of bile acids is provided by a Na^+/K^+- ATPase located on the basolateral membrane of the enterocyte. Approximately 500–700 mg are lost per day in the faeces. This is replaced by hepatic synthesis.

There is a total bile acid pool of 2–5 g in the liver. Twenty to 30 g per day of bile acid enters the duodenum, i.e. the bile acid pool recycles 6–10 times in 24 hours through the enterohepatic circulation.

Gall bladder

The gall bladder is around 7–10 cm long. It contains an average volume of 30 ml. The capacity ranges from 25–50 ml.

Functions

Storage and concentration of bile in the fasting or inter-digestive phase;

Evacuation by smooth muscle contraction in response to cholecystokinin;

Moderation of hydrostatic pressure within the biliary tract;

Absorption of organic components of bile;

Acidification of bile.

■ Exocrine pancreas

Structural features

Length: 12–15 cm; weight around 100 g

It is a compound acinar gland, with at least 85% of the gland being comprised of exocrine secretory cells.

The acinus is the functional unit. It consists of pyramidal shaped glandular cells with their apices facing the lumen of the acinus. The acinar cells are arranged in a semicircle around the lumen.

Acinar cells have the following characteristics:

Highly polarised, with functional and structural differences in the apical and basolateral plasma membrane domains;

Well developed Golgi complexes and rough endoplasmic reticulum, designed for the synthesis and storage of secretory proteins;

Zymogen or storage granules are found in the apical (luminal) side of the cytoplasm. These fuse with the luminal membrane of acinar cell at the time of secretion.

The pancreas secretes about 1 litre of juice per day, which consists of water, electrolytes and digestive enzymes. The secretion has two major functions, the intra-luminal digestion of macronutrients and the maintenance of a near neutral intra-luminal pH by the action of bicarbonate.

The pancreas is protected from **autodigestion** by its enzymatic products by virtue of the following mechanisms:

Synthesis of inactive proenzyme precursor zymogens;

Proteins secreted by the pancreas

Proteolytic enzymes
Endopeptidases:
Trypsinogen
Chymotrypsinogen
Proelastase

Exopeptidases
Procarboxypeptidases – carboxypeptidase A and B

Lipolytic enzymes
Lipase
Phospholipase A2
Carboxyesterase

Amylolytic enzymes
Alpha-amylase

Nucleases
DNAase
RNAase

Other enzymes
Procolipase
Trypsin inhibitor

Zymogen granules are sequestrated in acinar cells;

Acinar cells make trypsin inhibitor, which is co-packaged with trypsinogen in zymogen granules;

The activation site is within the duodenal lumen.

Pancreatic function assessment

Plasma amylase.

Secretin-CCK test: intravenous injection of secretin and CCK after an overnight fast, followed by sampling of gastric and pancreatic secretions using a double-lumen tube.

Lundh test meal: pancreatic stimulation by a carbohydrate, protein and fat meal.

■ Colon

The colon is lined with a dynamic and protective mucous gel layer. The components of the mucous gel are largely derived from the goblet cells, which are characterised by basolateral nuclei, rough endoplasmic reticulum, a large Golgi apparatus and condensing vacuoles. The gel layer includes mucin glycoproteins, trefoil factors, defensins, immunoglobulins, electrolytes, sloughed epithelial cells, phospholipids, commensal bacteria and other components. The colon receives 500–2000 ml of ileal effluent per day, requiring it to possess absorptive and storage functions.

Colonic motility

The types of **colonic motility** include:

Segmental non-propulsive movements. The colon is divided into segments called haustra by segmental contractions. Sequential contraction and relaxation of haustral contractions is the major colonic contractile activity. This leads to retrograde and antegrade movement of the contents within the segment.

One to four mass movements occur per day.

Retrograde propulsion movements.

There are two types of reflex control of colonic motility:

Colono-colic reflex.

Gastro-colic reflex: food in the duodenum, especially fat, induces segmental contractions and mass movement of faeces.

Functions of the colon

Storage of faecal content with periodic controlled evacuation.

Further reabsorption of water, sodium and chloride. Active transport of sodium is achieved with accompanying absorption of water.

Secretion of potassium by K^+/H^+ ATPase on the apical membrane.

Secretion of bicarbonate.

Maintenance of bacterial microflora.

Rapid metabolism of malabsorbed sugars and of dietary fibre (polysaccharide) to short-chain fatty acids by bacteria and absorption by passive diffusion.

Bacteria produce vitamin K.

Bacterial gas (flatus) produced by fermentation of undigested polysaccharides.

Functions of the colonic microflora

Conversion of bilirubin to urobilinogen.

Cholesterol catabolism.

The degradation of mucin.

Regulation of faecal trypsin activity.

Fermentation of malabsorbed carbohydrate (which includes dietary fibre) and protein to organic acids, including short-chain fatty acids, which include acetate and butyrate. The short-chain fatty acids serve as an essential energy source for the colonic epithelium. Their absorption acts as a primary stimulus for the absorption of salt and water by the colon.

Recycling of urea back into the host amino acid metabolism.

Functions of the rectum and anal canal

These include:

The preservation of faecal continence;

Allowing differentiation between solids, liquids and gas within the lumen;

A reservoir function, achieved by adaptive compliance, to allow controlled voluntary defaecation;

Maintenance of nocturnal control.

Defaecation

Defaecation is triggered by filling of the rectum from the sigmoid colon, leading to rectal distension. Reflex relaxation of the internal anal sphincter allows sampling of rectal contents and differentiation between flatus and faeces. Relaxation is mediated via stretch activation of descending inhibitory motor pathways, which stimulate the intrinsic inhibitory motor neurons to motor pathways, which stimulate the intrinsic motor neurons to release VIP and nitric oxide to relax the circular smooth muscle. The relaxation of the internal sphincter is transient as the sensory receptors in the rectal wall accommodate to distension.

Voluntary relaxation of the external anal sphincter allows commencement of defaecation. Defaecation is brought about by increased intra-abdominal pressure brought about by abdominal wall muscle contraction and pelvic floor muscle contraction, along with relaxation of the anal canal and contraction of the rectal wall.

Factors in the maintenance of anal continence

These include:

Stool volume and consistency: solidity of faeces.

Sphincteric function: internal and external anal sphincters. The internal anal sphincter measures 30 mm in length and 5 mm in thickness, and comprises smooth muscle fibres of the circular or inner muscle layer of the rectum.

Rectal sensation, allowing discrimination between flatus and faeces.

Mechanical factors:

Anorectal angle: about 90° angle between the long axes of the anal canal and rectum in the resting state, maintained by the puborectalis sling.

Flutter valve.

Flap valve action of the anterior rectal wall mucosa just above the anal canal.

Reservoir function of the rectum.

Coordinated pelvic floor muscular activity.

Investigation of function of anal sphincters, rectum and pelvic floor

Anorectal manometry
Closed balloon system;
Perfused fluid-filled open-tipped catheter.
At manometry, information can be obtained about maximum resting (tonic contraction of internal sphincter) and squeeze (voluntary contraction of external sphincter), rectal sensation, sphincter length and the inhibitory recto-anal reflex.

Imaging
Defaecography or evacuation proctography
Endorectal ultrasound
Balloon proctography

Electrophysiological studies
Electromyogram
Nerve stimulation techniques

BIBLIOGRAPHY

Bayliss, W. M. & Starling, E. H. The movements and innervation of the small intestine. *J. Physiol.*, **24** (1899), 99–143.

   The mechanism of pancreatic secretion. *J. Physiol.*, **28** (1902), 325–33.

Duthie, G. & Gardiner, A. *Physiology of the Gastrointestinal Tract*. London: Whurr Publishers Ltd, 2004.

Mittal, R. K. & Balaban, D. H. The oesophagogastric junction. *New Engl. J. Med.*, **336** (1997), 924–32.

O'Grady, J. G., Lake, J. R. & Howdle, P. D. *Comprehensive Clinical Hepatology*. Philadelphia: Mosby, 2000.

Rappaport, A. M. The microcirculatory acinar concept of normal and pathological hepatic structure. *Beitr Path*, **157** (1976), 215–43.

Sherlock, S. & Dooley, J. *Diseases of the Liver and Biliary System*, 11th edn. Oxford: Blackwell Publishing Co, 2002.

RECOMMENDED FURTHER READING

Berne, R. M., Levy, M. N., Koeppen, B. M. & Stoke, B. A. *Physiology*, 5th edn. St Louis: Mosby, 2004.

Ganong, W. F. *Review of Medical Physiology*, 21st edn. New York: The McGraw-Hill Companies, Inc., 2003.

Johnson, L. R. (ed.) *Essential Medical Physiology*, 3rd edn. San Diego: Academic Press (Elsevier), 2003.

Pocock, G. & Richards, C. *Human Physiology. The Basis of Medicine*, 2nd edn. Oxford: Oxford University Press, 2004.

Rhoades, R. A. & Tanner, G. A. *Medical Physiology*, 2nd edn. Baltimore: Lippincott, Williams & Wilkins, 2003.

Sherwood, L. *Human Physiology. From Cells to Systems*, 4th edn. Pacific Grove, California: Brooks/Cole, 2001.

Index

acid, production by the body 32, 33
acid–base abnormalities
  acidosis 38–40, 41–2
  alkalosis 40–1
  anion gap 39–40
  arterial blood gas analyser 37–8
  base excess or base deficit (negative base excess) 35, 37–8
  clinical effects of acidosis 42
  clinical effects of alkalosis 43
  compensatory mechanisms 41–2
  hypokalaemia and metabolic alkalosis 40–1
  ketoacidosis 40
  renal compensation mechanisms 36–7
  scheme for assessment and management 34–43
  Siggaard–Anderson curve nomogram 38
  sodium bicarbonate and metabolic acidosis 42
  standard bicarbonate 35, 37–8
  types of acid–base disorders 35–6
acid–base balance in the body
  buffer systems 33
  buffering capacity of the body 34
  factors affecting 32
  physiological buffer systems 34
  to control pH 31
acid–base reactions
  amphoteric substances 31–2
  Bronsted–Lowry definitions 31–2
acid strength, dissociation constant 31–2
acidosis 38–40, 41–2
ACTH 281–2, 284–5
activin (peptide hormone) 294
adipose tissue
  effects of glucagon 289–90
  effects of insulin 286–7
adrenal glands
  ACTH 281–2
  ACTH and adrenocortical disorders 284–5

adrenal cortex 279–80
adrenal medulla 279–80, 281
adrenaline and nonadrenaline secretion 280
adrenocortical disorders 284–5
adrenocortical function testing 285
aldosterone 284
catecholamine synthesis 280, 281
chromaffin cells 280
cortisol 280–1
Cushing's syndrome 283, 284–5
glucocorticoid deficiency 284
glucocorticoid excess 284
glucocorticoids 280–1, 281–2, 282–3
glucocorticoids, anti-inflammatory effects 283
hypothalamic–pituitary–adrenal axis 283
pregnenolone 281–2
primary hyperaldosteronism 284
structural features 279–80
adrenaline and nonadrenaline secretion 280
aldosterone 284
alkalosis 40–1, 41–2, 43
altitude acclimatisation, effects of 150
amino acids, reabsorption in the kidney 54
anaemia
  and erythropoietin deficiency 144–50
  evaluation for iron deficiency 152
androgens 292
  androgen actions 293
  modes of androgen action 293
  sources of androgen in the female 292
anion gap 39–40
anti-arrhythmic agents 114
anti-inflammatory effects of glucocorticoids 283
anticoagulants
  effects of aspirin 169
  heparin 166–7
  normal mechanisms in the body 168–9
  therapeutic 169
arginine vasopressin (antidiuretic hormone)

arginine vasopressin (antidiuretic hormone) (cont.)
  antidiuretic effects 24–5
  factors that control release 24
  properties of 23–4
arterial blood gas analyser 37–8
articular cartilage
  functions 314
  intra-articular fibrocartilaginous menisci 314
  structure and properties 313–14
  synovial membrane structure and functions 314
aspirin, anticoagulant activity 169
asthma, exercise-induced 131–2
ATP
  generation and uses in red blood cells 153, 154
  role in muscle contraction and relaxation 239
autonomic nervous system
  acetylcholine neurotransmission 225
  acetylcholine receptors 227
  adrenergic receptor stimulation 226
  autonomic function tests 228
  autonomic neuropathy 229
  catecholamine action at adrenergic receptors 226–7
  central autonomic network 223–4
  cholinergic nerves locations 228
  cholinergic-receptor antagonists 228
  cholinergic receptors classification 227
  components 222–3
  drugs acting on adrenergic receptors 227
  enteric nervous system 223
  functions of autonomic nervous system 222
  G-protein-linked receptors (cholinergic) 227
  muscarinic receptors (cholinergic) 227
  myenteric plexus of Auerbach 223
  neurotransmitters 225
  nicotinic receptors (cholinergic) 227
  non-adrenergic non-cholinergic (NANC) system 222–3
  noradrenaline neurotransmission 225
  parasympathetic (cholinergic) system 222–3
  parasympathetic system components 225
  predominant autonomic tone of various tissues 225
  submucosal plexus of Meissner 223
  sympathetic (adrenergic) system 222–3
  sympathetic system components 224–5
  Valsalva manoeuvre 229

basal ganglia
  disorders 213
  functions 213
base excess or base deficit (negative base excess) 35, 37–8
basophils 154–5, 155–6
Bell–Magendie law (spinal cord nerve roots) 218
bilirubin 340–1
biological rhythms, and the pineal gland 216
bladder function, urodynamic assessment of micturition 64–5
bleeding tendency
  screening for coagulation disorders 158
  screening for platelet disorders 158
  screening for vascular disorders 158
  screening with viscoelastic devices 158
blood see also haemoglobin
  acute phase reactant plasma proteins 142–3
  altitude acclimatisation effects 150
  bleeding tendency 158
  carbon dioxide transport 150
  causes of thrombophilic states 171
  cellular composition 140
  cholesterol 143–4
  coagulation cascade 163–4, 165, 166
  coagulation factors 166
  composition 140
  cytokines 142–3
  disseminated intravascular coagulation 170
  electrophoretic separation of plasma proteins 141–2
  erythropoietin 144–50
  fibrinolytic system 159–73
  haemostasis 157, 158, 161
  haemostatic defects 158
  haemostatic role of platelets 161
  heparin anticoagulant activity 166–7
  high density lipoproteins (HDL) 143–4
  inflammatory response 142–3
  lipid transport 143–4
  lipoprotein metabolism 144
  low density lipoproteins (LDL) 143–4
  mechanisms preventing intravascular coagulation 168–9
  normal blood volume 21
  plasma lipoproteins 143–4
  plasma protein synthesis 140
  plasma proteins functions 140–1
  plasmin 171, 172
  plasminogen activators 172
  protease inhibitors in human plasma 142
  protein C 168–9
  protein S 168–9

screening for thrombophilic states 170
spleen 173, 174–5
therapeutic anticoagulants 169
thrombin 163–4, 164, 165, 166
thrombosis 169–70, 170, 171
very low density lipoproteins (VLDL) 143–4
blood–brain barrier *see also* cerebrospinal
    fluid
blood–brain interfaces 203
brain areas outside of the barrier 204
carrier-mediated transport systems 203–4
circumventricular organs 204
disruption of function 203
electrolyte transport 203–4
immunological privilege of the brain 204–5
mechanisms of transport across 203–4
micronutrient transport 203–4
structure and function 202–3
types of cerebral oedema 208
blood cells
    ATP generation and uses in red blood cells
        153, 154
    basophils 154–5, 155–6
    eosinophils 154–5, 155–6
    lymphocytes 154–5, 155–6
    macrophages 155–6
    monocytes 154–5, 155–6
    neutrophils 154–5, 155–6
    red blood cell glucose metabolism in 153
    red blood cell membrane structure 154
    red blood cells 153, 154
    stem cells 153
    white blood cell classes 154–5
    white blood cells, functions 155–6
blood glucose homeostasis 288–9, 289–90
blood group antigens 156
blood loss, effects of 73–4
blood pressure
    angiotensin II 79–81
    antihypertensive agents, classification 82
    antihypertensive effects of beta blockers 82
    arterial blood pressure determinants 75
    AT2-receptor blockers 81
    control by reticular formation 217–18
    factors regulating blood pressure 75–7
    measurement 77
    pharmacological manipulation of
        renin–angiotensin mechanism 81, 81–2
    renin inhibition and secretion 79
    renin–angiotensin mechanism (autocrine
        system) 77–9
    systemic arterial blood pressure 74–5
    systolic blood pressure 75–9
    Valsalva manoeuvre 77

blood transfusion
    blood components used for 157
    principles 156
blood vessels
    arterio-venous shunts 96
    capillary exchange 96–7
    cerebral capillaries, unique features 202
    coronary circulation 93–4
    damping vessels (arteries) 95
    exchange vessels (capillaries) 95–6
    factors determining smooth muscle tone 97
    lymphatic vessels 97
    nitric oxide synthesis, functions and uses
        102–3
    normal artery wall 101
    resistance vessels (small arteries, arterioles)
        95
    tissue oedema 96–7
    vascular endothelial dysfunction 101
    vascular endothelium 98–9, 99–100
blood viscosity
    determinants of 103–4
    effects on circulatory system 103
    Fahraeus–Lindqvist effect 103–4
    hyperviscosity syndromes 103–4
    laminar flow 104, 105
    Laplace's law 106
    plasma skimming and axial streaming 104
    Poiseuille's equation 105–6
    Reynolds number 105
    shear rate of blood 103–4
    turbulent flow 105
    viscous properties of blood
blood volume
    control 72–3
    distribution 72
body fluid compartments 20
    measurement of volume 21
body fluids
    assessment of extracellular fluid volume
        status 22
    components of extracellular fluid 20
    daily fluid requirements 22
    extracellular fluid volume 21
    extracellular fluid volume replacement 22–3
    normal blood volume 21
    osmolality and tonicity 19–20
    water reabsorption 23–5
bone function
    and calcitonin 307
    and PTH (parathyroid hormone) 306–7
    biochemical markers of bone turnover
        312–13
    bone cells 311

bone function (cont.)
  bone fractures 311–12
  bone mineral density 312
  bone remodelling 310, 311
  components of bone 310
  components of the extracellular matrix 310
  functions of bone 309–10
  mechanism of bone repair 311–12
  osteoblasts 311
  osteoclasts 311
  osteocytes 311
  osteopenia 312
  osteoporosis and low bone mass 312
  structure of bone 309
brain *see also* basal ganglia; cerebellum;
    cerebral hemispheres; cranium;
    hypothalamus; limbic system; pineal
    gland; reticular formation; thalamus
  electroencephalogram (EEG) 220–1
  immunological privilege 204–5
brain ischaemia, and raised intracranial
    pressure 207
brain shift, and raised intracranial pressure
    207
Bronsted–Lowry definitions (acid–base
    reactions) 31–2
Brugada syndrome 11
buffer systems
  buffering capacity 34
  conjugate acid–base pairs 33
  dissociation constant (pK) 33
  Henderson–Hasselbach equation 33
  physiological 34

calcitonin 307
calcium
  Ca^{2+} second messenger system 266, 266–7
  calcium channels classification 112
  role in cardiac cycle 108–9
calcium metabolism
  and calcitonin 307
  and PTH (parathyroid hormone) 306–7
  body calcium pools 302
  calcium absorption 303, 304
  calcium abundance in the body 301–2
  calcium homeostasis 303–4, 305
  calcium reabsorption 303–4
  components of plasma calcium 302–3
  corrected calcium 302–3
  functions of calcium 302
  hypercalcaemia 304, 307
  hypocalcaemia 305
  plasma calcium homeostasis 301–2
  regulatory mechanisms 301–2

carbohydrate
  digestion 331
  effects of insulin on metabolism 287–8
carbon dioxide, transport in the blood 150
cardiac cycle
  cardiac contraction sequence 107
  contractile regulatory proteins 108
  contraction and relaxation mechanisms
    107–8
  left ventricular contraction 106
  left ventricular diastolic dysfunction 106–7
  left ventricular relaxation (diastole) 106–7
  myocardial energy consumption 108
  phases 106–9
  role of calcium 108–9
cardiac electrophysiology
  anti-arrhythmic agents 114
  cardiovascular calcium channels
    classification 112
  conduction system 111–12
  conduction velocities 113
  electrocardiograph 112–13
  factors affecting slope of phase 4
    depolarisation 112
  pacemaker potential 111
  phases of cardiac action potential 109–11
cardiac output
  adaptive mechanisms associated with heart
    failure 91–2
  control by reticular formation 217–18
  determinants of cardiac output 82–4
  determinants of venous return to the heart
    88–90
  Frank–Starling mechanism 86–7
  heart failure 91, 91–2
  measurement of 84–5, 86
  relationship of heart rate to contractility 90
  Starling's law of the heart (length–tension
    relationship) 86–7, 88
  ventricular function curves 86–7, 88
cardiovascular system *see also* blood vessels
  angiotensin II effects 79–81
  arterial blood pressure measurement 77
  blood loss effects 73–4
  blood pressure 74–5, 75–9, 79–81, 81–2
  blood volume control 72–3
  blood volume distribution 72
  cardiac cells 94
  cardiac muscle properties 94–5
  circulation of newborn 72
  components of 71
  coronary circulation 93–4
  factors affecting blood pressure 75–7
  fetal circulation 72

myocardial oxygen consumption 92–3, 93–4
pharmacological manipulation of
    renin–angiotensin mechanism 81, 81–2
renin inhibition and secretion 79
renin–angiotensin mechanism (autocrine
    system) 77–9
Valsalva manoeuvre 77
cardiovascular peptides, natriuretic peptides
    54–5, 55–6
catecholamine synthesis 280, 281
cell 1
cell adhesion molecules
    cell body to cell body adhesion 5
    cell to extracellular matrix adhesion 5
    roles 6
cell–cell signalling mechanisms 5
cell membrane
    adherent junction types 4, 5
    classification of membrane proteins 2–3
    fluid mosaic model of structure 2
    functions 1
    integral membrane proteins 3
    intercellular junctions 4, 5
    membrane protein functions 3
    structure 2
    transmembrane proteins 3
cell membrane receptors
    signal transduction mechanisms 3
    structural groups 3–4
    tyrosine kinase receptors 3–4
cell membrane transport mechanisms
    active transport 6–7, 8–9
    facilitated transport 6, 8–9
    ion channels 9–11
    osmosis 7
    passive diffusion 6, 7–8
    receptor-mediated endocytosis 7
    vesicular transport 7
cell polarity 18
cellular organelles 12–18
    cytoskeleton 15–17, 17–18
    Golgi apparatus 13
    lysosomes 14, 15
    mitochondria 13–14
    nucleus 12
    peroxisomes (microbodies) 15, 16
    rough endoplasmic reticulum 12–13
    smooth endoplasmic reticulum 12–13
CNS, evoked potentials 221–2
cerebellum
    anatomical portions 214
    functional subdivisions 214
    structure and functioning 214–15
cerebral blood flow

autoregulation capability 200–2
blood vessels and flow rates 198
causes of increased flow 202
causes of reduced flow 202
cerebral capillaries, unique features 202
cerebral ischaemia 200
cerebral metabolism 199–200
cerebral oxygen consumption 199
cerebral uptake of glucose 199
circle of Willis 198
Fick principle for measuring 198
high energy functions of the brain 199–200
ischaemic lesions and ischaemic penumbra
    200
regulation of 200–2
techniques for measuring 198
cerebral cortex, study of localisation of
    function 210
cerebral hemispheres
    association fibres 209
    basal ganglia disorders 213
    basal ganglia functions 213
    Brodmann's system of numbering areas 209
    frontal lobe functions 209–10
    frontal lobe lesions 211
    limbic system 213–14
    occipital lobe functions 212
    occipital lobe lesions 212–13
    parietal lobe functions 211
    parietal lobe lesions 212
    projection fibres 209, 210
    structure 209
    study of localisation of cortical function
        210
    temporal lobe functions 211
    temporal lobe lesions 212
cerebral ischaemia 200
cerebral metabolism 199–200
cerebrospinal fluid
    and intracranial pressure 205
    brain ischaemia and raised intracranial
        pressure 207
    brain shift and raised intracranial pressure
        207
    clinical effects of raised intracranial
        pressure 207
    compensation for increased intracranial
        pressure 206
    formation and circulation 205–6
    functions of 206
    hydrocephalus and raised intracranial
        pressure 207
    intracranial pressure measurement 208–9
    intracranial pressure range 207

cerebrospinal fluid (cont.)
  normal intracranial pressure waveform 208–9
  reducing intracranial pressure 208
  types of cerebral oedema 208
cholecystokinin 328
cholera, effects of cyclic AMP 266
cilia
  disorders of 18
  structure 17–18
Cl^- ion, reciprocal relationship with HCO_3 ion 41
coagulation cascade 163–4, 165, 166
coagulation disorders, screening for 158
colon
  colonic microflora functions 346
  colonic motility 345
  components of mucous gel layer 345
  defaecation 346–7
  functions 346
  investigation of anal sphincters, rectum and pelvic floor 347
  maintenance of anal continence 347
  rectum and anal canal functions 346–7
coronary circulation 93–4
cortisol 280–1
cranium
  brain ischaemia and raised intracranial pressure 207
  brain shift and raised intracranial pressure 207
  cerebrospinal fluid 205–6
  clinical effects of raised intracranial pressure 207
  compensation for increased intracranial pressure 206
  hydrocephalus and raised intracranial pressure 207
  intracranial pressure measurement 208–9
  intracranial pressure range 207
  Monroe–Kellie doctrine 205
  normal intracranial pressure waveform 208–9
  reducing intracranial pressure 208
Cushing's syndrome 283, 284–5
cyclic AMP (adenosine $3'$–$5'$-monophosphate) second messenger 264–6
cystic fibrosis 11
cytokines 142–3
cytoskeleton 15–17

diabetic ketoacidosis 289
diffusion across a membrane (Fick's Law) 7–8
digestion 331–2, 332–3

dissociation constant 31–2, 33
diuretics
  classes of 63
  mechanisms of action 62
DNA
  in the cell nucleus
  mitochondrial 13–14
2,3-DPG (2,3-diphosphoglycerate) 148–9

ear see hearing; vestibular function
electrocardiograph 112–13
electroencephalogram (EEG)
  abnormalities 221
  non-rapid eye movement sleep 220–1
  rapid eye movement sleep 220–1
  recording 220
  rhythms 220
  sleep phases 220–1
electrolytes, effects of insulin 287–8
endocrine pancreas
  blood glucose homeostasis 288–9, 289–90
  C peptide 286
  diabetic ketoacidosis 289
  glucagon effects on adipose tissue 289–90
  glucagon effects on gastrointestinal tract 289–90
  glucagon effects on the liver 289–90
  glucagon synthesis and actions 289–90
  hypoglycaemia 288–9
  insulin effects on adipose tissue 286–7
  insulin effects on carbohydrate metabolism 287–8
  insulin effects on cellular metabolism 286–7
  insulin effects on electrolytes 287–8
  insulin effects on fat metabolism 287–8
  insulin effects on liver 286–7
  insulin effects on protein metabolism 287–8
  insulin effects on skeletal muscle 286–7
  insulin metabolic effects 287–8
  insulin receptors 288
  insulin synthesis and release 286
  islets of Langerhans 285–6
  structure 285–6
endocrine physiology see also adrenal glands; articular cartilage; bone function; calcium metabolism; endocrine pancreas; hormones; hypothalamus; parathyroid glands; phosphorus metabolism; pituitary gland; reproductive system; thyroid gland; vitamin D
gastrointestinal tract as an endocrine organ 327

mechanisms of endocrine disease 260
regulatory systems 258
endocytosis 7
endogenous opioids
   endogenous opioid peptides 235
   functions 235
   opioid receptors 236
   types and modes of action 235
eosinophils 154–5, 155–6
erythropoietin 144–50
   and red blood cell production 46
Eustachian tube 255
evoked potentials 221–2
exocrine pancreas
   pancreatic function assessment 345
   proteins secreted 344
   secretions 344, 344–5
   structural features 343–4
exocytosis 7
extracellular fluid
   assessment of status 22
   components of 20
   options for replacement 22–3
   volume 21
eyes *see* vision

Fahraeus–Lindqvist effect 103–4
fat metabolism, effects of insulin 287–8
fever 70
fibrinolytic system
   inhibitors of fibrinolysis 159–73
   plasmin 171, 172
   plasminogen activators 172
   platelets 159–60, 161, 162
   tests for fibrinolysis 173
Fick principle, for measuring cerebral blood
     flow 198
Fick's law (diffusion across a membrane) 7–8
Fowler's method, measuring anatomical dead
     space 121
Frank–Starling mechanism 86–7
FSH, regulation by GnRH (gonadotrophin
     releasing hormone) 290–1

G-proteins (GTP-binding transducer proteins)
     262–3
   G-protein-coupled receptors 263, 264
gall bladder 343
gangliosidoses
gastrointestinal neuroendocrine tumours 329
gastrointestinal regulatory peptides
   cholecystokinin effects 328
   cholecystokinin production 328
   endocrine peptides 327

gastrointestinal hormone receptors 328
   hormonal functions 327
   neurocrine peptides 327
   paracrine peptide 327
   secretin effects 329
   secretin production 328
   somatostatin 329
   structural classification 328
   vasoactive intestinal peptide 329–30
gastrointestinal tract *see also* colon; exocrine
     pancreas; liver; small intestine; stomach
   as an endocrine organ 327
   barrier function 333–4
   effects of glucagon 289–90
   function 316
   gastrointestinal motility 334
   gastro-oesophageal competence 319, 320
   gastro-oesophageal reflux 320
   lower oesophageal sphincter 319, 320
   oesophagitis 320
   oesophagus 319, 320
   salivary function studies 318
   salivary functions 316–17
   salivary glands 316
   salivary production deficiency 317
   salivary protein families 317
   salivary secretion 317
   swallowing, oesophageal phase 318–19
   swallowing, oral phase 318
   swallowing, pharyngeal phase 318
   upper oesophageal sphincter 319
   vomiting reflex 320–1
GH (growth hormone) 276–7, 277–8
Gibbs–Donnan equilibrium 187–8
glucagon 289–90
glucocorticoids 280–1, 281–2, 282–3
glucose
   reabsorption in the kidney 54
   uptake by the brain (D-glucose) 199
GnRH (gonadotrophin releasing hormone)
     290–1
Goldman–Hodgkin–Katz equation (to predict
     equilibrium voltage or resting potential)
     187

H^+ ion, relationship with Na^+ and K^+ ions 41
   see also pH scale
haemoglobin 150
   action of erythropoietin 144–50
   allosteric properties 146–8
   'co-operative' oxygen binding 146–8
   2,3-DPG (2,3-diphosphoglycerate), and
     oxygen affinity 148–9
   molecular pathology 149

haemoglobin (cont.)
  oxygen carrying capacity 145
  oxyhaemoglobin dissociation curve 145–6,
    148
  Perutz mechanism 146–8
  structure of haemoglobin 144–5
  T and R structural states 146–8
  tissue oxygen delivery 145
haemostasis 157, 158
  coagulation cascade 163–4, 165, 166
  fibrinolytic system 159–73
  role of platelets 161
  role of vascular endothelium 100
  vascular endothelium-derived modulators
    of 99–100
haemostatic defects 158
HCO_3^- ion, reciprocal relationship with Cl^- ion
  41
hearing
  audiometry 252–3
  decibel scale 252–3
  function of the cochlea 251
  function of the organ of Corti 250–1
  functions of the ear 249–50
  hearing process 250–1
  inner ear 250
  middle ear 249–50
  outer ear 249–50
  output of sound amplification mechanisms
    250
  testing of 252–3
heart failure
  adaptive mechanisms to maintain output
    91–2
  causes 91
  pathophysiology 91
Heliox mixture, to reduce the work of
  breathing 126–7
Henderson–Hasselbach equation, for buffer
  solutions 33
heparin, anticoagulant activity 166–7
hormones
  Ca^{2+} second messenger system 266, 266–7
  characteristics 259
  classification 261
  classification of protein kinases 267
  cyclic AMP (second messenger) 264, 264–6
  effects on a target cell 259
  effects on gene transcription rates 261–2
  G-protein-coupled receptors 263, 264
  G-proteins (GTP-binding transducer
    proteins) 262–3
  hormone receptors 261–2
  in endocrine regulatory systems 258

inositol 1,4,5,-triphosphate (second
    messenger) 264, 266–7
  intracellular receptors 261–2
  magnitude of response to 259
  mechanisms of endocrine disease 260
  mechanisms of signal transduction 262
  membrane receptor protein super-families
    263
  phosphoinositide cascade and its effects
    266–7
  plasma membrane receptors 261–2
  positive feedback mechanisms 260
  receptors for molecules used in signalling 261
  regulation of hormone levels 259–60
  second messengers 264, 264, 266–7
  steroid-hormone receptor mechanism 267–8
hydrocephalus and raised intracranial
    pressure 207
hyperaldosteronism 284
hyperoxaluria type 1 16
hyperprolactinaemia 278
hypoglycaemia 288–9
hypokalaemia and metabolic alkalosis 40–1
hypophyseal portal venous system 275
hypothalamus
  hypothalamic–pituitary–adrenal axis 283
  hypothalamic–pituitary axis 274
  hypothalamic–pituitary–thyroid axis 271–2
  hypothalamic releasing and inhibitory
    hormones 274–5
  location and structure 215
hypothermia 69
hysteresis, in lung volume/pressure
    relationship 135–6

infantile Refsum disease 16
inflammation, vascular endothelium
    secretion caused by 100
inhibin (peptide hormone) 294
inositol 1,4,5,-triphosphate (second
    messenger) 264, 266–7
insulin
  and blood glucose homeostasis 288–9,
    289–90
  C peptide 286
  effects on adipose tissue 286–7
  effects on carbohydrate metabolism 287–8
  effects on cellular metabolism 286–7
  effects on electrolytes 287–8
  effects on fat metabolism 287–8
  effects on liver 286–7
  effects on protein metabolism 287–8
  effects on skeletal muscle 286–7
  insulin receptors 288

islets of Langerhans 285–6
  metabolic effects 287–8
  synthesis and release 286
intercellular junctions 4, 5
intracranial pressure *see* cranium
iodine, role in thyroid hormone synthesis 268, 268–9
ion channel transport across a membrane 9–11
  advantages of 9
  calcium channel blockers 10
  calcium channels 10, 11
  chloride channels 11
  gating mechanism 9
  ion channel disorders 11
  ion channels classification 10–11
  ion flow rates 9
  ligand (agonist)-gated ion channels 10
  potassium channels 10–11
  sodium channels 11
  study of ion channel structure 11
iron
  absorption and bioavailability 151–2
  body stores evaluation 152
  distribution and storage in the body 152
  enzymes containing iron 151
  functions of 151
  iron deficiency anaemia evaluation 152
  metabolism 150
isolated deafness syndrome 11

K^+ *see* potassium
ketoacidosis 40, 289

Laplace's law 106
LH, regulation by GnRH (gonadotrophin releasing hormone) 290–1
Liddle's syndrome 11
limbic system 213–14
  Papez circuit 213–14
lipid digestion 331–2
liver
  acinus units 337
  bile acids 342
  bile components 342
  bile salts functions 342–3
  bile salts production 342
  bile secretion 341–2
  bilirubin metabolism 340–1
  bilirubin production 340
  blood flow measurement 340
  cells of the liver 335–6, 336
  detoxification of drugs 341
  effects of glucagon 289–90
  effects of insulin 286–7

enterohepatic circulation 343
functions 334, 337–8
gall bladder 343
hepatocytes 336
Kupffer cells 336
links with gastrointestinal tract 334
liver function tests 338–40
lobule units 337
plasma proteins synthesised by 338
segmental anatomy 335
serum protein changes and liver disease 338
structural features 335–6, 336, 337
tests indicating bile flow obstruction 339
tests of synthetic function 339
tests of uptake, conjugation and excretion of anionic compounds 338–9
tests reflecting hepatocellular damage 339
units of the liver 337
vascular system 335
long QT syndrome 11
lung volumes and capacities *see also* respiratory system
  body plethysmography 132–3
  expiratory reserve volume 130–1, 131–2, 132–3
  flow–pressure relationship 135–6
  flow–volume relationship 133–5
  forced vital capacity (FVC) 131–2
  functional residual capacity (FRC) 131–2, 133
  helium dilution measurement method 132–3
  inspiratory capacity (IC) 131–2, 132–3
  inspiratory reserve volume (IRV) 130–1, 131–2
  lung function testing 136, 136–7, 138
  residual volume (RS) 130–1, 131–2
  spirometry 132–3, 133–5
  tidal volume (VT) 130–1, 131–2, 132–3
  total lung capacity (TLC) 131–2, 132–3
  vital capacity (VC) 130–1
lymphatic system
  functions of 97
  lymphatic vessels 97
lymphocytes 154–5, 155–6
lysosomal storage diseases 15

macrophages 155–6
magnesium (important intracellular cation)
  causes of hypomagnesaemia 30
  daily requirements 29
  functions of 30
  locations in the body 29
malignant hyperthermia 11
melatonin, and biological rhythms 216

memory, and the limbic system 213–14
micelles 332
micturition 63–5
mitochondria 13–14
monocytes 154–5, 155–6
Monroe–Kellie doctrine 205
motility, molecular motor proteins 15–17
motor system
    components of 230
    electromyogram 230–1
muscle *see also* skeletal muscle
    factors determining smooth muscle
        tone 97
myocardial oxygen consumption 92–3, 93–4

Na$^+$ *see* sodium
natriuretic peptides 54–5, 55–6
neonatal respiratory distress, surfactant
        therapy 122–3
nephrons (in the kidneys) 44–5
Nernst equation 180–2, 186–7
nerve fibres
    action potential generation 182–4
    action potential measurement 186
    effects of myelin sheath on action potential
        185
    Gibbs–Donnan equilibrium 187–8
    Goldman–Hodgkin–Katz equation 187
    membrane action potential 180–2
    membrane graded potential 180–2
    Nernst equation 180–2, 186–7
    patch clamping techniques 182
    potassium channels 186
    properties of the action potential 184–5
    saltatory conduction 185
    voltage clamp technique 181–2
nervous system
    astrocytes 178, 179
    cells of the nervous system 177–8, 178–9
    CNS components 177
    nerve fibre membrane potentials 180–2,
        182–4, 184–5
    neuroglial cells 177–8, 179
    neurons 177–8, 178–9
    oligodendrocytes 178, 179
    peripheral nerve fibre types 180
    peripheral nervous system components
        177
    physiological effects of membrane action
        potentials 185
    synapses 178–9
neurotransmission
    acetylcholine 188–9
    acetylcholine receptors 191–2

agents used to reverse non-depolarising
        blocking agents 190
    antimuscarinic agents 190
    autonomic nervous system 225
    known or postulated neurotransmitters
        192–3
    miniature end-plate potentials 189–90
    muscarinic acetylcholine receptors 191–2
    neuromuscular blockade types 191
    neuromuscular blocking agent, required
        characteristics 190–1
    neuromuscular blocking agents 190
    neuromuscular junction components 188
    neuromuscular junction transmission
        188–9
    neuropeptide Y 193
    neurotransmitter identification 192
    nicotinic acetylcholine receptors 191–2
    opioid receptors classification 193
    reflexes 196–7
    synapses 194–5, 195–6
    uses of neuromuscular blocking agents 191
neutrophils 154–5, 155–6
nitric oxide
    clinical uses 103
    functions 102–3
    synthesis in vascular endothelium 102–3
nose 116–17
    olfaction 256
    paranasal sinuses 116–17
    tests of nasal function 116–17

oedema, mechanisms of 96–7
oesophagus 319, 320
oestrogens
    hormonal effects of oestrogen levels 292
    oestrogen actions 291–2
olfaction 256
opioids, endogenous
    endogenous opioid peptides 235
    functions 235
    types and modes of action 235
    types of opioid receptors 236
osmotic threshold for thirst 23–4
osteopenia 312
osteoporosis
    and calcitonin 307
    and low bone mass 312
oxygen consumption in the brain 199
oxytocin 279

pain
    analgesic effects of counterirritation
        characteristics of 232

endogenous opioids 235, 236
fibres which convey pain 231
gate control theory
mechanisms of production 232
modulation 232
neurotransmitters involved 233, 234
nociceptors and pain perception 232, 233, 234
pathway to the CNS 233
pathways involved in pain perception 233
sensory unit 231
sites of sensory receptors 231
somatic sensation classification 230
steps leading to pain perception 232
the medial lemniscal system 234
the spinothalamic pathway 233, 234
transcutaneous electrical nerve stimulation 234–5
types of sensory receptors 231
pancreas see endocrine pancreas; exocrine pancreas
Papez circuit (limbic system) 213–14
parathyroid glands
calcitonin 307
PTH (parathyroid hormone) 306–7
structure and location 306
peroxisomal disorders 16
Perutz mechanism 146–8
pH scale 31–2
phosphoinositide cascade and its effects 266–7
phosphorus metabolism
functions of phosphate 305
phosphate absorption and reabsorption 305
phosphorus content in the body 305
pineal gland
location and structure 216
melatonin secretion and biological rhythms 216
pituitary gland
adenohypophysis (anterior pituitary) 273
anterior pituitary function testing 279
anterior pituitary hormones 276
anterior pituitary secretory cells 276
feedback to the hypothalamus 275
growth hormone (GH) structure and secretion 276–7
growth hormone actions 277–8
hyperprolactinaemia 278
hypophyseal portal venous system 275
hypothalamic releasing and inhibitory hormones 274–5
hypothalamic–pituitary axis 274
hypothalamic–pituitary–adrenal axis 283

hypothalamic–pituitary–thyroid axis 271–2
location and size 273
neurohypophysis (posterior pituitary) 273
oxytocin actions 279
oxytocin release 279
pituitary hormone release 274
prolactin actions 278–9
prolactin synthesis and secretion 278
structural components 273
platelets
coagulation cascade 163–4, 165, 166
contractile apparatus 159
disorders, screening for 158
features and function 158–9
glycoprotein receptors 160
granule types 159–60
haemostatic role 161
inhibiting and activating agents 160
inhibition of platelet function 161, 162
microanatomy 159
platelet factors 160
prothrombin time (clotting time) 162
role in haemostasis 157
role of vitamin K 163
Poiseuille's equation 105–6
potassium (major cation in intracellular fluid)
abnormalities in homeostasis 29
functions of 27–8
homeostatic mechanisms 28–9
K^+ ion, relationship with H^+ and Na^+ ions 41
regulation 27
pregnenolone 281–2
progestagens 293
hormonal effects of progestagen levels 294
progestagen actions 293–4
progesterone 293
prolactin 278–9
protein
digestion 332–3
insulin effects on metabolism 287–8
reabsorption in the kidney 54
prothrombin time (clotting time) 162
PTH (parathyroid hormone) 306–7

Rapoport–Leubering shuttle 148–9
reflex activity, effects of reticular formation 217–18
reflexes
general properties 197
neural components of the tendon jerk reflex (stretch or myotactic reflex) 197
pupillary light reflex 248–9
reflex arc 196–7

reflexes (cont.)
 reflex control of colonic motility 345
 vomiting reflex 320–1
renal aquaporins (water channel proteins) 24
 mediation of water reabsorption 23–4
renal circulation 46–8
 and urine production 47
 autoregulation mechanisms 47–8
 substances which affect renal vasculature 48
renal function, micturition 63–5
renal function tests
 glomerular filtration tests 60–1
 renal tubular function tests 61–2
renal physiology
 erythropoietin 46
 functional components of kidneys 44–5
 functions of the kidneys 46
 nephrons in the kidneys 44–5
 structure of kidneys 44
renal stone formation, mechanisms 62
renin–angiotensin mechanism (autocrine
  system) 77–9
 angiotensin II effects 79–81
 antihypertensive agents 82
 antihypertensive effects of beta blockers 82
 AT2-receptor blockers 81
 pharmacological manipulation 81–2
 renin inhibition and secretion 79
Renshaw internuncial neuron (Renshaw cell)
  243
reproductive system
 activin (peptide hormone) 294
 androgens 292, 293
 GnRH (gonadotrophin releasing hormone)
  290–1
 inhibin (peptide hormone) 294
 oestrogens 291–2
 progestagens 293–4
reproductive system (female)
 changes at puberty 297
 Fallopian tube functions 299
 fertilisation mechanisms 299
 functional constituents of the adult ovary
  296–7
 hormonal mediation of monthly ovarian
  cycle 297
 hypogonadism 299
 menopause 299
 menstruation 298, 299
 ovarian cycle 297–8
 phases of menstrual cycle 298
 physiological changes in pregnancy 300
 placental structure and circulation 300
 placental transfer of drugs 301

placental transport functions 300–1
reproductive system (male)
 components and normal function 294
 hypogonadism 299
 Leydig cells 294–5
 penile erection 296
 semen analysis 295
 semen components 295
 Sertoli cells 294–5
 smooth muscle activity in the penis 296
 testes products 294–5
 testis structure and endocrine control 294
 vascular phases of penile erection 296
respiration, mitochondria 13–14
respiratory rhythm, generation by reticular
  formation 217–18
respiratory system
 air–blood barrier 119–20
 alveolar dead space 121–2
 alveolar surface tension (action of
  surfactant) 122–3
 alveolar ventilation and perfusion 130
 alveoli 117–19
 body plethysmography 132–3
 Bohr's method (measuring physiological
  dead space) 121–2
 bronchial circulation 128
 bronchopulmonary segment 117–19
 capillary endothelial cell transport
  mechanisms 121
 cough reflex 124
 dead space (alveolar) 121–2
 dead space (anatomical) 121
 dead space (physiological) 121–2
 diffusing capacity measurement 120
 diffusion 119–21
 dyspnoea, pathophysiology of 127
 elastic properties of lungs and chest wall
  122–3
 expiration 115–16
 flow–pressure relationship in the lungs 135–6
 flow–volume relationship in the lungs 133–5
 Fowler's method (measuring anatomical
  dead space) 121
 functional components 115–19
 functional residual capacity (FRC) 131–2, 133
 functions of pulmonary circulation 129
 Heliox mixture to reduce the work of
  breathing 126–7
 helium dilution measurement method
  132–3
 Hering Breuer inhibitory reflex 124
 hysteresis in lung volume/pressure
  relationship 122–3, 135–6

immune defences 119
inspiration 115–16
larynx 116–17
lower respiratory tract 117–19
lung capacities 131–2, 133
lung compliance 135–6
lung disease detection and the flow–volume
    loop 133–5
lung function testing 136–7, 138
lung volumes 130–1, 132–3
nasal function tests 116–17
neonatal respiratory distress (surfactant
    therapy) 122–3
nose 116–17
paranasal sinuses 116–17
pharynx 116–17
pulmonary acinus (terminal respiratory
    unit) 117–19
pulmonary arterial hypoxia, causes 137
pulmonary circulation 127–8, 128–9, 129–30
pulmonary defence mechanisms 119
pulmonary interstitium 119–20
pulmonary oedema 129–30
pulmonary surfactant 122–3
pulmonary vasculature 127, 128–9
pulse oximetry 138
rate-limiting steps for oxygen diffusion 120
resistance to airflow 126–7
respiration (gas exchange) 115–16
respiratory epithelium 118–19
spirometry 132–3, 133–5
tracheo-bronchial tree 117–19
turbulent gas flow 126–7
upper respiratory tract 116–17
ventilation 115–16
ventilation control 123–6
work of breathing 126–7
reticular formation, structure and functions
    217–18
Reynolds number 105

secretin 328, 329
sensory system *see also* pain
    classification of somatic sensation 230
    olfaction 256
    sensory unit 231
    sites of sensory receptors 231
    taste 256
    types of sensory receptors 231
servomechanisms (feedback control) 243
Siggaard–Andersen curve nomogram 38
skeletal muscle
    endurance training effects 241
    exercise training effects 241

factors affecting muscle tension 240–1, 244
insulin effects 286–7
isometric muscle contraction 240
isotonic muscle contraction 240
muscle cell types (fast and slow twitch) 240
muscle contraction types 240
muscle fatigue 239–40
muscle fibre types 239–40
muscle metabolic systems 239
myofibril structure 237
myosin structure and biological activities
    237–8
pathophysiology of hyperpyrexia 237
role of ATP in contraction and relaxation 239
sarcotubular functional proteins 236–7
structural proteins of the sarcomere 237
structure 236
skeletal muscle contraction
    excitation-contraction coupling 238–9
    sliding filament theory 239
skeletal muscle spindle
    components 242–4
    Renshaw internuncial neuron (Renshaw
        cell) 243
    structure and function 242
sleep phases
    non-rapid eye movement sleep 220–1
    rapid eye movement sleep 220–1
small intestine
    barrier function 333–4
    bile acid absorption test 333
    carbohydrate absorption tests 333
    carbohydrate digestion 331
    components of 330
    digestion 331, 331–2, 332–3
    electrolyte transport proteins 330
    epithelial cell types 331
    epithelial characteristics 330
    fat absorption tests 333
    fat soluble vitamin absorption 332
    intestinal absorption tests 333
    lipid digestion 331–2
    micelles 332
    motility of 334
    protein digestion 332–3
    vitamin B12 absorption test 333
sodium (major cation in extracellular fluid)
    abnormalities in sodium metabolism 26–7
    homeostatic mechanisms 26
    Na^+ ion, relationship with H^+ and K^+ ions 41
    natriuretic peptides 54–5, 55–6
    physiological roles 25
    reabsorption in the kidney 52–4
    regulation 25

somatostatin 329
spinal cord
    Bell–Magendie law 218
    effects of spinal cord lesions 219
    structure and functions 218
    tracts in the white columns 219
spleen
    functions 174–5
    hyposplenism 175
    post-splenectomy blood picture 174
    structural features 173
standard bicarbonate 35, 37–8
Starling forces 73–4
    and capillary exchange 96–7
    and tissue oedema 96–7
Starling's law of the heart (length–tension
    relationship) 86–7, 88
stomach
    chief cells 324
    functions 321–2
    gastric acid secretion control mechanisms
        325
    gastric acid secretion mechanism 322–4
    gastric acid secretion phases 324–5
    gastric acid secretion tests 325
    gastric emptying 322
    gastric mucosal homeostasis 323
    gastrin cells 324
    gastrin effects 326
    gastrin secretion stimuli 326
    gastrin structures 326
    hypergastrinaemia 326
    parietal cells 324
    stomach cells 324
    structure 321
    vomiting reflex 320–1
synapses
    chemical transmission 194–5
    electrical transmission 194–5
    epsp (excitatory postsynaptic potential)
        195–6
    features of neuron-to-neuron transmission
        195
    generation of postsynaptic potentials 195–6
    genetropic postsynaptic potentials 196
    ionotropic postsynaptic potentials 196
    ipsp (inhibitory postsynaptic potential) 195–6
    metabotropic postsynaptic potentials 196
    post-tetanic facilitation 194
    properties of 194
    structure and classification 194
    synaptic delay 194
    synaptic fatigue 194
    synaptic transmission in the CNS 195

synaptic transmission modulation 195
synaptic vesicle exo-endocytic cycle 194–5
synaptic vesicle proteins 196
transmission modes 194–5
types of postsynaptic potentials in the
    CNS 196

taste 256
temperature regulation 66
    cold response 68
    core temperature measurement 66
    factors affecting metabolic rate 69
    fever 70
    heat loss mechanisms 67
    heat production measurement 68–9
    heat production sources 68–9
    heat stress response 67–8
    hypothermia 69
    thermoregulatory mechanisms 67
thalamus, structure and functions 217
thermoregulation see temperature regulation
thirst, osmotic threshold for 23–4
thrombosis 169–70, 170, 171
thyroid gland
    causes of high TSH levels in the serum 272
    causes of low TSH levels in the serum 272
    components of serum thyroxine 271
    hypothalamic–pituitary–thyroid axis 271–2
    mechanisms of hyperthyroidism 272–3
    mechanisms of hypothyroidism 272, 273
    regulation of thyroid hormone production
        271–2
    role of iodine in thyroid hormone synthesis
        268–9
    the iodide pump 270
    thyroid function tests 272
    thyroid gland structure and functions 268
    thyroid hormone actions and effects 270–1
    thyroid hormone secretion 269
    thyroid hormone synthesis 268–9, 270
tyrosine kinase receptors 3–4

urine production
    clearance techniques to measure
        glomerular filtration rate 50–1
    Cockcroft–Gault formula (creatinine
        clearance) 51
    concentrated urine production 60
    effects of renal circulation 47
    endogenous creatinine clearance
        measurement 50–1
    glomerular balance 56–7
    glomerular filtration 48, 49–51
    inulin clearance measurement 50–1

loop of Henle 57–60
micturition 63–5
natriuretic peptides 54–5, 55–6
processes involved 48, 49–51, 51–4
renal epithelial co-transporters and
    antiporters 54
sodium reabsorption mechanisms 52–4
tubular function 51–4
tubular reabsorption functions 52–4

Valsalva manoeuvre 77, 229
vascular disorders, screening for 158
vascular endothelium
    characteristics of endothelial cells 99
    endothelial dysfunction 101
    modulators of haemostasis 99–100
    products of 99
    role in haemostasis 100
    secretion in acute inflammation 100
    structure and functions 98–9
vasoactive intestinal peptide 329–30
vasopressors 101
ventricular function curves 86–7, 88
vestibular function
    balance mechanisms 254–5
    body movement detection 254
    central vestibular pathways 253–4
    Eustachian tube functions 255
    factors involved in equilibrium 254
    functions of the vestibular system 254
    inner ear structure 253
    labyrinthine stimulation effects 255
    otolith organs (utricle, saccule) 253–4
    proprioceptive system 254
    semicircular canals 253–4
    statokinetic system 254
    vestibular apparatus 253–4
    vestibular function testing 255
    vestibular nuclei 253–4
    warm caloric test 255

Virchow's triad 169–70
vision
    astigmatism 245
    blood–eye barrier 246
    central visual pathways 248
    eye compartments 245
    eye movement by extra-ocular muscles 246
    eye movement systems 246
    hypermetropia (long-sightedness) 245
    lens properties 244–5
    myopia (near-sightedness) 245
    optical characteristics of the eye 244–5
    pre-corneal tear film 245
    pupillary light reflex 248–9
    refractive defects 245
    refractive power of the eye 244–5
    retinal light-sensitive pigment 247–8
    retinal rods and cones 246–8
    structural features of the eye 244
    visual cycle 246–8
vitamin B12 absorption test 333
vitamin D
    actions 308
    disorders 309
    receptor 309
    synthesis 307–8
vitamin K 163
vitamins, fat soluble vitamin absorption 332

water balance
    homeostatic mechanisms 19
    osmolality and tonicity of body fluids
        19–20
    sources of intake and output 19
water reabsorption 23–5, 54

X-linked adrenoleukodystrophy 16

Zellweger syndrome (cerebro-hepato-renal
    syndrome) 16